Gastrointestinal Surgical Techniques in Small Animals

Gastrointestinal Surgical Techniques in Small Animals

Edited by

Eric Monnet DVM, PhD, FAHA, DACVS, DECVS
Department of Clinical Sciences
College of Veterinary Medicine and Biomedical Sciences
Colorado State University
Fort Collins, CO, USA

Daniel D. Smeak DVM, DACVS
Department of Clinical Sciences
College of Veterinary Medicine and Biomedical Sciences
Colorado State University
Fort Collins, CO, USA

WILEY Blackwell

Registered Office
John Wiley & Sons, Inc., 111 River Street, Hoboken, NJ 07030, USA

Editorial Office
111 River Street, Hoboken, NJ 07030, USA

For details of our global editorial offices, customer services, and more information about Wiley products visit us at www.wiley.com.

Wiley also publishes its books in a variety of electronic formats and by print-on-demand. Some content that appears in standard print versions of this book may not be available in other formats.

Library of Congress Cataloging-in-Publication Data

Names: Monnet, Eric, author, editor. | Smeak, Daniel D., author, editor.
Title: Gastrointestinal surgical techniques in small animals / edited by
  Eric Monnet, Dan Smeak.
Description: Hoboken, NJ : John Wiley & Sons, 2020. | Includes
  bibliographical references and index.
Identifiers: LCCN 2019056768 (print) | LCCN 2019056769 (ebook) | ISBN
  9781119369202 (hardback) | ISBN 9781119369226 (adobe pdf) | ISBN
  9781119369233 (epub)
Subjects: MESH: Digestive System Surgical Procedures–veterinary |
  Dogs–surgery | Cats–surgery | Surgery, Veterinary–methods
Classification: LCC SF911 (print) | LCC SF911 (ebook) | NLM SF 911 | DDC
  636.089/743–dc23
LC record available at https://lccn.loc.gov/2019056768
LC ebook record available at https://lccn.loc.gov/2019056769

Cover Design: Wiley
Cover Images: Courtesy of Eric Monnet

Set in 9.5/12.5pt STIXTwoText by SPi Global, Pondicherry, India
Printed and bound in Singapore by Markono Print Media Pte Ltd

10 9 8 7 6 5 4 3 2 1

Contents

List of Contributors

Chad Lothamer, DVM, DAVDC
Dentistry and Oral Surgery
College of Veterinary Medicine
University of Tennessee
Knoxville, TN, USA

Eric Monnet, DVM, PhD, DACVS, DECVS
Department of Clinical Sciences
College of Veterinary Medicine and Biomedical
Sciences
Colorado State University
Fort Collins, CO, USA

Jennifer Rawlinson, DVM, DAVDC
Department of Clinical Sciences
College of Veterinary Medicine and Biomedical
Sciences
Colorado State University
Fort Collins, CO, USA

Bernard Séguin, DVM, MS, DACVS
Department of Clinical Sciences
College of Veterinary Medicine and Biomedical
Sciences
Colorado State University
Fort Collins, CO, USA

Daniel D. Smeak, DVM, DACVS
Department of Clinical Sciences
College of Veterinary Medicine and Biomedical
Sciences
Colorado State University
Fort Collins, CO, USA

Preface

Small animal general surgery has evolved rapidly in the past decade. Procedures have become increasingly complex, including the expansion of minimally invasive surgery options. Gastrointestinal conditions requiring surgical therapy are very common in small animal practice. Therefore, we have created this gastrointestinal surgery textbook to serve as a current and comprehensive reference tool for general practitioners, surgery residents in training, and surgeons.

In this textbook, current techniques for gastrointestinal surgery are thoroughly described with detailed illustrations embedded in the text. With this in mind we chose to work closely with Molly Pullen (www.mborman.com) for her expert pen-and-ink illustrations. In addition, when necessary, surgical techniques are supplemented with intraoperative images.

For each technique described, tips are included by the authors to explain the surgeon's preferences among all the techniques depicted, and to give details to help the reader perform the procedures effectively. Our intent for adding tips was to allow chapter authors the ability to express their preferences in technique, many of which are not evidence-based.

In this textbook we placed a strong emphasis on description of surgical techniques. We chose not to delve heavily in the pathophysiology or the diagnostic workup for the different surgical conditions mentioned because those topics are well described in other textbooks.

We would like to thank all the authors who assisted us during the arduous process of developing this new textbook. In the future, this textbook will be updated as needed to follow the progress and advances in veterinary gastrointestinal surgery.

About the Companion Website

Don't forget to visit the companion website for this book:

www.wiley.com/go/monnet/gastrointestinal

There you will find valuable material designed to enhance your learning, including:

- Illustrations
- Video clips

Scan this QR code to visit the companion website

Section I

General Concepts

1

Gastrointestinal Healing

Eric Monnet and Daniel D. Smeak

Department of Clinical Sciences, College of Veterinary Medicine and Biomedical Sciences, Colorado State University, Fort Collins, CO, USA

The gastrointestinal tract heals as any other tissue in an orderly manner, with an inflammatory phase, a debridement phase, a granulation phase, and a maturation phase. However, there are some characteristics very specific to the gastrointestinal tract that sets it apart from other healing tissues.

The healing process of the gastrointestinal tract should not only re-establish the anatomical integrity of the tract but also its function. Healing should happen with minimal scaring and stricture formation that could impede the motility of the gastrointestinal tract. Additionally, the formation of adhesions, even though rare in small animal surgery, could deteriorate gastrointestinal motility and should be minimized.

1.1 Anatomy

The wall of the gastrointestinal tract has a mucosa, a submucosa, a muscularis, and a serosa, except the esophagus and the distal rectum.

The mucosa has three distinct layers: the epithelium, the lamina propria and the muscularis mucosa. The lamina propria layer is made of vessels, lymphatics, and mesenchymal cells whereas the muscularis mucosa is a thin muscle layer. After completing the anastomosis, the mucosa heals very fast by epithelial cells migration over the defect providing a rapid barrier from the intestinal content. For intestinal healing to occur, a good surgical apposition of layers is required; everting or inverting patterns interfere with mucosal healing.

The submucosa layer, incorporating the bulk of the collagen, is the holding layer in intestinal surgery. Type I collagen (68%) predominates in the submucosa,

followed by type III (20%) and finally collagen type V (12%) (Thornton and Barbul 1997). It is a loose connective tissue with lymphatic, nerve fibers, ganglia, and blood vessels that should be preserved during surgery. The muscularis layer consists of an inner circular muscle layer, a longitudinal outer muscle layer and collagen fibers. The serosal surface is made of connective tissue with mesothelial cells, lymphatics, and blood vessels. The serosa is important in the healing process because it helps prevent leakage of the gastrointestinal content in the immediate post-operative period.

1.2 Phases of Wound Healing

1.2.1 Partial Thickness Injury

A partial thickness injury affecting only the mucosa or the serosa heals with epithelial cells and mesothelial cells proliferation without scaring. A full-thickness trauma of the gastrointestinal tract results in an inflammatory reaction and a non-epithelial cell proliferation that can result in scaring secondary to fibroblast activity (Thornton and Barbul 1997; Thompson et al. 2006).

1.2.2 Full-Thickness Injury

As soon as the wall of the gastrointestinal tract is incised, hemorrhage occurs but it is rapidly controlled by an intense vasoconstriction. Following this initial phase, vasodilation occurs with migration of neutrophils, macrophages, platelets, and liberation of inflammatory mediators which characterizes the inflammatory phase. The platelets, by releasing diverse platelet-derived growth factors (PDGF) and cytokines, contribute to hemostasis

Gastrointestinal Surgical Techniques in Small Animals, First Edition. Edited by Eric Monnet and Daniel D. Smeak.
© 2020 John Wiley & Sons, Inc. Published 2020 by John Wiley & Sons, Inc.
Companion website: www.wiley.com/go/monnet/gastrointestinal

and cell recruitment like macrophages and fibroblasts. The neutrophils predominate during the first 24 hours but then macrophages become predominant past 48 hours following the initial injury. The macrophages play an important role in healing of the gastrointestinal tract by controlling local infection with phagocytosis, production of oxygen radicals, and nitric oxide. They also participate in debridement with phagocytosis and production of collagenase and elastase. The macrophages also regulate matrix synthesis and cell recruitment and activation. They release several growth factors (PDGF, transforming growth factor (TGFβ), fibroblast growth factor (FGF), IGF) and cytokines (TNFα, IL-1) important for tissue healing. The macrophages recruit lymphocytes that liberate interleukin (IL-6) and interferon (IFN) and promote angiogenesis with production of VEGF (Vasculogenic Endothelial Growth Factor). Finally, the capillary permeability is increased resulting in inflammation and edema on the edges of the incision that can persist for two weeks. Care should be taken initially when the sutures are placed to not induce tissue strangulation and necrosis. A fibrin seal develops over the serosa very quickly to provide a leakage protection of the surgical site (Pascoe and Peterson 1989; Thornton and Barbul 1997; Thompson et al. 2006).

Overlapping with the inflammatory phase is the debridement phase, with removal of injured tissue by macrophages. The debridement phase should not exceed 1–2 mm from the edges of the incision. During this process, collagen is resorbed by collagenase and synthesized by smooth muscle and fibroblast. The smooth muscles are the major contributor in collagen production within the gastrointestinal tract. The collagen degrade by the collagenase activity weakens the strength of the anastomosis. In the colon, the collagenase activity is increased over the entire length of the colon while in the small intestine, it is increased only at the site of the anastomosis (Hawley 1970; Jiborn et al. 1978a). The risk of dehiscence is high between 3 and 10 days after surgery. Usually, after 4 to 5 days, collagen synthesis is superior to lysis and the anastomosis regains strength. This collagenase activity can be increased by the amount of trauma induced by tissue manipulation at the time of surgery or the presence of a foreign body, and by the degree of contamination. The amount of collagen synthesized is affected by hypotension, hypovolemia, shock, and certain medications.

The granulation tissue appears at the beginning of the proliferative phase of intestinal healing. Fibroblast is the major cell type present past day 4 after surgery. The fibroblasts migrate under the control of PDGF, TGFβ and FGF. Fibroblast and smooth muscle lay down collagen fibers and new capillaries appear in the field.

After one to two weeks following the anastomosis, the epithelial layer is fully restored. The epithelialization of the anastomosis reduces the formation of excessive fibrosis tissue secondary to inflammation. The excessive fibrosis could lead to stricture formation. During the maturation phase, the collagen fibers are reorganized and the anastomosis is becoming thinner.

In summary, an intestinal anastomosis loses bursting strength during the first 3 to 5 days to finally regain 50–70% of the initial bursting strength in 2 to 3 weeks (Jiborn et al. 1978a, 1978b; Thompson et al. 2006; Munireddy et al. 2010).

1.3 Factors Affecting Gastrointestinal Tract Healing

1.3.1 Ischemia and Tissue Perfusion

Ischemia interferes with healing of any tissue and especially the gastrointestinal tract. The oxygen delivery to the peripheral tissue depends on the anatomy of the capillaries, vasomotor control, and oxygen saturation. The tissue perfusion depends on the amount of soft tissue trauma and especially trauma to the blood supply of the loop of intestine. The placement of tight sutures interferes with tissue perfusion and may increase the risk of dehiscence, especially in the colon and esophagus (Shikata et al. 1982; Chung 1987; Jonsson and Hogstrom 1992; Thornton and Barbul 1997). Hypovolemia and hypotension are critical factors that divert blood flow to essential organs, and oxygen delivery is also very important for collagen synthesis. A partial pressure of oxygen of at least 40 mmHg is required for collagen synthesis. During a hypovolemic event, the gastrointestinal tract downregulates its own blood flow. Anemia does not interfere with healing as long as the patient has a good cardiac output to compensate (Thompson et al. 2006).

1.3.2 Suture Intrinsic Tension

Incising oral and visceral tissues stimulate an initial vasoconstriction, followed by secondary vasodilation and increased vascular permeability mediated largely by kinins, ultimately causing edema and swelling of tissue edges. This should be kept in mind when tensioning suture lines or stitches because ischemic necrosis may develop as the suture strangulates the swelling tissue. In general, sutures in viscera of the digestive tract should be tensioned such that the incision edges are held firmly together without crushing or cutting through the needle purchase. When inverting suture patterns are used, the suture line is firmly tensioned such that the incised edges are fully inverted and minimal suture is exposed on the surface of the organ (Thornton and Barbul 1997).

1.3.3 Surgical Technique

A simple apposition of the submucosa of the gastrointestinal tract is desired to achieve primary healing because it is associated with the least amount of fibrous tissue and better function. An apposition of the submucosa is important for the rapid healing of the mucosa and preventing migration of microorganisms within the surgical site. An eversion or inversion of the mucosa has been shown to interfere with primary healing (Jiborn et al. 1978a, 1978c; Jansen et al. 1981; Ellison et al. 1982; Jonsson et al. 1985; Pascoe and Peterson 1989; Thornton and Barbul 1997). Stapled anastomoses are becoming commonplace in veterinary surgery (Hansen and Smeak 2015; Duell et al. 2016; Snowdon et al. 2016). Staples do not promote better healing of the gastrointestinal tract when sepsis or ischemia are present (Thornton and Barbul 1997). Sutureless anastomoses have been performed with devices working by compressing two inverted ring of bowel (Maney et al. 1988; Corman et al. 1989; Ryan et al. 2006; Bobkiewicz et al. 2017).

1.3.4 Nutrition

The nutritional support of the patient is paramount for the healing of the gastrointestinal tract. Malnourished patients are at increased risk for dehiscence. The addition of a feeding tube is very important to support the anorectic patient in the post-operative period as the enterocytes are getting their nutrients mostly from the intestinal content traveling in the lumen. Vitamin A, C, and B6 are required for collagen synthesis. Iron and copper are also important for the cross-linking of protein and tissue healing. The enteral nutrition is beneficial for the integrity of the gastrointestinal tract and prevent bacterial translocation (Thornton and Barbul 1997; Marks 2013).

1.3.5 Blood Transfusion

A blood transfusion has been associated with an increased risk of leakage after gastrointestinal surgery. It has been postulated that blood transfusion is affecting the inflammatory phase and the migration of macrophages (Apostolidis et al. 2000; Munireddy et al. 2010).

1.3.6 Local Infection

A local infection increases protease activity, which delays epithelialization because protease resorbs growth factors required for healing. A braided suture should be avoided even if they received an antimicrobial treatment as bacteria adhere to them more than to monofilament (Chu and Williams 1984; Masini et al. 2011). Polydioxanone seems to have the lowest affinity for bacteria (Chu and Williams 1984).

1.3.7 Intraperitoneal Infection

A septic peritonitis interferes with healing of an intestinal anastomosis because it reduces collagen content at the level of the anastomosis. The combination of bacterial and neutrophil collagenases increases the collagen fibers breakdown. The collagen synthesis and deposition are reduced by the peritonitis (Ahrendt et al. 1996; Munireddy et al. 2010). The septic exudate present in the anastomosis prevents synthesis and deposition of collagen and angiogenesis (Thornton and Barbul 1997).

1.3.8 Medications

In an experiment in rats, it was shown that the administration of methylprednisolone did not affect the mechanical strength of colonic anastomosis (Mastboom et al. 1991a). However, the effect of steroids on the healing of the gastrointestinal tract is controversial (Thornton and Barbul 1997; Thompson et al. 2006).

The administration of NSAIDs after gastrointestinal surgery is also very controversial (Mastboom et al. 1991b; Gorissen et al. 2012; Bhangu et al. 2014; Collaborative 2014). The non-selective cyclo-oxygenase inhibitors seem to increase the risk of leakage after colorectal surgery (Gorissen et al. 2012). Two meta-analyses in human patients reported opposite results (Bhangu et al. 2014; Collaborative 2014). However, both of those studies have focused on colorectal surgery, which is not performed frequently in small animal surgery. In one of the studies, animal experiments were reviewed and showed that NSAID administration in the post-post-operative period increased the risk of leakage (Bhangu et al. 2014). The NSAIDs affect production of VEGF and angiogenesis. They also interfere with collagen formation and cross-linking (Inan et al. 2006; Gorissen et al. 2012). After administration of

NSAIDs, hydroxyproline concentration was significantly reduced after resection and anastomosis of the ileum. This effect was mostly present three days after surgery. Seven days after surgery, the concentration of hydroxyproline had risen again (Mastboom et al. 1991b). In a study on rats, NSAIDs increased the morbidity and mortality rates without necessarily leading to an increased risk of leakage (Mastboom et al. 1991b).

The chemotherapy drugs because of their immunosuppressant effect can negatively affect the healing of the gastrointestinal tract (Thornton and Barbul 1997).

1.3.9 Disease

There is very little evidence that diabetes interferes with gastrointestinal healing. In a rat model of diabetes, collagen synthesis was not affected. However, the bursting pressure of the intestinal anastomosis was reduced on day 3 after surgery, but this effect did not persist past day 7 (Verhofstad and Hendriks 1994; Thornton and Barbul 1997). Icterus has been shown to interfere with tissue healing (Bayer and Ellis 1976; Muftuoglu et al. 2005).

1.3.10 Large Intestine

The colon is considered by most surgeons as a rather "unforgiving" structure when it is incised and repaired, largely because of its unique healing qualities, and when leakage occurs, the results are often devastating to the animal (Williams 2012). An understanding of colonic healing is important, and incorporation of all the principles of repair are critical to reduce life-threatening anastomotic dehiscence. Healing of the colon undergoes similar phases of wound healing to those found in the skin and other tissue layers but with a number of important differences (Agren et al. 2006). During the inflammatory phase, a fibrin clot forms over the site and, although this clot has minimal strength, it is important to achieve an early "seal," and it is vital that it remains to act as a scaffold for fibroblast migration during the early repair phase. For the first three to four days, nearly all support for the colonic repair comes from the suture or staple line. Angiogenesis and migration of fibroblasts occurs and eventually replaces the fibrin clot scaffold during days 3 and 4. It is during this stage of repair that breakdown is most likely to occur (Williams 2012).

Although a fragile mucosal bridge also occurs within the first three to four days, depending on the size of the defect, substantive wound strength occurs only when local recruited smooth muscle cells and fibroblasts from the colonic submucosa and muscularis bridge the incision and begin producing collagen. Appropriate-sized tissue bites are particularly important when repairing the colon because a zone of active collagen lysis occurs in a 1–3 mm zone immediately adjacent to the incised colon edge. The activity of matrix metalloproteases that cause collagen degradation peaks during the debridement phase through day 3 (Agren et al. 2006). Provided there is ample vascular supply after this time, collagen synthesis is accelerated, coupled with a rapid gain in wound strength. Aggressive tissue handling and excess contamination of the colonic wound can greatly increase the debridement activity at the sutured wound edge and this increases the risk of early tissue disruption, leading to dehiscence and leakage (Williams 2012). Return of strength at the healing site reaches about 75% of normal strength at four months after surgery, which is considerably slower than in the small intestine (Thornton and Barbul 1997). Surgeons can influence uncomplicated colonic healing by ensuring adequate tissue perfusion, eliminating any tension on the repair, accurately apposing colonic edges without inducing excess trauma, containing contamination, and avoiding increased intraluminal pressures by eliminating any distal obstruction (Holt and Brockman 2003; Williams 2012). Omental pedicle wraps have been advocated to reinforce the gastrointestinal repairs and support the local healing environment. Omentum may stimulate and augment angiogenesis and may also help maintain the vital fibrin clot and seal during the early phases of wound healing. The benefit of omental wraps in colonic surgery have not been proven in recent human clinical studies of colonic resection and anastomosis. However, most surgeons still recommend covering colonic repairs with omentum (Hao et al. 2008).

References

Agren, M.S. et al. (2006). Action of matrix metalloproteinases at restricted sites in colon anastomosis repair: an immunohistochemical and biochemical stud`. *Surgery* 140 (1): 72–82.

Ahrendt, G.M. et al. (1996). Intra-abdominal sepsis impairs colonic reparative collagen synthesis. *Am. J. Surg.* 171 (1): 102–107; discussion 107–108.

Apostolidis, S.A. et al. (2000). Prevention of blood-transfusion-induced impairment of anastomotic healing by leucocyte depletion in rats. *Eur. J. Surg.* 166 (7): 562–567.

Bayer, I. and Ellis, H. (1976). Jaundice and wound healing: an experimental study. *Br. J. Surg.* 63 (5): 392–396.

Bhangu, A. et al. (2014). Postoperative nonsteroidal anti-inflammatory drugs and risk of anastomotic leak: meta-analysis of clinical and experimental studies. *World J. Surg.* 38 (9): 2247–2257.

Bobkiewicz, A. et al. (2017). Gastrointestinal tract anastomoses with the biofragmentable anastomosis ring: is it still a valid technique for bowel anastomosis? Analysis of 203 cases and review of the literature. *Int. J. Color. Dis.* 32 (1): 107–111.

Chu, C.C. and Williams, D.F. (1984). Effects of physical configuration and chemical structure of suture materials on bacterial adhesion. A possible link to wound infection. *Am. J. Surg.* 147 (2): 197–204.

Chung, R.S. (1987). Blood flow in colonic anastomoses. Effect of stapling and suturing. *Ann. Surg.* 206 (3): 335–339.

Collaborative, S.T. (2014). Impact of postoperative non-steroidal anti-inflammatory drugs on adverse events after gastrointestinal surgery. *Br. J. Surg.* 101 (11): 1413–1423.

Corman, M.L. et al. (1989). Comparison of the valtrac biofragmentable anastomosis ring with conventional suture and stapled anastomosis in colon surgery. Results of a prospective, randomized clinical trial. *Dis. Colon Rectum* 32 (3): 183–187.

Duell, J.R. et al. (2016). Frequency of dehiscence in hand-sutured and stapled intestinal anastomoses in dogs. *Vet. Surg.* 45 (1): 100–103.

Ellison, G.W. et al. (1982). End-to-end approximating intestinal anastomosis in the dog – a comparative fluorescein dye, angiographic and histopathologic evaluation. *J. Am. Anim. Hosp. Assoc.* 18 (5): 729–736.

Gorissen, K.J. et al. (2012). Risk of anastomotic leakage with non-steroidal anti-inflammatory drugs in colorectal surgery. *Br. J. Surg.* 99 (5): 721–727.

Hansen, L.A. and Smeak, D.D. (2015). In vitro comparison of leakage pressure and leakage location for various staple line offset configurations in functional end-to-end stapled small intestinal anastomoses of canine tissues. *Am. J. Vet. Res.* 76 (7): 644–648.

Hao, X.Y. et al. (2008). Omentoplasty in the prevention of anastomotic leakage after colorectal resection: a meta-analysis. *Int. J. Color. Dis.* 23 (12): 1159–1165.

Hawley, P.R. (1970). Collagenase activity and colonic anastomotic breakdown. *Br. J. Surg.* 57 (5): 388.

Holt, D.E. and Brockman, D. (2003). Large intestine. In: Textbook of Small Animal Surgery (ed. D. Slatter), 665–682. Philadelphia: Saunders.

Inan, A. et al. (2006). Effects of diclofenac sodium on bursting pressures of anastomoses and hydroxyproline contents of perianastomotic tissues in a laboratory study. *Int. J. Surg.* 4 (4): 222–227.

Jansen, A. et al. (1981). The importance of the apposition of the submucosal intestinal layers for primary wound healing of intestinal anastomosis. *Surg Gynecol. Obstet.* 152 (1): 51–58.

Jiborn, H. et al. (1978a). Healing of experimental colonic anastomoses. I. Bursting strength of the colon after left colon resection and anastomosis. *Am. J. Surg.* 136 (5): 587–594.

Jiborn, H. et al. (1978b). Healing of experimental colonic anastomoses. II. Breaking strength of the colon after left colon resection and anastomosis. *Am. J. Surg.* 136 (5): 595–599.

Jiborn, H. et al. (1978c). Healing of experimental colonic anastomoses. The effect of suture technic on collagen concentration in the colonic wall. *Am. J. Surg.* 135 (3): 333–340.

Jonsson, T. and Hogstrom, H. (1992). Effect of suture technique on early healing of intestinal anastomoses in rats. *Eur. J. Surg.* 158 (5): 267–270.

Jonsson, K. et al. (1985). Comparison of healing in the left colon and ileum. Changes in collagen content and collagen synthesis in the intestinal wall after ileal and colonic anastomoses in the rat. *Acta Chir. Scand.* 151 (6): 537–541.

Maney, J.W. et al. (1988). Biofragmentable bowel anastomosis ring: comparative efficacy studies in dogs. *Surgery* 103 (1): 56–62.

Marks, S.L. (2013). Enteral and parenteral nutrition. In: Canine and Feline Gastroenterology (eds. R.J. Washabau and M.J. Day), 429–444. St Louis: Elsevier.

Masini, B.D. et al. (2011). Bacterial adherence to suture materials. *J. Surg. Educ.* 68 (2): 101–104.

Mastboom, W.J. et al. (1991a). Influence of methylprednisolone on the healing of intestinal anastomoses in rats. *Br. J. Surg.* 78 (1): 54–56.

Mastboom, W.J. et al. (1991b). The influence of NSAIDs on experimental intestinal anastomoses. *Dis. Colon Rectum* 34 (3): 236–243.

Muftuoglu, M.A. et al. (2005). Effects of high bilirubin levels on the healing of intestinal anastomosis. *Surg. Today* 35 (9): 739–743.

Munireddy, S. et al. (2010). Intra-abdominal healing: gastrointestinal tract and adhesions. *Surg. Clin. North Am.* 90 (6): 1227–1236.

Pascoe, J.R. and Peterson, P.R. (1989). Intestinal healing and methods of anastomosis. *Vet. Clin. North Am. Equine Pract.* 5 (2): 309–333.

Ryan, S. et al. (2006). Comparison of biofragmentable anastomosis ring and sutured anastomoses for subtotal colectomy in cats with idiopathic megacolon. *Vet. Surg.* 35 (8): 740–748.

Shikata, J. et al. (1982). The effect of local blood flow on the healing of experimental intestinal anastomoses. *Surg Gynecol. Obstet.* 154 (5): 657–661.

Snowdon, K.A. et al. (2016). Risk factors for dehiscence of stapled functional end-to-end intestinal anastomoses in dogs: 53 cases (2001–2012). *Vet. Surg.* 45 (1): 91–99.

Thompson, S.K. et al. (2006). Clinical review: healing in gastrointestinal anastomoses, part I. *Microsurgery* 26 (3): 131–136.

Thornton, F.J. and Barbul, A. (1997). Healing in the gastrointestinal tract. *Surg. Clin. North Am.* 77 (3): 549–573.

Verhofstad, M.H. and Hendriks, T. (1994). Diabetes impairs the development of early strength, but not the accumulation of collagen, during intestinal anastomotic healing in the rat. *Br. J. Surg.* 81 (7): 1040–1045.

Williams, J.M. (2012). Colon. In: Veterinary Surgery Small Animal, 2e (eds. K.M. Tobias and S.A. Johnston), 1542–1563. St Louis: Elsevier.

2

Suture Materials, Staplers, and Tissue Apposition Devices

Daniel D. Smeak

Department of Clinical Sciences, College of Veterinary Medicine and Biomedical Sciences, Colorado State University, Fort Collins, CO, USA

Suture remains the most common means of achieving apposition of wound edges to promote optimal healing (Booth 2003, Smeak 1998). Ideally, sutures should provide support until the repair has regained sufficient strength to withstand tensile forces. When this has been achieved, the suture material should ideally disintegrate in a predictable fashion to prevent further tissue reaction and inhibition of wound healing. Sutures should not create undue tissue reaction because inflammation can prolong the lag phase of wound healing, and delay return to strength. In general, monofilament and synthetic nonabsorbable sutures induce the least amount of tissue reaction, whereas multifilament sutures that are made from natural materials such as silk or chromic catgut are some of the most reactive suture materials. Monofilament absorbable suture materials are often the first choice for surgeons because they are relatively inert and have good to excellent tensile strength, and most have very predictable absorption profiles when exposed to contamination and variable pH environments. Multifilament suture materials have been used successfully in a variety of visceral repairs, however, because most have inherent capillarity (or the drawing up of fluid between the fine woven strands of suture) and high affinity for bacterial adherence, these sutures have fallen out of favor (Chih-Chang and William 1984). Wicking up of contaminated fluid into multifilament suture filaments from the lumen of hollow organs can contribute to increased tissue reaction, and the bacterial load within the material may be difficult to clear by normal host defenses. For these reasons and others mentioned later, monofilament absorbable sutures are favored and are now used more often in oral and gastrointestinal surgeries.

It should be emphasized that the surgeon's technique (the manner of needle and suture placement, and tissue handling) likely has a greater influence on the generation of tissue inflammation at the repair site than the choice of suture material used in the repair. Needles should be carefully introduced and removed from the tissue "along the curve of the needle" to reduce tissue damage and minimize the size of the needle "track." Tissue should be well-apposed with suture without being crushed and handled atraumatically if instruments are required. Forcibly tied sutures and aggressive instrument handling cause tissue damage that impedes healing and inhibits proliferation of new blood vessels, increasing the risk of repair dehiscence (Hoer et al. 2001).

2.1 Suture Materials

Sutures are classified as absorbable or nonabsorbable, and monofilament or multifilament (Table 2.1). Absorbable sutures are desirable in gastrointestinal surgery since they eventually are degraded and removed by the body over days to months. Nonabsorbable sutures do not lose significant strength over 60 days, and remain in the tissues to some degree for years. Monofilament sutures are composed of a single smooth strand, whereas multifilament sutures are braided or woven from multiple strands.

Suture is selected for a specific digestive organ wound repair considering the physical characteristics of the suture material (tensile strength and knot security, absorption rate, surface qualities, capillarity, tissue reactivity), and the environment and healing rate of the

Gastrointestinal Surgical Techniques in Small Animals, First Edition. Edited by Eric Monnet and Daniel D. Smeak.
© 2020 John Wiley & Sons, Inc. Published 2020 by John Wiley & Sons, Inc.
Companion website: www.wiley.com/go/monnet/gastrointestinal

Table 2.1 Characteristics of suture materials used in digestive system procedures.

Absorbable Suture	Nonabsorbable Suture	Trade Name	Type	Degradation Process	Foreign Body Response	Tensile Strength Retention (%)	Relative Knot Security	Mass Absorption Time (days)	Comments
Chromic Catgut		Surgical gut; chromic gut	Rapid to Intermediate absorbable multifilament	Phagocytosis and proteolytic enzymes	Moderate	Unpredictable	Fair	Variable; 45–60 d or longer	Degradation and tissue reactivity related to where implanted; knots imbibe fluid and unravel if knot ears are cut short
Polyglactin 910		Vicryl Rapide	Rapid absorbable multifilament	Hydrolysis	Mild	50% after 5 d; 0% after 14 d	Fair to good	42	Irradiated to aid in dissolving
		Vicryl, Coated Vicryl Plus	Intermediate absorbable multifilament	Hydrolysis	Mild	75% after 14 d; 50% after 21 d	Fair to good	56–70	Plus designates triclosan (antibacterial) impregnated
Lactomer		Polysorb (coated)	Intermediate absorbable multifilament	Hydrolysis	Mild	80% after 14 d; 30% after 21 d	Fair to good	56–70	Improvements in braid construction and coating reduce drag and improve knot security
		Velosorb (coated)	Rapid absorbable multifilament	Hydrolysis	Mild	60% at 5 d; 0% at 14 d	Fair to good	40–50	Irradiated to aid in dissolving; similar to Vicryl Rapide
Polyglycolic Acid		Dexon S (uncoated), Dexon II (coated)	Intermediate absorbable multifilament	Hydrolysis	Mild	65% after 14 d; 35% after 21 d	Fair to good	60–90	Coated Dexon II helps reduce drag, but decreases knot security
Polyglytone 6211		Caprosyn	Rapid to intermediate absorbable monofilament	Hydrolysis	Minimal	60% after 5 d; 20–30% after 10 d	Fair	56	Knots have been known to untie spontaneously when incubated in serum; supple easy to handle for monofilament; fastest mass absorption of absorbable monofilaments
Polygliocaprone 25		Monocryl	Rapid to intermediate absorbable monofilament	Hydrolysis	Minimal	50–60% after 7 d; 20–30% after 14 d; 0% after 21 d	Good	91–119	Supple easy to handle for monofilament.

Category	Product	Type	Degradation	Tissue reaction	Tensile strength retention		Absorption (days)	Notes
Polyglycolic Acid/ Polycaprolactone	Quill Monoderm	Intermediate absorbable monofilament barbed	Hydrolysis	Slight	42–76% at 7d; 36–52% at 14d	N/A	90–120	Uni- and bidirectional barbed suture; choose one size larger due to strength loss from barbs. Slightly higher tissue reaction than V-Loc 90.
	Stratafix PGA-PCL Plus (barbed)	Rapid to intermediate absorbable monofilament barbed	Hydrolysis	Minimal	50–60% after 7 d; 20–30% after 14d; 0% after 21 d	N/A	90–120	Stratafix Monocryl comes with spiral barbs; uni- or bidirectional. Plus – antibacterial
Glycomer 631	Biosyn	Intermediate absorbable monofilament	Hydrolysis	Minimal	75% after 14d; 40% after 21 d	Average	110	Knots occasionally untie spontaneously
	V-Loc 90	Intermediate absorbable monofilament barbed	Hydrolysis	Minimal	90% at 7d; 75% at 14d	N/A	90	Unidirectional barbed suture; equivalent to strength of suture one size smaller – choose size as you would conventional suture
Polyglyconate	Maxon	Prolonged absorbable monofilament	Hydrolysis	Minimal	81% after 14d; 59% after 28d; 30% after 42d	Good	180	Similar to PDS II; tends to have slightly more memory in larger sizes
Polydioxanone	PDS II; PDS Plus	Prolonged absorbable monofilament	Hydrolysis	Minimal	74% after 14d; 58% after 28d; 41% after 42d	Good	180	Plus designates triclosan (antibacterial) impregnated
	V-Loc 180	Prolonged absorbable monofilament barbed	Hydrolysis	Negligible	80% at 7 d; 75% at 14d; 65% at 21 d	N/A	180	Unidirectional barbed suture; equivalent to strength of suture one size smaller-choose size as you would conventional suture.
	Stratafix PDO, PDO Plus	Prolonged absorbable monofilament barbed	Hydrolysis	Negligible	80% at 7d; 75% at 14d; 65% at 21 d	N/A	120–180	Stratafix comes in uni- and bidirectional strands with symmetrical or spiral barbs. Symmetrical unidirectional barbed sutures are recommended for high tension repairs. PDS plus is antibacterial

(Continued)

Table 2.1 (Continued)

Absorbable Suture	Nonabsorbable Suture	Trade Name	Type	Degradation Process	Foreign Body Response	Tensile Strength Retention (%)	Relative Knot Security	Mass Absorption Time (days)	Comments
		Quill PDO	Prolonged absorbable monofilament barbed	Hydrolysis	Negligible	67–80% at 14 d; 50–80% at 28 d	N/A	180	Uni- and bidirectional barbed suture; choose one size larger due to strength loss from barbs
	Polyamide	Ethilon; Dermalon; Surgilon	Nonabsorbable monofilament	N/A	Minimal	15–20% loss in 365 d; retains 80% indefinitely	Fair	N/A	Slowly loses strength over years by process of hydrolysis
		Nurolon	Nonabsorbable multifilament	N/A	Minimal	15–20% loss in 365 d; retains 80% indefinitely	Fair	N/A	Slowly loses strength over years by process of hydrolysis
		Quill Nylon	Nonabsorbable monofilament barbed	N/A	Minimal	Similar to conventional nylon	N/A	N/A	Similar to conventional nylon
	Polybutester	Novafil	Nonabsorbable monofilament	N/A	Negligible	N/A	Good	N/A	Handles well for monofilament; stretchy
		V-Loc PBT	Nonabsorbable monofilament barbed	N/A	Negligible	N/A	N/A	N/A	Unidirectional barbed suture; permanent soft tissue approximation; equivalent to strength of suture one size smaller – choose size as you would conventional suture
	Polypropylene	Prolene; Surgipro; Surgipro II	Nonabsorbable monofilament	N/A	Negligible	N/A	Good	N/A	Does not lose appreciable strength over long periods of time; one of most inert suture besides steel
		Quill Polypropylene	Nonabsorbable monofilament barbed	N/A	Negligible	N/A	N/A	N/A	Uni- and bidirectional barbed suture; choose one size larger due to strength loss from barbs
		Stratafix Polypropylene	Nonabsorbable monofilament barbed	N/A	Negligible	N/A	N/A	N/A	Uni- or bidirectional spiral barb configuration. Similar characteristics otherwise with conventional polypropylene

Material	Product(s)	Classification	Degradation	Tissue Reaction	Tensile Strength Retention	Handling	Tissue Absorption	Comments
Hexafluoropropylene VDF	Pronova	Nonabsorbable monofilament	N/A	Negligible	N/A	Good to very good	N/A	Good alternative to polypropylene; better handling and strength
Stainless Steel	Surgical Stainless Steel (mono); Steel	Nonabsorbable monofilament	N/A	Negligible	N/A	Excellent	N/A	Difficult to handle; may tend to cut through soft tissues
	Surgical Stainless Steel (Multi); Flexon	Nonabsorbable multifilament	N/A	Negligible	N/A	Excellent	N/A	Multifilament improves handling; excellent knot security
Silk	Permahand; Sofsilk	Nonabsorbable multifilament	Proteolytic enzymes	Moderate to severe	70% after 14d; 50% after 30d	Fair	Gradual encapsulation by fibrous tissue	Considered one of the best handling sutures available
Polyester	Mersilene (uncoated); Ethibond Excel (coated); Ticron; Surgidac	Nonabsorbable multifilament	N/A	Mild to moderate	N/A	Fair	Gradual encapsulation by fibrous tissue	Strong, relatively good handling; knot security is a concern

NA = Not Applicable.
Chu et al. (1997) and Capperauld (1989).
http://www.medtronic.com/covidien/en-us/products/wound-closure.html.
http://woundclosure.ethicon.com/traditional-suture-search.

tissue involved in the repair. As a rule, more pliable and smaller diameter sutures have favorable handling properties in gastrointestinal surgery compared to larger, stiffer suture materials.

2.1.1 Predictable Absorption Profile

Suture materials are manufactured from natural and synthetic sources. Natural absorbable sutures mentioned in this chapter include catgut and chromic catgut. Absorption of catgut is unpredictable because it is degraded by proteolytic enzymes and phagocytosis and causes a marked tissue inflammatory response that may be detrimental to healing. Pre-existing tissue inflammation and enzymatic digestion from gastric enzymes can lead to rapid catgut suture degradation. These aforementioned suture characteristics have nearly made natural sutures made of catgut obsolete in small animal surgery.

Synthetic absorbable monofilament suture materials are preferred for gastrointestinal surgery. Synthetic sutures are degraded by controlled hydrolysis making their absorption from tissue highly predictable. The degradation of most synthetic sutures is accelerated in alkaline environments, except for polydioxanone. This suture degrades rapidly in highly acidic environments, so, theoretically, other synthetic absorbable sutures may be better choices when exposed to gastric contents (Freudenberg et al. 2004). The stomach generally heals quickly, so more rapid absorption of polydioxanone from the wall may not be clinically important.

2.1.2 Tensile Strength and Knot Security

Most suture materials out of the package have adequate strength to hold gastrointestinal wound edges together until adequate wound strength is regained (Table 2.1). Knot security is influenced by suture diameter, coefficient of friction, and, most of all, quality of the tied knot. In general, braided suture materials have greater tensile strength than monofilament sutures. Coating of braided sutures negatively affects knot security. Some sutures, particularly glycomer (Biosyn) and polyglytone 6211 (Caprosyn), may been found to have decreased knot security when incubated in canine serum for 24 hours (Marturello et al. 2014). For most sutures within the size range of 3-0 and 4-0, at least four square throws are necessary to secure knots effectively. Care should be taken when tying monofilament sutures, particularly nylon, that the knots are pulled tight enough to cause "plastic deformation."

Tightening monofilament suture materials to ensure security by "plastic deformation" is important, but overtightening of the stitch can occur due to their slippery, smooth surface. With multifilament suture materials, on the second square throw, the knot is set when snugged firmly. Therefore, the tightness of the first throw is locked in place when the second throw is snugged down. Subsequent square throws are placed to ensure permanent knot security. For monofilament sutures, however, tightening the second throw to create plastic deformation will continue to tighten down the stitch because the smooth suture strands slip somewhat. Therefore, use this characteristic when tensioning throws on monofilament suture. The first throw is left somewhat loose, the second throw is tightened until the stitch apposes the tissue edges (but the knot is still not fully plastically deformed), and subsequent throws are firmly tensioned to deform and lock the throws securely together (Zimmer et al. 1991).

2.1.3 Low Capillarity and Bacterial Adhesion

The degree of fluid and bacteria transport along suture fibers is determined by the fluid absorption and capillarity of the suture material. Multifilament sutures that penetrate contaminated areas have the potential to wick bacteria and toxic fluid into adjacent sterile areas, and this can increase tissue inflammation and delay wound healing. In addition, the interstices within capillary multifilament sutures can help shield or slow bacteria clearance from the material (Osterberg 1983). Bacteria adhere more readily to the increased surface area around and within multifilament sutures. For these reasons, multifilament sutures are falling out of favor in gastrointestinal surgery (Thornton and Barbul 2014).

2.1.4 Handling Characteristics

Much of the desirable handling properties of suture are associated with the degree of "stiffness" or inherent memory of the suture material. As a rule, multifilament sutures handle better than the monofilaments because they are softer and more flexible. Smaller, more pliable sutures tend to hold their position when inserted and knotted in soft tissues, just as the surgeon intended. Sutures with "memory" that are stiff can force or shift stitches away from their intended path in tissue as they are secured, and this can cause unwanted malapposition and gap formation. The cut ends of stiff sutures can also result in significant mechanical irritation of adjacent tissues, and this can increase adhesion formation, and even cause erosion of adjacent friable tissue. A suture's handling quality is also related to its elasticity, or its tendency to elongate under tensile force. Smaller, more elastic suture materials are desirable because they can elongate with increased tensile loads, and this may help reduce suture cut-out in tissue.

Multifilament sutures have rough surfaces compared to monofilaments, and they may cause considerable friction and trauma when pulled through tissues, particularly when used in continuous suture lines. Coating is often applied to help smooth out the surface of multifilament sutures so they pass through tissue without "drag." However, suture coating causes other less desirable handling qualities as it tends to increase the stiffness of the material, and it often reduces its knot security. Braided suture should be avoided even if they received an antimicrobial treatment because bacteria adhere to them more than to monofilament (Chu and Williams 1984; Masini et al. 2011).

2.1.5 Rate of Strength Gain in GI Surgery

Under a normal healing environment, intestinal repair strength rapidly increases by the fifth day, and about 50% of strength return occurs by 10–14 days (see Chapter 1 for a review of intestinal healing). Since intermediate to prolonged absorbable sutures possess similar absorption rates (strength loss rate), they are preferred for most gastrointestinal repairs.

2.1.6 Suture Needles

Surgical needles are constructed of surgical grade stainless steel, and they have three basic parts, the suture attachment (swag), body, and needle point (Table 2.2). Needles chosen for use in gastrointestinal surgery are of the swaged-on variety (permanently crimped to the suture material).

The body of needles used for most gastrointestinal surgeries are curved. The "flatter" curve of the 3/8 circle needle is best for suturing on surfaces that are superficial and readily exposed to the surgeon. Curved needles with great arc (1/2 and 5/8) are more suited for suturing small, deeper wounds in more confined areas.

Needle points can be divided into cutting, taper, or taper-cut types. Cutting needles possess sharp points (two opposing cutting edges and a third edge along the outer curvature (reverse cutting) or the inside of the curvature (conventional cutting)). Both types of cutting needles are triangular on cross-section, but the reverse cutting is most popular because it is 32% stronger, and it resists cut-out during tissue passage due to the flat nature of the inner curvature. Cutting needles readily penetrate tough, heavily collagenous tissues such as gingiva. Taper point needles are round on cross-section, and result in less tissue trauma, and smaller tissue punctures than cutting point needles. They are the preferred needle type for most gastrointestinal procedures. Taper-cut needles combine the cutting action of the triangular shaped point, and the round body of the taper needle for atraumatic passage through delicate tissues. These needles are often chosen for mucogingival repairs, or when a friable tissue edge is sutured to tough skin or mucoperiosteum (Domnick 2014).

2.1.7 Directional Barbed Suture

Recently, use of directional or barbed suture materials have been documented in gastrointestinal procedures (Table 2.1) (Hansen and Monnet 2012; Erhart et al. 2013). Barbed sutures are manufactured by making small cuts in the surface of smooth suture, creating spurs. They are specifically designed to be used in continuous suture patterns. The barbs catch within collagenous tissue as each suture pass is taken. Unlike conventional sutures, previously placed tissue bites grab and remain secure in tissue, spreading tension throughout the line. Intestinal anastomosis performed with the unidirectional barbed suture seems to have a higher leakage pressure than anastomosis performed with regular monofilament sutures (Hansen and Monnet 2012). Each suture pass cannot "back out" due to the directional barbs. These sutures make it possible to secure a suture line without a knot. The suture is placed through a loop at the beginning of the suture line and then at the end of the suture line for gastrointestinal surgery two extra bites are made at 180° to lock the suture.

Barbed sutures have tensile strength comparable to their unbarbed equivalents when factoring size by their inner diameter at the depth of the barb cut versus outer diameter of conventional suture (Arbaugh et al. 2013; Ferrer-Marquez and Belda-Lorano 2009).

Both unidirectional suture and bidirectional sutures are available. Unidirectional sutures have a loop at one end and a needle on the other. The first needle bite is taken in tissue, and instead of creating a knot, the needle is passed through the loop to secure the end. With bidirectional barbed sutures, barbs are cut toward each end, starting mid-strand with needles swaged on both ends.

Barbed sutures are more efficient to place than conventional sutures. They have been documented to reduce operative time and in some cases intraoperative bleeding, likely due to maintained consistent tightness

Table 2.2 Suture, staple recommendations for GI surgery in small animals.

Tissue/Procedure	Suture Recommendations	Needle Recommendations	Suture Size Range	Stapling Equipment, Cartridge Size	Comments
Mucoperiosteal Flap, Cleft Palate, Oronasal Fistula Repair	Intermediate to prolonged absorbable suture; nonabsorbables are acceptable	Superficial closures 3/8 circle, deeper closures 1/2 circle; keratinized layers – reverse cutting or taper-cut (skin, mucoperiosteum, gingiva); 5/8 circle needles may aid in suture placement for deep wounds in confined areas.	5-0 for small dogs and cat, 4-0 larger animals	NA	Choose the smallest-sized suture comfortably possible to minimize trauma from suture placement, and to reduce foreign body reaction. Removal of nonabsorbable sutures can be difficult from deeper regions of the mouth without sedation.
Gingiva, Oral Mucosa, Labial, Tongue Repair	Rapid to intermediate absorbable sutures	3/8 circle, taper needles for mucosa; taper-cut for gingiva	5-0 for small dogs and cat, 4-0 larger animals	NA	Oral mucosa heals quickly. Be sure knots are firmly and squarely applied since knot ears have a tendency to untie prematurely particularly with multifilament absorbable sutures.
Esophagus/ Anastomosis, Esophagotomy, Muscular Patch	Monofilament prolonged absorbable sutures	3/8 to 1/2 circle taper needle. Deeper layers or hard to reach areas choose 1/2 circle	4-0	Circular stapling, EEA 21, 25 mm	Circular stapler size is a limitation for small dogs and cats. Tissue thickness must be more than 1 mm and less than 2.5 mm for proper staple engagement and formation.
Stomach wall/ Gastrotomy, Gastrectomy, Diversions; Gastric Wall Invagination	Monofilament, intermediate to prolonged absorbable suture	1/2 circle, taper needle	3-0 to 4-0	Linear stapling GIA (green cartridge) or TA (green cartridge)	Monocryl, Biosyn, or Maxon are recommended. Polydioxanone loses strength rapidly in acidic environments, so avoid if suture penetrates stomach lumen.
Gastropexy	Monofilament intermediate to prolonged absorbable suture	1/2 circle, taper needle	2-0 to 3-0	Skin stapler (wide); GIA (3.5 mm)	Larger suture size is recommended due to tension on the gastropexy suture line. Skin staplers have been used successfully for gastropexy. A limited number of dogs have undergone gastropexy using a GIA linear stapler.
Pancreas, Marsupialization	Monofilament, intermediate to prolonged absorbable suture	1/2 circle, taper needle	4-0	NA	
Liver/Lobectomy, Partial Lobectomy, Laceration, Biopsy	Monofilament, intermediate absorbable	3/8 to 1/2 circle, taper	4-0	Hilar resection TA 30; partial resection TA (3.5 mm)	Some surgeons prefer multifilament suture for guillotine biopsy. Monofilaments are recommended for laceration repair since smooth surface does not cut friable tissue. Blue linear staple lines may not control all hemorrhage during partial lobectomy; electrocoagulate or skeletonize and ligate remaining bleeders.

Procedure	Suture material	Needle	Suture size	Stapler	Comments
Common Bile Duct, Gall Bladder/ Cholecystotomy, Choledocotomy, Anastomosis	Monofilament intermediate to prolonged absorbable sutures	Fine 3/8 to 1/2 circle taper	4-0 to 5-0	NA	Multifilament sutures can be used successfully. Nonabsorbable sutures may act as a nidus of infection or calculus formation.
Small Intestine/ Anastomosis, Enterotomy, Serosal Patch, Enteroplication	Monofilament, intermediate to prolonged absorbable suture	1/2 circle taper needle	3-0 to 4-0	GIA (3.5 mm), TA (3.5 mm), skin stapler (regular)	Multifilament sutures can be successfully used for intestinal surgery but they cause more tissue drag and may potentiate infection in the presence of contamination. Monofilament nonabsorbable sutures are an acceptable alternative. Avoid nonabsorbable sutures in continuous lines because suture migration – linear foreign body formation is possible.
Large Intestine/ Colotomy, Colostomy, Typhlectomy	Monofilament, intermediate to prolonged absorbable suture	1/2 circle taper needle	3-0 to 4-0	Circular stapling 21, 25 mm; GIA (3.5 mm), TA (3.5 mm)	Multifilament sutures can be successfully used for intestinal surgery but they cause more tissue drag and may potentiate infection in the presence of contamination. Monofilament nonabsorbable sutures are an acceptable alternative. Circular stapler size is a limitation for small dogs and cats. Tissue thickness must be more than 1 mm and less than 2.5 mm for proper staple engagement and formation.
Colopexy	Monofilament prolonged absorbable suture	1/2 circle taper needle	2-0 to 3-0	NA	Larger suture size is recommended due to tension on the colopexy suture line.
Rectum/Partial Resection, Anastomosis	Monofilament, intermediate to prolonged absorbable suture	1/2 circle taper needle	3-0 to 4-0	Circular stapling 21, 25 mm (3.5 to 4.8 mm)	Multifilament sutures can be successfully used for intestinal surgery but they cause more tissue drag and may potentiate infection in the presence of contamination. Monofilament nonabsorbable sutures are an acceptable alternative. Circular stapler size is a limitation for small dogs and cats. Tissue thickness must be more than 1 mm and less than 2.5 mm for proper staple engagement and formation.
Anus/Anal Mass Resection, Mucosal Repair	Rapid to intermediate absorbable sutures	3/8 to 1/2 circle taper or taper-cut	4-0	NA	Healing of anal mucosa is rapid, so intermediate absorbable sutures are preferred. Multifilament sutures may not irritate sensitive anal mucosa compared to more rigid multifilament knot ears.

NA = Not Applicable.

throughout the continuous suture line. When used on hollow viscera, bursting pressures were comparable between barbed suture lines and conventional ones (Hansen and Monnet 2012; Erhart et al. 2013). Comparable outcomes following gastric, enteric, and biliary duct repairs using barbed suture have been reported (Denyttenaera et al. 2009). When using barbed suture for intra-abdominal visceral repair, the exposed rough suture end from the final pass can create adhesion formation and possibly adjacent tissue erosion. It is recommended when terminating barbed suture placed for viscera, two final needle passes in opposing directions should be completed and the end should be cut short against the tissue to avoid excessive adhesion formation.

2.1.8 Biofragmentable Anastomosis Ring

The Bowel Anastomosis Ring (BAR) (Valtrac, Medtronic, Minneapolis, MN) is a biofragmentable medical device made of two interconnecting half-shells made of polyglycolic acid and barium sulfate (Figure 2.1). The device is designed to facilitate anastomosis of the inverted ends of bowel without suturing. The device is placed without an incision in the cecum or retrograde placement through the rectum. It has been reported for use in human and veterinary colonic anastomoses, but also in small bowel and esophagogastric anastomoses (Corman et al. 1989; Thiede et al. 1998; Ryan et al. 2006). Its size range (21–34 mm) generally limits its use in small animal surgery for colonic and rectal anastomosis in larger

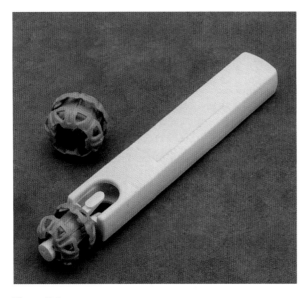

Figure 2.1

breed dogs. Purse-string sutures are placed with a Furniss clamp at the ends of bowel to be connected and the affected bowel is resected. The purse-string sutures are tightened individually over the middle of the two interconnecting half-shells of the BAR. The half-shells are compressed together and intestinal continuity is restored. The rings gradually dissolve and are shed into the bowel for evacuation. The rate of leakage and stricture formation associated with the BAR is comparable to that reported in the literature for stapled and hand-sewn colon repairs in humans (Corman et al. 1989). The BAR has been used with success in cats with megacolon (Ryan et al. 2006). The presence of the megacolon allows placement of a 25 mm BAR with 1.5 mm gap between the two-half after compression. Relaxation of the wall of the colon to facilitate placement of the BAR can be induced with warm saline irrigation, application of topical 1% lidocaine or with IV glucagon (Hardy et al. 1987).

2.2 Staplers, Linear, Circular, Skin Staples

Surgical staples have been used in virtually all aspects of gastrointestinal surgeries.

Staple height is the length of the legs of the staple after trigger closure. Choosing the proper staple leg length is critical because staple legs that are too short do not engage the opposing tissue plane properly or may occlude the intramural blood supply, and choosing legs that are too long may produce ineffective closure, with subsequent leakage of bowel contents or hemorrhage. Surgeons should inspect the thickness of the tissues before choosing the appropriate stapler cartridge (staple height), since edema, and thickened and inflamed intestinal wall, may prevent proper tissue closure with staples. Different stapler configurations have been developed for gastrointestinal stapling by lot of different companies. The author is mostly familiar with the stapling from Medtronics therefore will refer to their product for the remaining of the chapter.

Surgical staplers are classified as "skin" staplers, linear staplers, and circular or end-to-end staplers. Skin staplers have been successfully used in single-layer, noncrushing appositional small intestinal anastomosis, enterotomy closure, and gastropexy techniques (Coolman et al. 2000). For intestinal use, regular-size disposable skin staplers using stainless steel staples (4.7 mm H × 3.5 mm W) (Autosuture Premium 35, Medtronics, Minneapolis, MN) (Figure 2.2) have been

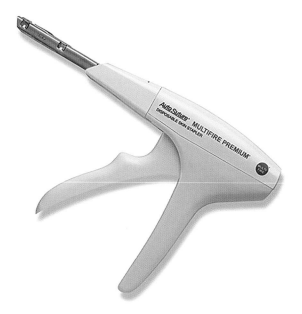

Figure 2.2

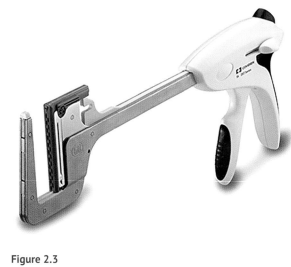

Figure 2.3

reported. For gastropexy, a wide skin stapler has been recommended (Royal 12 W 6.5 mm × 4.1 H) (Coolman et al. 1999).

Linear stapling devices come in a variety of lengths and staple rows. Most linear staplers for veterinary medicine have staple height that is predetermined based on cartridge selection. Some are disposable while others come with reloadable handles with disposable cartridges. In veterinary medicine linear staplers are used most frequently for liver lobectomy, gastrotomy, gastrectomy, and bowel closure. Thoraco-abdominal staplers (TA stapler, Medtronic, Minneapolis, MN) are common linear staplers supplied with double or triple staple rows (Figure 2.3). Non-cutting linear staplers are used for partial hilar lobectomy and pancreatectomy, for gastrotomies, or to staple off intestinal ends during functional end-to-end stapled intestinal anastomoses. TA stapler 30 V3 fires three rows of fine staples (2.5 mm open to 1 mm closed) for secure hemostatic vascular closures at the hilus of organs (lobectomies). The double-row TA 55 and 90 mm long (3.5 mm open to 1.5 mm closed) cartridge linear staplers are most used for intestinal surgery and partial liver or partial lung lobectomy. Double-row TA 55 or 90 (4.8 mm open to 2.0 mm closed) staplers are used nearly exclusively for partial gastrectomies or Billroth 1 procedures. Newer DST TA linear staplers use reloadable linear cartridges with directional staple technology titanium staples. This technology uses a cross-sectional rectangular staple wire that bends

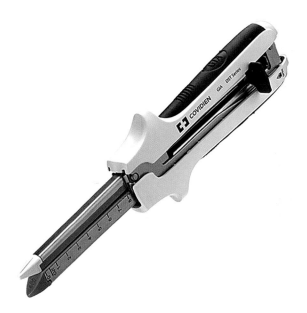

Figure 2.4

more reliably into a fully formed "B"-shaped secure staple (http://www.medtronic.com/covidien/en-us/products/surgical-stapling/open-staplers.html).

Cutting linear staplers have a cutting blade that divides the tissue after two rows of staggered staples are fired on either side of line. The gastrointestinal staplers (GIA, Medtronic, Minneapolis, MN) are commonly used in veterinary surgery and they are 60, 80, or 100 mm long (Figure 2.4).

Linear cutting and stapling devices are often used for pulmonary, cardiac, gastrointestinal, hepatobiliary, or

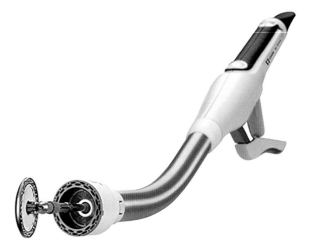

Figure 2.5

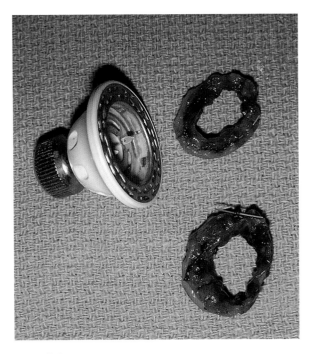

Figure 2.6

reproductive applications. The staplers allow occlusion and division of tissue in a single surgical maneuver. GIA 4.8 mm staplers (4.8 mm open to 2.0 mm closed) are often used for partial gastrectomy during GDV surgery, and GIA 3.8 mm staplers (3.8 mm open to 1.5 mm closed) are used for intestinal anastomosis. Gastrointestinal staplers (Endo GIA, Medtronic, Minneapolis, MN) are used during endoscopic procedures. These cutting linear staplers have staples that continue past the cutting blade limit to ensure that incomplete incisions into vessels or hollow organs do not leak.

Circular stapling devices are used to perform end-to-end, end-to-side, or side-to-side anastomoses in the gastrointestinal tract. It fires a circular staggered double-row staple line, and an inner circular cutting device creates a stoma within the circular staple line (Figure 2.5). Circular staplers create an inverted anastomosis. Circular staplers need to be sized correctly according to the diameter of the organ, and should not be used when the combined tissue thickness is less than 1 mm or more than 2.5 mm. In small animal surgery, the 21 and 25 mm EEA devices with 3.5 or 4.8 mm staples are used most often in gastrointestinal surgeries. The device diameter must fit inside the lumen of the organ to be stapled without tension. Patient size is a limiting factor for circular staplers in small animal surgery. Generally EEAs can be used in large bowel of most small animals and only medium- to large-breed dogs for the small bowel. A Furniss device is used to place a purse-string of monofilament sutures on either side of the tubular organ ends to be anastomosed. A detachable anvil is secured with one purse-string suture. The other end is secured in a similar fashion to the stapler head. The anvil is connected to the head and the ends are firmly brought together. After the stapler is fired a circular cutting blade cuts a donut of tissue within the circular staple line (Figure 2.6). Always inspect the donut to be sure all layers of the bowel have been cut and there is a patent lumen.

References

Arbaugh, M. et al. (2013). Biomechanical comparison of glycomer 631 and glycomer 631 knotless for use in canine incisional gastropexy. *Vet. Surg.* 42 (2): 205–209.

Booth, H.W. (2003). Suture materials, tissue adhesives, staplers, and ligating clips. In: *Textbook of Small Animal Surgery*, 3e (ed. D. Slatter), 234–244. Philadelphia: Saunders.

Capperauld, I. (1989). Suture materials: a review. *Clin. Mater.* 4 (1): 3–12.

Chih-Chang, C. and Williams, D.F. (1984). Effects of physical configuration and chemical structure of suture materials on bacterial adhesion: A possible link to wound infection. *Am. J. Surg.* 147 (2): 147–204.

Chu, C.C., Von Franhofer, J.A., Greisler, H.P. et al. (eds.) (1997). *Wound Closure Biomaterials and Devices*. New York: CRC Press.

Chu, C.C. and Williams, D.F. (1984). Effects of physical configuration and chemical structure of suture materials on bacterial adhesion. A possible link to wound infection. *Am. J. Surg.* 147 (2): 197–204.

Coolman, B.R. et al. (1999). Evaluation of a skin stapler for belt-loop gastropexy in dogs. *J. Am Anim. Hosp. Assoc.* 35 (5): 440–444.

Coolman, B.R. et al. (2000). Comparison of skin staples with sutures for anastomosis of the small intestine in dogs. *Vet. Surg.* 29 (4): 293–302.

Corman, M.L. et al. (1989). Comparison of the valtrac biofragmentable anastomosis ring with conventional suture and stapled anastomosis in colon surgery. Results of a prospective, randomized clinical trial. *Dis. Colon Rectum* 32 (3): 183–187.

Denyttenaera, S.V. et al. (2009). Barbed suture for gastrointestinal closure: A randomized control trial. *Surgical Innovation.* 16 (3): 237–242.

Domnick, E.D. (2014). Suture material and needle options in oral and periodontal surgery. *J. Vet. Dentistry* 31 (3): 204–211.

Erhart, N.P. et al. (2013). In vivo assessment of absorbable knotless barbed suture for single layer gastrotomy and enterotomy closure. *Vet. Surg.* 42 (2): 210–216.

Ferrer-Marquez, M. and Belda-Lorano, R. (2009). Barbed sutures in general and digestive surgery. *Cirugia Espanola.* 94 (2): 65–69.

Freudenberg, S. et al. (2004). Biodegradation of absorbable sutures in body fluids and pH buffers. *Eur. Surg. Res.* 36 (6): 376–385.

Hansen, L.A. and Monnet, E.L. (2012). Evaluation of a novel suture material for closure of intestinal anastomoses in canine cadavers. *Am. J. Vet. Res.* 73 (11): 1819–1823.

Hardy, T.G. Jr. et al. (1987). Initial clinical experience with a biofragmentable ring for sutureless bowel anastomosis. *Dis. Colon Rectum* 30 (1): 55–61.

Hoer, J., et al. (2001). Influence of suture technique on laparotomy wound healing: An experimental study in the rat. *Langenbeck's archives of surgery/Deutsche Gesellschaft fur Chirurgie* 386 (3): 218–223.

Masini, B.D. et al. (2011). Bacterial adherence to suture materials. *J. Surg. Educ.* 68 (2): 101–104.

Marturello, D.M. et al. (2014). Knot security and tensile strength of suture materials. *Vet. Surg.* 43 (1): 73–79.

Osterberg, C.A. (1983). Enclosure of bacteria within capillary multifilament sutures as protection against leukocytes. *Acta Chir. Scand.* 149 (7): 663–668.

Ryan, S. et al. (2006). Comparison of biofragmentable anastomosis ring and sutured anastomoses for subtotal colectomy in cats with idiopathic megacolon. *Vet. Surg.* 35 (8): 740–748.

Smeak, D.D. (1998). Selection and use of currently available suture materials and needles. In: *Current Techniques in Small Animal Surgery*, 4e (eds. M.J. Bojrab et al.), 19–26. Philadelphia: Williams and Wilkins.

Thiede, A. et al. (1998). Overview on compression anastomoses: biofragmentable anastomosis ring multicenter prospective trial of 1666 anastomoses. *W. J. of Surg.* 22 (1): 78–87.

Thornton, F.J. and Barbul, A. (2014). Healing in the gastrointestinal tract. *Surg. Clin. N. Am.* 77 (3): 549–573.

Zimmer, C.A. et al. (1991). Influence of knot configuration and tying technique on the mechanical performance of sutures. *J. Emerg. Med.* 9 (3): 107–113.

3

Suture Patterns for Gastrointestinal Surgery
Daniel D. Smeak

Department of Clinical Sciences, College of Veterinary Medicine and Biomedical Sciences, Colorado State University, Fort Collins, CO, USA

3.1 One- or Two-Layer Closure

Although this is still a controversial topic, both techniques have potential downfalls that could endanger an anastomosis. One would think two-layer closures are better than one-layer since they might provide added strength initially. However, they increase the inflammatory response in the early stages of visceral healing owing to the extra tissue handling, suture material, and ischemia of the inverted tissue cuff (Orr 1969; McAdams et al. 1970; Goligher et al. 1977). Excess inflammation at the healing site results in a weaker anastomosis as more collagen is broken down during the inflammatory and debridement phases of healing. Advocates of single-layer closures argue that this technique results in a larger lumen with less damage to the tissue edges (Thornton and Barbul 1997). Currently, in most conditions, a single-layer closure for most gastrointestinal repairs is considered adequate (Sajid et al. 2012). Provided the lumen is not compromised, double-layer repairs are sometimes elected when the surgeon expects higher intraluminal pressures, or when the tissue edge is considered extra friable or when sutures in the first layer tend to cut through the tissue.

3.2 Tissue Inversion, Eversion, or Apposition

Inverting suture patterns cause greater initial narrowing of the intestinal lumen (Bellenger 1982) but their main advantage is that these patterns provide more consistent initial leak-proof closures (higher leak pressures). Everting patterns elicit greater adhesion formation to exposed mucosal edges, and provide the least leak-proof closures, and therefore they are not currently recommended for gastrointestinal closure (Hamilton 1967). In theory, approximating (appositional) patterns accurately align tissue layers compared to inverting and everting patterns, and therefore, these patterns are now preferred for gastrointestinal closures. However, in practice, consistent tissue apposition with approximating suture patterns infrequently occurs when anastomoses were evaluated histologically. Nevertheless, direct apposition of all intestinal layers, particularly the submucosal layer, has been found to result in the most rapid direct bridging of the repair (Jansen et al. 1981).

3.3 Stapled or Hand-Sutured Anastomosis

Stapled anastomoses are technically easier and faster but they do not replace adherence to the principles of good surgical technique for successful intestinal healing (Chassin et al. 1984). Regardless of technique, an adequate blood supply and absence of contamination or tension is paramount to successful repair. Linear staples in thicker visceral tissue may not purchase the strength holding layer on both sides of the staple line leading to a weakened repair (Snowden et al. 2016). It is critical that the correct staple leg length is chosen when visceral edges are edematous or inflamed. In most situations, linear staple cartridges with 3.5 mm staples are acceptable for most intestinal repairs in dogs and cats. Linear staples with 4.8 mm staples are chosen for thicker intestinal edges and for stomach repairs. Stapled anastomoses

Gastrointestinal Surgical Techniques in Small Animals, First Edition. Edited by Eric Monnet and Daniel D. Smeak.
© 2020 John Wiley & Sons, Inc. Published 2020 by John Wiley & Sons, Inc.
Companion website: www.wiley.com/go/monnet/gastrointestinal

were not at more risk for dehiscence when performed in the face of septic peritonitis, unlike what has been encountered in hand-sewn repairs in multiple retrospective studies (Snowden et al., 2016; Davis et al. 2018).

3.4 Appositional Suture Patterns

3.4.1 Simple Interrupted

The major advantage of simple interrupted suture patterns is the ability to precisely control tension at each stitch along the wound with variable spreading forces along the margins (Moy et al. 1992). Another advantage is that each interrupted stitch is a separate entity, and failure of the single suture or knot may be inconsequential. Interrupted suture patterns take longer to place and knot, the individual knots increase the volume of foreign material in repairs, and suture economy suffers. A retrospective study comparing simple interrupted and continuous appositional patterns for enterotomy and anastomosis in dogs and cats found a low and comparable rate of enteric leakage with either pattern (Weisman et al. 1999).

3.4.2 Simple Continuous

The major advantage of simple continuous patterns is the speed of placement, and they generally create a more leak-proof closure when compared to their interrupted counterparts. Continuous lines use less suture and minimize exposure of knots that can untie or cause tissue reaction. Surgeons have less precise control of suture tension and wound approximation throughout the repair. Insecure knots, lack of adequate needle purchase of the strength holding layer, or suture breakage can have disastrous effects on gastrointestinal repairs.

3.4.3 Patterns to Reduce Excess Mucosal Eversion

After gastric and intestinal incision, it is common that muscle fibers within the wall contract, causing retraction and spasm. The underlying loosely attached mucosa aggressively everts and rolls over the incised edge of intestine or stomach. When simple interrupted or simple continuous sutures are placed while the mucosa is remains everted, true apposition of intestinal layers cannot be attained. Everted mucosa is caught between the incised edges. Intestinal healing in this instance is slowed, when compared to accurately aligned intestinal layers. Excess mucosal eversion also lowers leak pressure of the repair and may increase the incidence of adhesion formation. The Gambee and modified Gambee patterns help reduce mucosal eversion.

3.4.3.1 Gambee

In the Gambee pattern on the first side, the needle is inserted 3–4 mm away from the cut edge of serosa directly through the full-thickness wall of the intestine into the lumen (Figure 3.1a). The needle is backed up just enough to advance and pierce the middle of the cut surface of the everted mucosal edge. The second purchase on the opposite side begins with the needle inserted in the cut edge of the everted mucosa down into the lumen of the bowel. The needle is then advanced and driven full thickness directly from the bowel lumen to the serosa, catching 3–4 mm of wall. The advantage of this suture over the modified Gambee stitch (below) is that since the needle pierces the bowel wall full thickness, a good purchase of submucosa is guaranteed to be included with each needle bite.

3.4.3.2 Modified Gambee

In this suture pattern, the needle penetrates the serosa, muscularis, and submucosa, but the everting mucosal layer is not incorporated (Figure 3.1b). On the opposite side a mirror image of the needle purchase is taken; the needle incorporates the submucosa, muscularis, and serosa only. When the suture is pulled snuggly, the mucosa is buried within the lumen. This pattern can be used as a simple interrupted pattern or in a continuous fashion. Caution should be taken when considering this pattern. The downside to this modification is that the serosa and muscularis layers may be included, but because mucosal eversion hides the incised bowel edge, either the submucosa may not be included or too small of purchase if this layer is included, rendering the suture line susceptible to premature dehiscence (Kieves et al. 2014).

3.4.3.3 Luminal Interrupted Vertical Mattress Pattern

During intestinal anastomosis and other tubular anastomoses, occasionally the deep side of the bowel edges are difficult to mobilize and expose. In this instance, surgeons may elect to use vertical mattress suture patterns placed within the lumen on the deep side of the anastomosis. The sutures are generally preplaced and tied such that the knots are within the lumen of the tubular organ. This results in cut edges that are sealed and inverted within the lumen. No knots are exposed on the serosal surface. The remaining anastomosis on the exposed near side is closed with an appositional suture pattern.

(a)

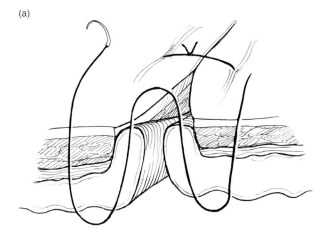

(b)

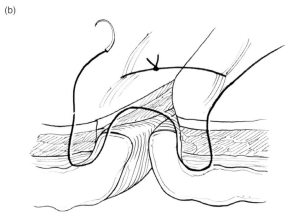

Figure 3.1

3.5 Inverting Suture Patterns

3.5.1 Halsted

This is an interrupted inverting suture pattern that is occasionally chosen by some surgeons when trying to purchase friable tissue edges in hollow organ incisions (Figure 3.2). The needle is passed into the hollow organ wall perpendicular and about 5 mm from the edge, through the serosa, muscularis, and submucosa and exits 2 mm from the edge on the same side. Across the incision, the needle is passed through the serosa perpendicular and about 2 mm from the edge into the serosa, muscularis, and submucosa before exiting 5 mm from the cut edge. Next the needle is reversed and identical bites are taken in the opposite direction about 5 mm from the first bite sequence. The free suture ends are tied to complete the stitch.

3.5.2 Cushing and Connell

These continuous patterns are often used to close hollow organs because they cause tissue inversion and provide a reliable leak-proof seal. The Cushing and Connell patterns are similar except that the Cushing

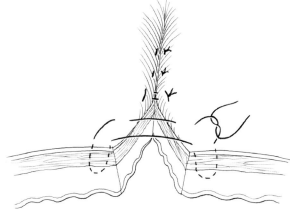

Figure 3.2

pattern is placed so that the suture purchases the serosa, muscularis, and submucosa, but it does not pierce the mucosa so it is not exposed to the lumen of the organ (Figure 3.3). For the Connell pattern, suture extends into the organ lumen (Figure 3.4). Some surgeons choose to avoid penetrating the lumen of hollow viscera to help reduce the potential for contamination from the needle track in highly contaminated visceral organs. The author prefers to begin these two inverting lines with a Lembert stitch which helps to begin tissue inversion with the first stitch. Subsequent bites are more readily inverted after the Lembert stitch is placed. The suture line is continued taking alternating 5 mm bites of tissue, 3 mm away and parallel to the incision line. Once the needle exits the bite, it is passed directly across the incision and another similar parallel bite of tissue is taken. This suture line is repeated until the incision is closed. The suture strand is pulled firmly to create inversion and to reduce suture exposure on the serosal surface.

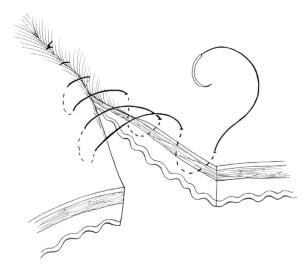

Figure 3.3

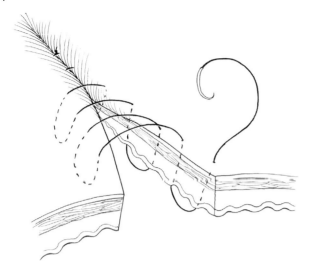

Figure 3.4

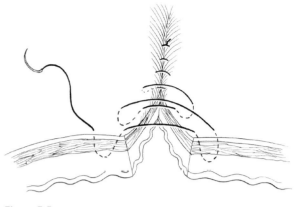

Figure 3.5

3.5.3 Lembert

This interrupted or continuous pattern results in aggressive inversion of hollow visceral edges (Figure 3.5). It may be used to help bury considerable eversion of mucosa. The needle penetrates through serosa and muscularis and purchases submucosa about 8–10 mm away from the incision edge and exits 3–4 mm from the wound margin on the same side. After the needle passes over the incision, it penetrates 3–4 mm from the wound margin and exits about 8–10 mm away from the incision. The further away from the incision the needle passes, the more inversion is formed. When placing continuous inverting suture lines, the surgeon must be aware of the

location of the cut edge at all time. As the cut edge inverts when the line is tightened, there is a tendency to take bites progressively further from the visceral wound edge which can result in an undesirable deep inverted stump of tissue at the end of the suture line.

3.5.4 Parker–Kerr Oversew

This continuous inverting pattern is used to "blind end" a tubular organ such as bowel or uterine stumps (Figure 3.6). To reduce contamination and aid in needle purchase, a large hemostatic clamp is first placed perpendicular to the long axis of the tubular organ. Any remaining organ tissue extending past the jaws of the clamp is removed. Starting at either the mesenteric or antimesenteric surface, a loose continuous Cushing suture pattern is placed catching 3–4 mm of bowel wall with each needle bite and running at least 3 mm from

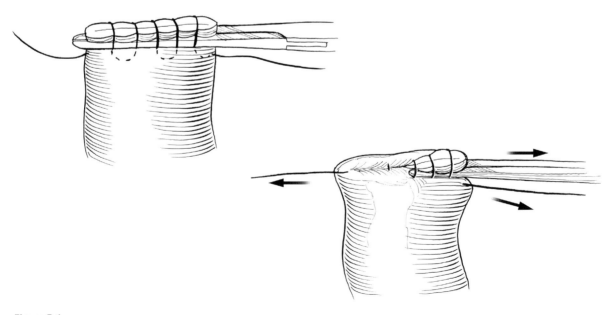

Figure 3.6

Figure 3.7

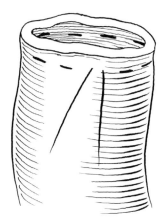
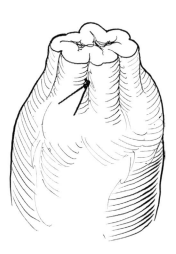

the edge of the clamp. Once the loose Cushing pattern is complete, the jaws of the clamp are partially opened releasing the incised bowel edges, while the suture end with the needle is slowly tensioned away from the side closest to the clamp hinge. The clamp is removed and the suture line is tensioned from both sides to completely invert the stump edges. The needle is then reversed and a Lembert pattern is placed and tied to the original free suture end to form a leak-proof double inverted stump.

3.6 Special Supplementary Patterns: Purse-String

This suture pattern is intended to close a hollow organ opening or body aperture, such as the anal opening, or around a tube entrance in viscera (Figure 3.7). It is often utilized around the anal opening to prevent fecal contamination during perineal surgery, and to create a seal around a feeding tube placed in hollow viscera, as in a gastrostomy tube procedure. As the suture is placed around the site, tension on the suture end will tighten the continuous pattern much like a purse being pulled together at its neck with a string. The suture pattern is begun with parallel 3–4 mm bites of tissue about 3–5 mm away from the opening or cut edge. Each successive bite is advanced no more than 2–3 mm from the exit site of the last purchase. This forms a circular pattern around the centrally located opening. At the end of the pattern, both beginning and ending suture strands are in close apposition to each other. The strands are pulled firmly to form a tight cuffed rim of tissue around the tube or orifice, preventing leakage.

Bibliography

Bellenger, C. (1982). Comparison of inverting and appositional methods of anastomosis of the small intestines in cats. *Vet. Rec.* 110: 265–268.

Chassin, J.L., Rifkind, K.M., and Tumer, J.W. (1984). Errors and pitfalls in stapling gastrointestinal tract anastomoses. *Surg. Clin. North Am.* 64: 441–459.

Chung, R.S. (1987). Blood flow in colonic anastomoses. Effect of stapling and suturing. *Ann. Surg.* 206: 335–339.

Davis, D.D., Demianiuk, R.M., Musser, J. et al. (2018). Influence of preoperative septic peritonitis and anastomotic technique on the dehiscence of enterectomy sites in dogs. A retrospective review of 210 anastomoses. *Vet. Surg.* 47: 125–129.

Ellison, G. (1989). Healing in the gastrointestinal tract. *Semin. Vet. Med. Surg. (Small Anim.)* 4: 287–293.

Getzen, L.C., Roe, R.D., and Holloway, C.K. (1966). Comparative study of intestinal anastomotic healing in inverted and everted closures. *Surg. Gynecol. Obstet.* 123: 1219–1227.

Goligher, J.C., Lee, P.W., Simpkins, K.C. et al. (1977). A controlled comparison of one- and two-layer techniques of suture for high and low colorectal anastomoses. *Br. J. Surg.* 64: 609–614.

Graham, M.F., Diegelmann, R.F., Elson, C.O. et al. (1988). Collagen content and types in the intestinal strictures of Crohn's disease. *Gastroenterology* 94: 257–264.

Halstead, W.S. (1887). Circular suture of the intestine. An experimental study. *Am. J. Med. Sci.* 94: 436–461.

Hamilton, J.E. (1967). Reappraisal of open intestinal anastomoses. *Ann. Surg.* 165: 917–924.

Hogstrom, H., Haglund, U., and Zederfeldt, B. (1990). Tension leads to increased neutrophil accumulation and decreased laparotomy wound strength. *Surgery* 107: 215–219.

Hunt, T.K., Cederfeldt, B., and Goldstick, T.K. (1969). Oxygen and healing [review]. *Am. J. Surg.* 118: 521–525.

Jansen, A., Becker, A.E., Brummelkamp, W.H. et al. (1981). The importance of apposition of the submucosal intestinal layers for primary wound healing of intestinal anastomoses. *Surg. Gynecol. Obstet.* 152: 51–58.

Kieves N., Thompson D.A. and Krebs A.I. (2014). Comparison of ex vivo leak pressures for single-layer enterotomy closure between novice and trained participants in a canine model. Scientific Presentation Abstracts: 2014 ACVS Surgery Summit October 16–18, San Diego, CA.

McAdams, A.J., Meikle, A.G., and Taylor, J.O. (1970). One layer or two layer colonic anastomoses? *Am. J. Surg.* 120: 546–550.

Moy, R.L., Waldman, B., and Hein, D.W. (1992). A review of sutures and suturing techniques. *J. Dermatol. Surg. Oncol.* 18: 785–795.

Orr, N.W.M. (1969). A single-layer intestinal anastomosis. *Br. J. Surg.* 56: 771–774.

Sajid, M.S., Siddiqui, M.R.S., and Baig, M.K. (2012). Single layer versus double layer suture anastomosis of the gastrointestinal tract. *Cochrane Database Syst. Rev.* 18 (1): CD005477. https://doi.org/10.1002/14651858. CD005477.

Snowden, K.A., Smeak, D.D., and Chiang, S. (2016). Risk factors for dehiscence of stapled functional end-to-end intestinal anastomoses in dogs: 53 cases (2001–2012). *Vet. Surg.* 45: 91–99.

Thornton, F.J. and Barbul, A. (1997). Healing in the gastrointestinal tract. *Surg. Clin. N. Am.* 77: 549–573.

Udenfriend, S. (1966). Formation of hydroxyproline in collagen [review]. *Science* 152: 1335–1340.

Weisman, D.L., Smeak, D.D., Birchard, S.J. et al. (1999). Comparison of a continuous suture pattern with a simple interrupted pattern for enteric closure in dogs and cats: 83 cases (1991–1997). *J. Am. Vet. Med. Assoc.* 214: 1507–1510.

4

Feeding Tubes

Eric Monnet

Department of Clinical Sciences, College of Veterinary Medicine and Biomedical Sciences, Colorado State University, Fort Collins, CO, USA

Enteral feeding is an important component of the treatment of critically ill patients, and for the support of patients with anorexia related to chronic conditions. Different type of feeding tubes are available to the surgeons to support the patients according to their need and underlying conditions (Armstrong et al. 1990a; Abood and Buffington 1992; Marks 1998).

Each of those feeding tubes has its advantages and disadvantages. The choice of feeding tube is based on the underlying disease, the goal of the enteral nutrition, and the length of time the tube will be needed. Combination of tubes is also possible. It is not rare to combine a gastrostomy tube with a jejunostomy tube to support a patient in the short term and the long term. The jejunostomy tube will be used in the short term to support the patient in the recovery phase of the surgery, especially if the patient is vomiting, while the gastrostomy tube will be used in the long term to support the patient if still anorexic.

Enteral feeding is also very important to support the integrity of the gastrointestinal tract. The enterocytes are getting their nutrient directly from the metabolite present in the lumen of the gastrointestinal tract.

4.1 Nasoesophageal and Nasogastric Tubes

Nasogastric or nasoesophageal feeding tubes can be used in dogs and cats. Since the tubes are of a small diameter they can be advanced in the stomach without increasing the risk of gastric reflux and esophagitis (Crowe 1986; Armstrong et al. 1990a; Abood and Buffington 1991; Yu et al. 2013; Herring 2016).

4.1.1 Indications

Nasoesophageal and nasogastric tubes are mostly used for the short-term support of a patient. It is an interesting tube for a patient that may not tolerate general anesthesia since it can be placed with only local anesthesia.

It can be used to feed a patient with a liquid diet since the tubes are of a small diameter. This tube is more efficient for small dogs and cats than for large-breed dogs, since only liquid can be used.

It can also be used to keep the stomach decompressed or empty to prevent gastroesophageal reflux, regurgitation, and/or vomiting (Crowe 1986).

Nasoesophageal tubes are contraindicated if the patient has esophageal motility disorders. Nasogastric tubes are contraindicated for patients with esophageal strictures.

Feeding with these tubes should not be attempted if the patient is vomiting or lateral recumbent because it will increase the risk of aspiration pneumonia. However, a nasogastric tube can still be used to keep the stomach decompressed as mentioned above.

4.1.2 Materials and Equipment

Feeding tube of small diameter is required. Size 5 or 6 Fr is commonly used in dogs and cats. Polyurethane or silicone tubes are used. The tube needs to be long enough to reach the stomach. Weighted tubes can be used to facilitate their migration in the stomach (Figure 4.1). Because of the size of the tube only liquid diet can be used.

Local anesthetic mixed with a lubricant is needed to facilitate the placement of the tube. Usually 1 ml of 0.5% bupivacaine can be mixed with 1 ml of water-soluble lubricant.

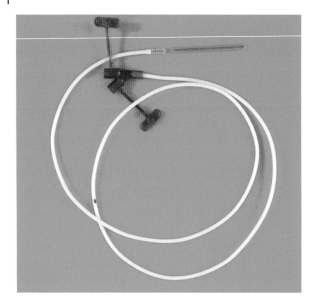

Figure 4.1

General anesthesia is not required to place a nasoesophageal or nasogastric tube. Heavy sedation might be required.

4.1.3 Surgical Techniques

Local anesthesia is applied in the ventral meatus of the nasal cavity. The extremity of a nasoesophageal tube is usually sitting in the middle of the thoracic esophagus. The length of the tube is measured from the tip of the nose to the level of the 8th or 9th rib. If a nasogastric tube is placed, it is measured from the tip of the nose to the last rib. The tube is introduced in the ventral meatus of the nasal cavity after the nares are gently pushed dorsally with the thumb while the hand is holding the head of the dog or cat. The tube is advanced and when it reaches the nasopharynx the dog or cat will start swallowing, which will facilitate the passage of the tube in the esophagus. The tube is then advanced to the desired length to reach the middle of the thoracic esophagus or the stomach (Figure 4.2).

If the patient is coughing, the tube should be withdrawn because it is progressing into the larynx and the trachea.

After placement of the tube it is stabilized on the side of the nares with a simple interrupted suture. Another suture is placed on the side of the lips and cheeks to stabilize the tube.

It is paramount that appropriate placement of the tube is confirmed before it is used to provide nutrition to the patient. Since the tubes are small it may not be possible to palpate the tube in the neck. First aspiration of the tube should generate negative pressure if it is in the esophagus or gastric content if it is in the lumen of the stomach. If air is aspirated it has been placed in the airway. If the tube is in the stomach, injection of 5 ml of air should induce borborygm, easily detected with a stethoscope placed over the stomach. Injection of 5 ml of sterile saline will induce coughing reflex if the tube is in the airway. Finally, since the feeding tubes are radiodense a lateral radiograph should confirm the accurate placement of the tube (Figure 4.2).

4.1.4 Utilization

Nasoesophageal and nasogastric feeding tubes can be used immediately to support the patient. Only liquid diet can be used. After calculating the daily calorie

Figure 4.2

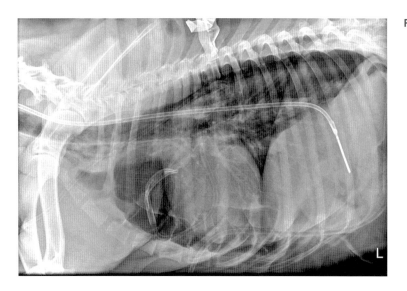

requirement of the patient the diet is delivered in six feedings very slowly. The tube is then flushed with saline to prevent obstruction.

The nasogastric tube can also be used to keep the stomach decompressed in case of severe ileus after abdominal surgery.

4.1.5 Tips

The administration of a long-acting local anesthesia in the nasal cavity every four to six hours greatly improves the tolerance of the tube by the patient.

4.1.6 Complications

Nasoesophageal and nasogastric tubes can be dislodged if the patient is vomiting. Epistaxis and sneezing can occur with a nasoesophageal or nasogastric tube. Local anesthesia reduces the risk of sneezing. Nasogastric tubes may trigger gastroesophageal reflux and regurgitation. In this case it is then recommended to convert the tube into a nasoesophageal tube by pulling the tube into the esophagus. Obstruction of the tube can occur. It is important to regularly flush the tube with saline.

4.2 Esophagostomy Tube

4.2.1 Indications

Esophagostomy tubes are used to provide long-term support to the patients. Esophagostomy tube can be maintained for several weeks to months. They are mostly used to support anorexic patients with chronic systemic disease. They are also used for patients with severe trauma to the head, after surgery of the oral cavity, or to keep the stomach decompressed (Crowe and Devey 1997a; Devitt and Seim 1997; Levine et al. 1997; Kanemoto et al. 2017).

Esophagostomy tubes are contraindicated for dogs or cats with esophageal disease. Megaesophagus, esophagitis, esophageal stricture, and reflux are contradictions for the placement of an esophagostomy tube. However, an esophagostomy tube has been used to keep a megaesophagus decompressed to reduce the risk of aspiration pneumonia in one dog (Kanemoto et al. 2017). Esophagostomy tubes have also been advanced to the jejunum to support dogs with pancreatitis or anorexia (Cummings and Daley 2014).

The main advantage of an esophagostomy tube is that a diet modified into a gruel can be used to support the patient. The nutrition is delivered three or four times a day. Diet is blenderized with enough water and delivered slowly and warm to the patient. Also, dogs and cats can eat orally even if the tube is in place. The tube is then used for complement if the caloric intake is not sufficient.

4.2.2 Materials and Equipment

Esophagostomy tubes are usually 16–20 Fr in diameter. A red rubber tube, a polyvinyl chloride tube, a polyurethane tube, or a silicone tube can be used for an esophagostomy tube (Figure 4.3). The holes at the extremity of the tube need to enlarged to prevent clogging of the tube with the gruel (Crowe and Devey 1997b; Devitt and Seim 1997).

The dog or the cat needs to be placed under general anesthesia and intubated for the placement of an esophagostomy tube. The patient is positioned in right lateral recumbency and the left side of the neck is clipped and surgically prepared and draped.

4.2.3 Surgical Techniques

The length of the tube is measured from the proximal part of the esophagus to the level of the 8th or 9th rib. The appropriate length is marked on the tube.

A long curved forceps is introduced through the oral cavity in the proximal esophagus (Figure 4.4a). The tip of the forceps is palpated percutaneously in the proximal part of the neck.

A small skin incision is made over the tip of the forceps (Figure 4.4b). It is important to tent the soft tissue of the neck while the instrument is tipped up in the neck. This minimizes the risk of stabbing the jugular vein or the carotid artery. The tip of the forceps is then

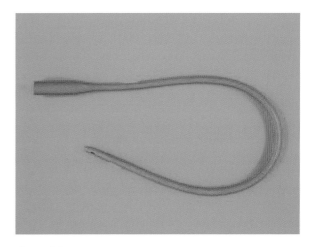

Figure 4.3

(a)

(b)

(c)

(d)

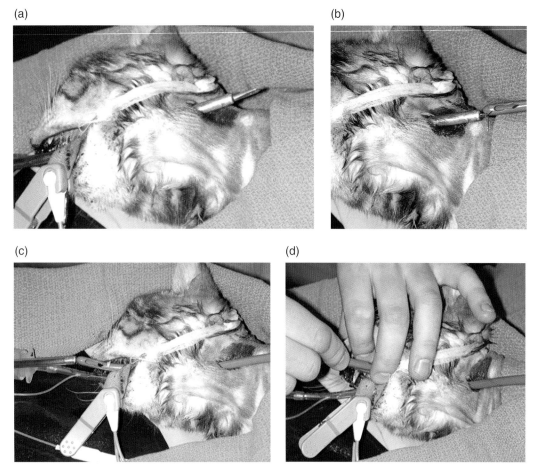

Figure 4.4

exposed after incising the wall of the esophagus. The incision should be long enough to advance the tip of the forceps through the wall of the esophagus. A large incision will result in leakage of saliva around the tube in the subcutaneous area, inducing cellulitis.

The tip of the esophagostomy tube is then grabbed and pulled in the oral cavity (Figure 4.4b and c). The tube is then reinserted in the esophagus (Figure 4.4d). It is important not to wrap the esophagostomy tube around the endotracheal tube. The tube is advanced until it passes the point of insertion in the esophagus. Then it can be pushed in the esophagus to the desired length.

As an alternative technique a special trocar can be used to place the esophagostomy tube. The tube is first introduced in the esophagus through the mouth (Figure 4.5a). Then the distal end of a special curved trocar is advanced in the proximal esophagus. The skin and the wall of the esophagus are incised over the tip of the trocar (Figure 4.5b). The esophagostomy tube is attached to the distal end of the trocar (Figure 4.5c).

The trocar is then pulled through incision in the neck, dragging the esophagostomy tube with it (Figure 4.5d–g).

The tube is secured in placed with 2-0 nylon suture as a Chinese finger trap (Song et al. 2008).

It is paramount that the placement of the tube is confirmed prior to feeding of the patient. A lateral radiograph is used to confirm the placement of the tip of the esophagostomy tube in the distal esophagus (Figure 4.5g). If the tube is in the stomach, it needs to be pulled back in the esophagus.

The tube can be removed eight days after placement if it is not needed. The finger-trap suture is just cut and the tube is pulled out. The stoma is left to heal by second intention. The dog or cat can eat immediately.

4.2.4 Tips

It is important to have an endotracheal tube to prevent placement of the tube in the airway. A long curved forceps greatly facilitates the placement of the esophagostomy tube, especially in large obese dogs. The tube

(a)

(b)

(c)

(d)

(e)

(f)

(g)

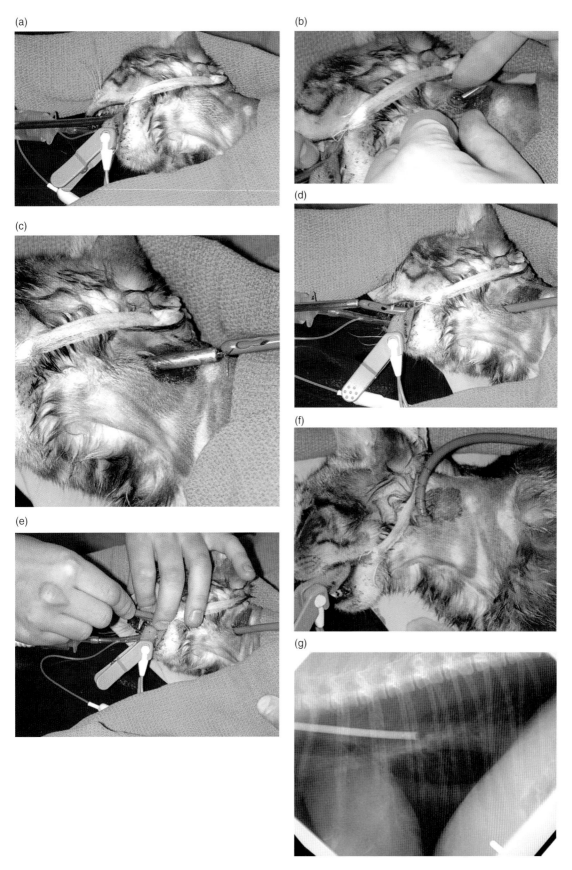

Figure 4.5

should be easy to advance in the esophagus. If the tube is forced in the esophagus, there is a significant risk of perforating the esophagus at the base of the heart.

4.2.5 Utilization

Esophagostomy tube can be used right away to feed the patient. After calculation of the daily caloric requirement, the amount of food is divided in four feedings. Any diet transformed in a gruel can be used with an esophagostomy tube. The gruel is delivered slowly over 5–10 minutes to prevent vomiting. The tube is then flushed with saline to prevent obstruction.

4.2.6 Complications

Esophagostomy tubes can be dislodged or kinked if the patient is vomiting. Laceration of the jugular vein and/or the carotid artery can happen with sharp dissection. Inflammation at the stoma is frequent. It may result in mild exudate. Obstruction of the tube can occur. It is important to flush the tube with saline regularly.

4.3 Gastrostomy Tube

4.3.1 Indications

Gastrostomy tubes are used in anorexic patients. They are used to bypass the oral cavity and the esophagus because of disease process, trauma, or obstruction (Armstrong et al. 1990a; Armstrong and Hardie 1990b; Bright et al. 1991; Marks 1998).

Gastrostomy tube can be kept for long-term support of dogs and cats. It is not unusual to have tube in place for four months. Low-profile gastrostomy tubes are then very appropriate for long-term support. Low-profile gastrostomy tubes are less bulky and have more likely less chance to be pulled accidentally by the dog or the cat (Yoshimoto et al. 2006).

4.3.2 Materials and Equipment

Large-bore feeding tube can be used for gastrostomy tube. Usually a 20–30 Fr tube can be placed. Either a Foley catheter or a mushroom-tipped tube are used in dogs and cats (Figure 4.6). The balloon of a Foley catheter has a tendency to rupture quickly because of the acidic environment. Mushroom-tipped tubes are commonly use if long-term utilization is anticipated. A low-profile gastrostomy tube with a mushroom-tipped can also be used.

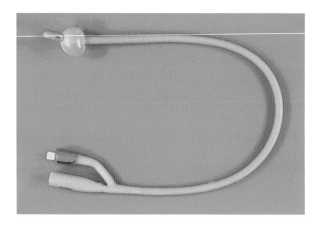

Figure 4.6

Gastrostomy feeding tubes can be placed surgically during a laparotomy or percutaneously with endoscopy (Armstrong et al. 1990a, Armstrong and Hardie 1990b, Bright et al. 1991, Marks 1998). General anesthesia is required for the placement of a gastrostomy tube. The tubes are placed in the left side of the abdominal cavity into the body of the stomach.

4.3.3 Technique

4.3.3.1 Endoscopic Placement
Endoscopic placement of gastrostomy is recommended for patients not undergoing laparotomy. Endoscopic placement is contraindicated for patients with esophageal stricture.

The patient is placed in right lateral recumbency. A flexible endoscope is advanced in the stomach. After sufficient insufflation of the stomach an 18 gauge over-the-needle catheter is placed percutaneously in the lumen of the stomach. A suture is then threaded in the catheter. A snare or a grasping forceps can grab the suture in the lumen of the stomach. The suture is then pulled out through the esophagus and the mouth of the patient. The suture has to be long enough to exit in the oral cavity and still be present through the abdominal wall. Another over-needle catheter is threaded over the suture and the gastrostomy tube securely attached to the suture. The proximal end of the gastrostomy tube is wedged in the flared end of the over-needle catheter. A mushroom-tipped catheter is used. The suture is then pulled from the abdominal wall to bring the gastrostomy tube in the lumen of the stomach. A small skin incision is made to facilitate the passage of the catheter through the abdominal wall. A Chinese finger-trap suture with 2-0 nylon is then used to secure the gastrostomy tube to the skin (Song et al. 2008). The endoscope can be reintroduced to confirm appropriate placement of the gastrostomy tube.

4.3.3.2 Surgical Placement

4.3.3.2.1 *Laparoscopically Assisted* A single-access port is inserted in the left side of the abdominal cavity caudal to the last rib. The port is placed lateral to the rectus abdominal muscle. After insufflation of the abdominal cavity a 5 mm rigid endoscope and 5 mm grasping forceps are used to visualize and grab the wall of the body of the stomach toward the fundus between the lesser and greater curvature. The stomach is brought against the abdominal wall and the single-access port is removed. Small Gelpy retractors are used to keep the incision through the abdominal wall opened. A stay suture is placed in the wall of the stomach. A 3-0 monofilament absorbable suture is then used to place a purse-string suture in the wall of the stomach. A #11 blade is used to puncture the center of the purse-string suture. The gastrostomy tube is then introduced in the lumen of the stomach. The purse-string suture is tightened around the tube. If a Foley catheter has been used, the balloon is inflated with 5 ml of saline. Four pexy sutures are placed between the wall of the stomach and the transverse abdominalis muscle. A 3-0 monofilament absorbable suture is used for the pexy. Another purse-string suture is placed in the transverse abdominalis muscle around the tube to prevent its displacement. The subcutaneous tissue and skin are closed in a routine fashion around the tube. A Chinese finger-trap suture with 2-0 nylon is placed on the skin to secure the tube (Song et al. 2008).

4.3.3.2.2 *Laparotomy* Gastrostomy tubes are frequently placed during a laparotomy. A purse-string suture with 3-0 monofilament absorbable suture is placed in the wall of the body of the stomach close to the junction with the fundus between the lesser and the greater curvature (Figure 4.7a–f).

A #11 blade is then used to penetrate the abdominal wall from the skin surface. The blade is introduced caudal to the last rib lateral to the rectus abdominalis muscle. A large size forceps grabs the blade in the abdominal cavity. The blade is withdrawn from the abdominal wall with the forceps. The forceps then grabs the feeding tube and pulls it inside the abdominal cavity. A puncture is made in the center of the purse-string in the wall of the stomach. The gastrostomy tube is then introduced in the lumen of the stomach and the purse-string is tightened. If a Foley catheter has been used, the balloon is inflated with 5 ml of saline. Four pexy sutures are placed between the wall of the stomach and the transverse abdominalis muscle around the gastrostomy tube. A 3-0 monofilament absorbable suture is used for

the pexy sutures. A Chinese finger-trap suture with 2-0 nylon is placed on the skin to secure the tube.

The laparotomy is closed in a routine fashion.

4.3.4 Tips

The utilization of the #11 blade and the forceps to go through the abdominal wall minimizes the size of the incision made in the abdominal wall for the placement of the gastrostomy tube. It minimizes the risk of peristomal inflammation.

4.3.5 Utilization

Gastrostomy tubes are not used in the first 24 hours after placement to allow a seal to form between the stomach wall and the abdominal wall. Feedings are then conducted four times a day with a blenderized diet. The total daily caloric requirements are calculated and divided in four feedings. The amount of food is delivered over 5–10 minutes. The tube should be flushed with water after each feeding to prevent obstruction of the tube.

4.3.6 Complications

Gastroesophageal reflux and vomiting can occur if the gruel is delivered too fast or cold. Increasing the frequency of the feeding and reducing the volume of each feeding might also help reduce the risk of vomiting. Peristomal inflammation can happen if leakage occurs around the tube.

Gastrostomy tubes can be dislodged accidentally or pulled by the dog. Premature removal of the tube may result in leakage and peritonitis. If the tube has been pulled accidentally it is usually possible to replace it immediately with heavy sedation. A new Foley catheter can be introduced into the stoma. A radiograph with water-soluble iodine is used to confirm placement of the new tube in the stomach. Obstruction of the tube can occur. It is important to regularly flush the tube with saline. If the tube cannot be cleared the tube will need to be replaced.

4.4 Jejunostomy Tube

4.4.1 Indications

Jejunostomy tubes are indicated when feeding in the stomach is not possible. It is used to bypass a diseased upper gastrointestinal tract, resulting in chronic vomiting. It is also indicated in surgery to bypass an enterotomy or

(a)

(b)

(c)

(d)

(e)

(f)

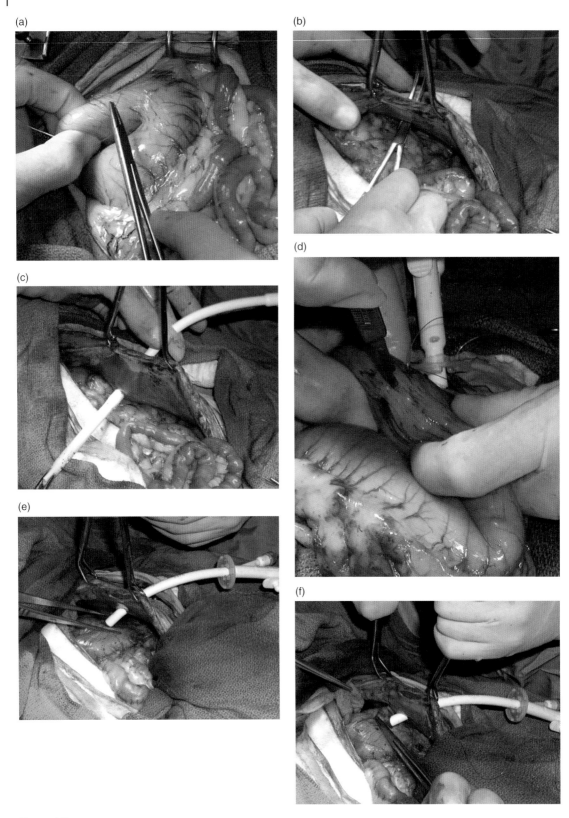

Figure 4.7

enterectomy. Jejunostomy tubes are often placed during the surgical treatment of peritonitis to be able to provide nutrients to a hyper-metabolic patient without increasing of gastroesophageal reflux and aspiration pneumonia (Marks 1998; Daye et al. 1999; Heuter 2004; Hewitt et al. 2004).

4.4.2 Materials and Equipment

A small long bore feeding is used for a jejunostomy tube. Usually tube from 5 to 9 Fr are used (Figure 4.8). The tubes are 50–89 cm long.

General anesthesia is required for the placement of a jejunostomy tube.

4.4.3 Technique

4.4.3.1 Laparoscopically Assisted

Three separate cannulas are used. One cannula is placed where the jejunostomy tube is placed in the right side of the abdominal cavity (Figure 4.9). A single-access port can also be used and it is inserted in the middle of the right side of the abdominal cavity. The port is placed lateral to the rectus abdominalis muscle.

After insufflation of the abdominal cavity a 5 mm rigid endoscope and two 5 mm grasping forceps are used to visualize and manipulate the loop of jejunum. After identifying the most proximal loop of jejunum it is brought against the abdominal wall and the single-access port is removed (Figure 4.9a). The oral and aboral orientation of the loop of jejunum should be identified. A stay suture is placed in the wall of the jejunum. A 4-0 monofilament absorbable suture is then used to place a purse-string suture in the wall of the jejunum (Figure 4.9b). A #11 blade is used to puncture the center of the purse-string suture. The jejunostomy tube is then introduced in the lumen of the jejunum in the aboral

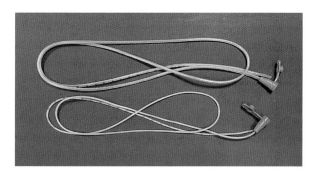

Figure 4.8

direction (Figure 4.9c). Usually 15–20 cm of the tube is placed in the jejunum. The purse-string suture is tightened around the tube. Four pexy sutures are placed between the wall of the jejunum and the transverse abdominalis muscle (Figure 4.9d and e). A 4-0 monofilament absorbable suture is used for the pexy. The subcutaneous tissue and skin are closed in a routine fashion around the tube (Figure 4.9f and g).

4.4.3.2 Laparotomy

Jejunostomy tubes are frequently placed during a laparotomy. During laparotomy the tubes are placed either very proximal in the jejunum or distal to a surgical site to bypass it.

A #11 blade is then used to penetrate the abdominal wall from the skin surface on the right or left side of the abdominal cavity. The blade is introduced in the middle of the abdominal wall lateral to the rectus abdominalis muscle. A mosquito forceps grabs the blade in the abdominal cavity. The blade is withdrawn from the abdominal wall with the forceps. The forceps then grabs the feeding tube and pulls inside the abdominal cavity (Figure 4.10a).

A purse-string suture with 4-0 monofilament absorbable suture is placed in the wall of the jejunum.

A puncture is made in the center of the purse-string in the wall of the jejunum (Figure 4.10b). The jejunostomy tube is then introduced in the lumen of the jejunum in the aboral direction. The tube is advanced over 20 cm and the purse-string is tightened (Figure 4.10c). Four pexy sutures are placed between the wall of the jejunum and the transverse abdominalis muscle around the jejunostomy tube (Figure 4.10d and e). A 4-0 monofilament absorbable suture is used for the pexy sutures. A finger-trap suture with 3-0 nylon is placed on the skin to secure the tube (Figure 4.10f).

The laparotomy is closed in a routine fashion.

4.4.4 Tips

An 8 Fr feeding tube can be used in cats as well as in small breed dogs. The larger tube will have less change to get occluded. It is important to flush the tube regularly.

The author has not been created a tunnel between the sero-muscularis and the submucosa to place the jejunostomy tube.

A interlock box suture technique has been described to pexy the jejunum to the abdominal wall (Daye et al. 1999).

(a)

(b)

(c)

(d)

(e)

(f)

(g)

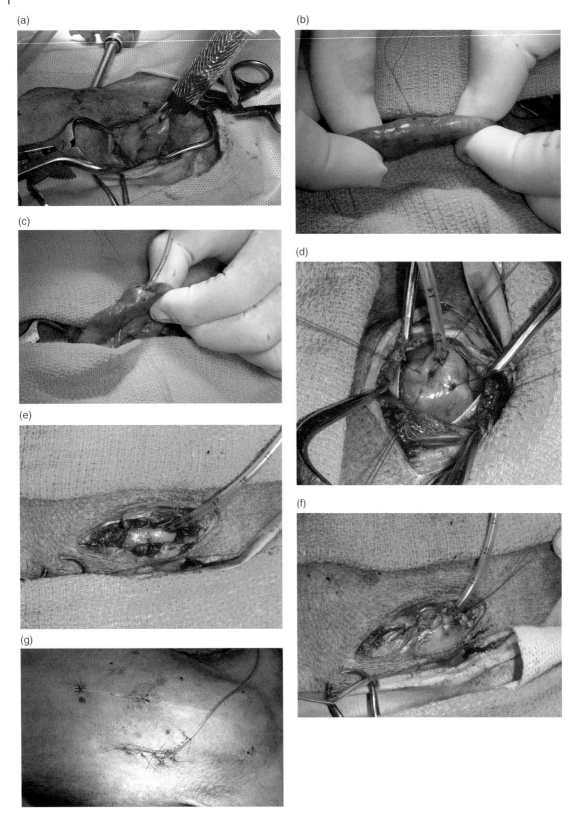

Figure 4.9

(a)

(b)

(c)

(d)

(e)

(f)

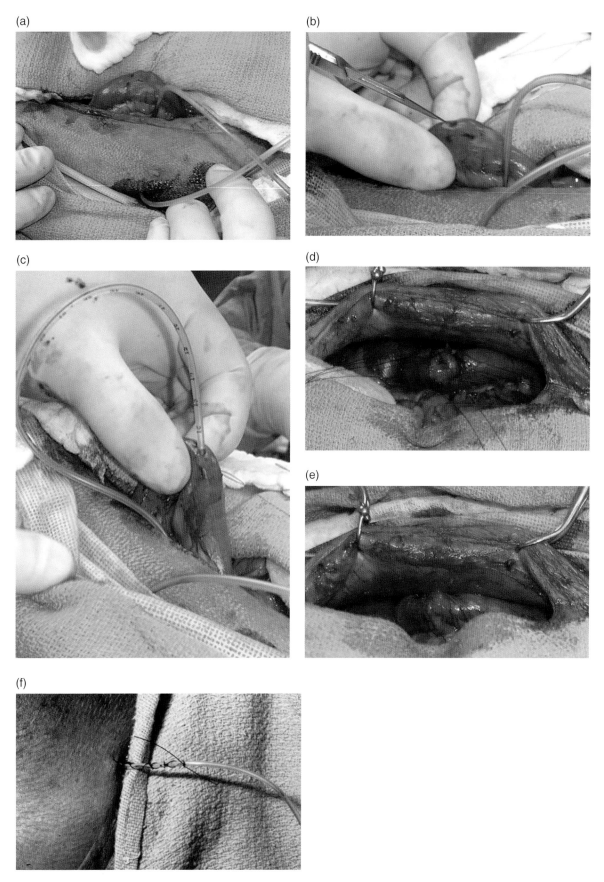

Figure 4.10

4.4.5 Utilization

A jejunostomy feeding tube can be used immediately even if the patient is heavily sedated. A liquid diet is required. After calculating the daily requirement the diet is delivery over 24 hours with a pump. The tube can be removed four days after its implantation.

An esophagojejunostomy tube can be placed also if an abdominal surgery is not indicated or possible (Cummings and Daley 2014).

4.4.6 Complications

Complications with jejunostomy tube are not frequent. The most common problem is obstruction of the tube. Also if the concentration of the liquid diet is too high it might induce diarrhea. Usually it is recommended to start with 1/4 to 1/3 of the daily maintenance and increase by 1/4 or 1/3 every day the amount of feeding.

4.5 Gastrojejunostomy Tube

4.5.1 Indications

The combination of a jejunostomy tube and gastrostomy tube is very common during the surgical treatment to septic peritonitis and during the reconstruction of the upper gastrointestinal tract (Cavanaugh et al. 2008). The jejunostomy tube is used first to support the patient while vomiting is occurring or the patient is lateral recumbent. The gastrostomy tube is used first to keep the stomach decompressed in an attempt to minimize gastroesophageal reflux, vomiting, and aspiration pneumonia. The gastrostomy is used later to provide more long-term support to the patient when the vomiting episodes have subsided.

Instead of placing two separate tubes, it is possible to surgically place a gastrotomy tube and then advance within the gastrostomy tube a jejunostomy tube that is directed through the pylorus into the duodenum and the proximal jejunum. A gastrojejunostomy tube can be placed percutaneously (Jergens et al. 2007).

4.5.2 Materials and Equipment

A large diameter (28 Fr) gastrostomy (Kangaroo gastrostomy feeding tube, Medtronics, Minneapolis, MN) and a

9 Fr jejunal feeding tube 89 cm long (Kangaroo jejunostomy feeding Tube, Medtronics, Minneapolis, MN) are used. The jejunostomy tube is weighted.

4.5.3 Technique

The gastrostomy tube is placed first as described above. A flexible tip wire is advanced in the jejunostomy tube. The wire-jejunostomy tube construct is then advanced in the gastrostomy tube and manually directed through the wall of the stomach in the pylorus and the duodenum. The jejunostomy tube is advanced in the proximal jejunum (Figure 4.11). The wire is removed and the jejunostomy tube is flushed to make sure there is no resistance due to a kink. The jejunostomy tube and the gastrotomy tube connect together with a special adaptor in the hub of the gastrostomy tube.

4.5.4 Tips

To facilitate the placement of the jejunostomy tube it is very helpful to advance the gastrostomy tube first through the pylorus. The gastrostomy tube can be manipulated through the stomach wall to be directed into the pylorus. Then it is easier to feed the jejunostomy tube with its wire in the duodenum. It is also very important not to let the jejunostomy tube make a loop in the stomach. If a loop of the jejunostomy tube is in the stomach, it might kink and occlude the jejunostomy tube. Also, if there is a loop in the stomach the jejunostomy tube might migrate back and coil in the lumen of the stomach.

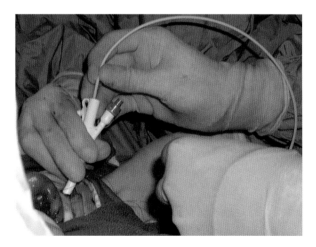

Figure 4.11

References

Abood, S.K. and Buffington, C.A. (1991). Improved nasogastric intubation technique for administration of nutritional support in dogs. *J. Am. Vet. Med. Assoc.* 199 (5): 577–579.

Abood, S.K. and Buffington, C.A. (1992). Enteral feeding of dogs and cats: 51 cases (1989–1991). *J. Am. Vet. Med. Assoc.* 201 (4): 619–622.

Armstrong, P.J. and Hardie, E.M. (1990b). Percutaneous endoscopic gastrostomy – a retrospective study of 54 clinical cases in dogs and cats. *J. Vet. Intern. Med.* 4 (4): 202–206.

Armstrong, P.J. et al. (1990a). Enteral nutrition by tube. *Vet. Clin. North Am. Small Anim. Pract.* 20 (1): 237–275.

Bright, R.M. et al. (1991). Percutaneous tube gastrostomy for enteral alimentation in small animals. *Compend. Contin. Educ. Pract. Vet.* 13: 15–22.

Cavanaugh, R.P. et al. (2008). Evaluation of surgically placed gastrojejunostomy feeding tubes in critically ill dogs. *J. Am. Vet. Med. Assoc.* 232 (3): 380–388.

Crowe, D.T. Jr. (1986). Use of a nasogastric tube for gastric and esophageal decompression in the dog and cat. *J. Am. Vet. Med. Assoc.* 188 (10): 1178–1182.

Crowe, D.T. and Devey, J.J. (1997a). Esophagostomy tubes for feeding and decompression: clinical experience in 29 small animal patients. *J. Am. Anim. Hosp. Assoc.* 33: 393–403.

Crowe, D.T. and Devey, J.J. (1997b). Esophagostomy tubes for feeding and decompression: clinical experience in 29 small animal patients. *J. Am. Anim. Hosp. Assoc.* 33 (5): 393–403.

Cummings, F. and Daley, C.A. (2014). Esophagojejunostomy feeding tube placement in 5 dogs with pancreatitis and anorexia. *Vet. Med. Int.* 2014: 197294.

Daye, R.M. et al. (1999). Interlocking box jejunostomy: a new technique for enteral feeding. *J. Am. Anim. Hosp. Assoc.* 35 (2): 129–134.

Devitt, C.M. and Seim, H.B. (1997). Clinical evaluation of tube esophagostomy in small animals. *J. Am. Anim. Hosp. Assoc.* 33 (1): 55–60.

Herring, J.M. (2016). A novel placement technique for nasogastric and nasoesophageal tubes. *J. Vet. Emerg. Crit. Care* 26 (4): 593–597.

Heuter, K. (2004). Placement of jejunal feeding tubes for post-gastric feeding. *Clin. Tech. Small Anim. Pract.* 19 (1): 32–42.

Hewitt, S.A. et al. (2004). Evaluation of laparoscopic-assisted placement of jejunostomy feeding tubes in dogs. *J. Am. Vet. Med. Assoc.* 225 (1): 65–71.

Jergens, A.E. et al. (2007). Percutaneous endoscopic gastrojejunostomy tube placement in healthy dogs and cats. *J. Vet. Intern. Med.* 21 (1): 18–24.

Kanemoto, Y. et al. (2017). Long-term management of a dog with idiopathic megaesophagus and recurrent aspiration pneumonia by use of an indwelling esophagostomy tube for suction of esophageal content and esophagogastric tube feeding. *J. Vet. Med. Sci.* 79 (1): 188–191.

Levine, P.B. et al. (1997). Esophagostomy tubes as a method of nutritional management in cats: a retrospective study. *J. Am. Anim. Hosp. Assoc.* 33 (5): 405–410.

Marks, S.L. (1998). The principles and practical application of enteral nutrition. *Vet. Clin. North Am. Small Anim. Pract.* 28 (3): 677–708.

Song, E.K. et al. (2008). Comparison of different tube materials and use of Chinese finger trap or four friction suture technique for securing gastrostomy, jejunostomy, and thoracostomy tubes in dogs. *Vet. Surg.* 37 (3): 212–221.

Yoshimoto, S.K. et al. (2006). Owner experiences and complications with home use of a replacement low profile gastrostomy device for long-term enteral feeding in dogs. *Can. Vet. J.* 47 (2): 144–150.

Yu, M.K. et al. (2013). Comparison of complication rates in dogs with nasoesophageal versus nasogastric feeding tubes. *J. Vet. Emerg. Crit. Care* 23 (3): 300–304.

5

Drainage Techniques for the Peritoneal Space

Eric Monnet

Department of Clinical Sciences, College of Veterinary Medicine and Biomedical Sciences, Colorado State University, Fort Collins, CO, USA

5.1 Indications

Drainage of the peritoneal space has been mostly performed for the treatment of peritonitis (Salisbury and Hosgood 1989; Hosgood 1990; Hosgood et al. 1991; Ludwig et al. 1997; Staatz et al. 2002; Buote and Havig 2012; Adams et al. 2014). Septic peritonitis and chemical peritonitis are the two most common conditions that are treated with some form of drainage. The main goal of the drainage is to decrease the bacterial load and/or to reduce the amount of chemical present in the pleural space.

Drainage is mostly indicated for generalized septic peritonitis. Drainage is also indicated if the cause of the peritonitis could not be totally controlled at the time of surgery (pancreatitis). Drainage is also indicated for a septic peritonitis associated with severe contamination with foreign materials (rupture of colon). The risk versus benefit of drainage has not been evaluated in a prospective trial to demonstrate the true benefit of drainage. "Drains provide a false sense of security and re-assurance; we have all seen the moribund post-operative patient with an abdomen crying to be reexplored while his surgeon strongly denies any possibility of intraperitoneal catastrophe because the tiny drains he inserted in each abdominal quadrant are 'dry' and nonproductive. We cannot produce high-level evidence to support our aversion to drains, but the generations of surgeons who used drains for many years also never succeeded in proving their advantage" (Schein 2002).

Open drainage has been historically used mostly during the treatment of generalized septic peritonitis with either presence of lot of foreign materials in the pleural space or bile. Bile salts are very caustic and potentiate the virulence of bacteria. Open drainage of the peritoneal

cavity is rarely recommended in human medicine for the treatment of peritonitis (Schein 2002).

Drainage of the peritoneal space should also reduce the risk of compartment syndrome resulting from the accumulation of abdominal effusion in the close space of the abdominal cavity. It might be the major benefit of the drainage of the peritoneal space (Schein et al. 1995; Schein 2002).

Drainage of a uroabdomen due to a ruptured urethra or bladder is an important component of the stabilization for the patient before abdominal surgery. Drainage of the urine present in the abdominal cavity is an important component of the treatment of hyperkalemia present with a uroabdomen. After placement of a percutaneous drain diuresis can be started to help lower the potassium level.

5.2 Techniques

Drainage of the peritoneal cavity can be achieved with either a closed suction drain, a negative pressure drainage system, or an open abdomen (Salisbury and Hosgood 1989; Hosgood 1990; Hosgood et al. 1991; Ludwig et al. 1997; Staatz et al. 2002; Buote and Havig 2012; Adams et al. 2014). Drains can be placed percutaneously with a local block or surgically during a laparotomy.

5.2.1 Percutaneous Placement of an Abdominal Drain

Drains that are placed percutaneously are usually temporary because they are getting wrapped in the omentum within 12–24 hours. Those drains should only be used for draining a uroabdomen to diurese the patient

Gastrointestinal Surgical Techniques in Small Animals, First Edition. Edited by Eric Monnet and Daniel D. Smeak.
© 2020 John Wiley & Sons, Inc. Published 2020 by John Wiley & Sons, Inc.
Companion website: www.wiley.com/go/monnet/gastrointestinal

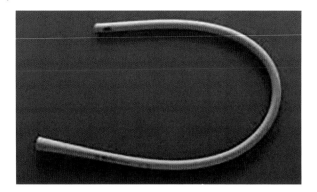

Figure 5.1

and help control hyperkalemia to be able to safely induce general anesthesia. Different drains have been used.

5.2.1.1 Passive Drain

A simple red rubber feeding tube can be used (Figure 5.1). The red rubber feeding tube can be wrapped in a fenestrated Penrose drain to protect the red rubber feeding tube from the omentum.

The patient is placed in right lateral recumbency. After surgically preparing the left caudal abdominal wall, a local block with bupivacaine is performed in the skin and the abdominal wall where the drain is going to be inserted. A bolus of fentanyl can be given to the patient also. The puncture in the abdominal wall is 2–3 cm cranial to the skin incision. A small skin incision is performed with a #15 blade where the local block was performed. A 2–3 cm subcutaneous tunnel is created with a curved Carmalt forceps in a cranial direction toward the local block in the abdominal wall. The tip of the red rubber feeding tube is then grabbed by the curved Carmalt and advanced in the tunnel. The abdominal wall is then punctured with the Carmalt and the red rubber feeding tube. The tube is then advanced in the abdominal cavity.

The red rubber feeding tube is then secured to the skin with a Chinese finger trap with 2-0 nylon. The tube is then connected to a passive collection system.

If a fenestrated Penrose drain is placed around the red rubber feeding tube it is inserted in a similar fashion than the simple red rubber feeding tube.

5.2.1.2 Closed Suction Drain

The patient is prepared as described above for the placement of a passive drain.

Usually a Seldinger technique is used to place a closed suction drain percutaneously. An 18G catheter is tunneled under the skin into the abdominal cavity. A wire

is then advanced in the catheter into the abdominal cavity. The 18G catheter is then removed and the closed suction drain is advanced over the wire into the abdominal cavity.

The drain is secured to the skin with a Chinese finger trap with 2-0 Nylon. The drain is then connected to a suction device and a reservoir. The device generates a negative pressure close to 10 mmHg. Usually the reservoir can be 100–400 ml depending on the size of the animal and the amount of effusion that is expected to be produced.

5.2.2 Surgical Placement of a Closed Suction Drain

According to the dynamic of fluids in the abdominal cavity, abdominal effusion moves from the caudal to cranial toward the diaphragm (Hosgood et al. 1989). Therefore drains need to be placed in the cranial part of the abdominal cavity between the liver lobes and the diaphragm. In this position the drain should be more efficient for collecting in the abdominal cavity and also it should keep the drain away from the omentum.

A Jackson–Pratt system, commonly made with a flat silicon drain, is placed in the abdominal cavity as described above (Figure 5.2). The flat silicon drain

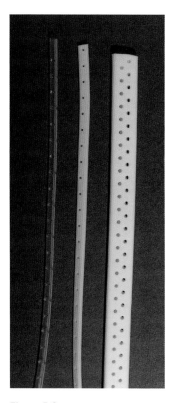

Figure 5.2

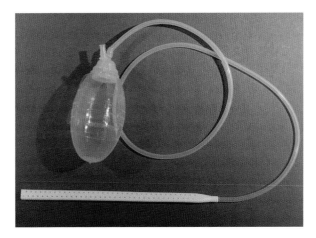

Figure 5.3

comes in different diameters. The tube is tunneled throughout the abdominal wall and the skin with a sharp trocar. A trocar is used to create a tight seal of the abdominal wall, subcutaneous tissue, and skin around the tube. Usually the exit point is in the left or right caudal abdomen.

A Chinese finger trap is used to secure the drain to the skin. The drain and the reservoir have to be well protected to prevent accidental removal of the drain by the patient. A suction device with a reservoir is connected to the drain (Figure 5.3). The device generates a negative pressure close to 10 mmHg. Usually the reservoir can be 100–400 ml, depending on the size of the animal and the amount of effusion that is expected to be produced. The reservoir has to be emptied as needed to maintain constant negative pressure in the abdominal cavity.

The drain needs to be inspected daily to reduce the risk of contamination and ascending infection.

5.2.3   Open Abdomen

An open abdomen allows passive drainage of the abdominal effusion in a sterile bandage applied over the midline incision of the laparotomy (Staatz et al. 2002; D'Hondt et al. 2007; Madback and Dangleben 2015). This technique allows daily lavage of the peritoneal space while the bandage is changed (Staatz et al. 2002; D'Hondt et al. 2007). It can also be associated to a vacuum-assisted bandage to actively drain the peritoneal space (Buote and Havig 2012; Madback and Dangleben 2015).

At the end of a laparotomy a 2-0 monofilament non-absorbable suture is placed loosely across the linea alba (Figure 5.4a). The linea alba should be maintained open on the entire length of the incision. Several loops of sutures are placed 3–5 cm from the edges of the skin incision and 3–4 cm from each other. Loop areas are

placed at the cranial and caudal ends of the incision (Figure 5.4a see arrow).

The laparotomy incision is then covered with two to three layers of sterile laparotomy sponges. Umbilical tape is then laced through the loop of suture over the laparotomy sponges. A sterile sticky plastic drape is then placed over the bandage and the skin to isolate the bandage from the environment (Figure 5.4b and c). If the patient is a male dog, a urinary catheter should be placed to prevent contamination of the bandage with urine.

Bandage is changed on a daily basis in the operating room. At each bandage change the abdominal cavity is flushed with sterile saline. A cytology is performed daily, and when cytology is improved, with a reduction of the number of bacteria and degenerative neutrophils, the abdominal cavity is closed over a closed suction drain.

5.2.4   Vacuum-Assisted Drainage of the Abdominal Cavity

Vacuum-assisted bandage has been used instead of an open abdomen drainage technique to actively drain the peritoneal space (Hondt et al. 2011; Buote and Havig 2012; Cioffi et al. 2012; Spillebeen et al. 2017).

The linea alba is partially closed. Foam used for vacuum-assisted wound therapy is then applied on the part of the incision left open. A drain and sticky bandage are applied over the foam to establish a water and airtight seal. The drain is connected to the vacuum generator. A negative pressure of 75–125 mmHg is generated through the catheter in the foam in a continuous fashion. Fluids drained out of the peritoneal cavity is collected in a reservoir and the bandage does not need to be changed daily.

5.3   Tips

It is paramount to keep any of those drains well protected from the environment to prevent ascending infection. Sticky drapes can be used to cover the exit site of the closed suction drain. It should also be well covered to prevent any accidental removal by the patient. An E collar should be placed on the patient.

Cytology of the abdominal fluid should be performed daily basis to follow the progression of the disease process in the abdominal cavity. Fluid can be collected from the reservoir if a closed suction drain has been used, or at each bandage change if the abdomen has been left open. Measurement of lactate and glucose from the abdominal fluid can help determine if septic peritonitis

(a)

Figure 5.4

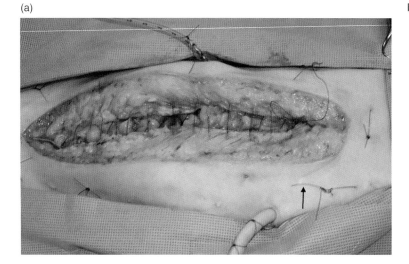

(b)

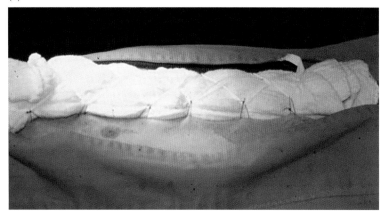

(c)

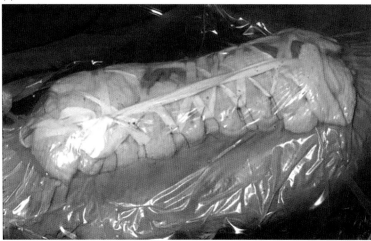

is still present. If septic peritonitis is present, the difference between the concentration of glucose in the fluid and blood is more than 20 units or the difference between the concentration of lactate in the fluid and blood is more than 2 units. Those results are 100% sensitive and specific in dogs and 86 and 100% respectively in cats (Bonczynski et al. 2003). However, if the fluid is collected from the closed suction drain and the reservoir and not the abdomen, those differences are not accurate (Szabo et al. 2011).

With an open abdomen, it is paramount that the bandage change and the lavage of the peritoneal space are performed under anesthesia in an operating room (Staatz et al. 2002). The surgical site is inspected at each bandage change. If needed, the additional sutures can be added to an enterotomy, or a resection anastomosis. Also it is important to perform enteral feeding for dogs and cats with open abdomen. A gastrostomy feeding tube is used to aspirate stomach content to prevent reflux, vomiting, and aspiration pneumonia. A jejunostomy feeding tube is used to feed the patient while under heavy sedation with an open abdomen. Enteral feeding is an efficient technique to maintain protein and albumin levels. Open abdomen drainage is usually used for 24 or 48 hours. The abdomen is then closed on a closed suction drain. Negative pressure therapy might be superior to passive abdominal drainage because the abdominal fluid is better contained (Spillebeen et al. 2017).

5.4 Complications and Aftercare

Since patients with abdominal drainage have some form of peritonitis, it is important to monitor those patients with electrocardiogram and arterial pressure measurement.

Hypovolemia, hypotension, arrhythmias, and disseminated intravascular coagulation are the common complications related to abdominal drainage and peritonitis. Monitoring urine production with a urinary catheter and a close collection system is important to adjust fluid therapy. Evaluation of electrolytes, glucose, and lactate are paramount to monitor and support the patients.

During abdominal drainage it is important to replace the losses to prevent hypovolemia. It is then important to add either synthetic colloids or plasma to maintain oncotic pressure.

Intra-abdominal compartment syndrome affects cardiac function, respiratory function, kidney function, and intracranial pressure (Diebel et al. 1992; Schein et al. 1995; Ivatury et al. 2001; Madback and Dangleben 2015). Abdominal drainage should therefore help to prevent this syndrome, which aggravates the clinical status of the patient. Monitoring intra-abdominal pressure is possible with a urinary catheter and a water manometer (Way and Monnet 2014; Madback and Dangleben 2015).

Septic peritonitis in dogs and cats is associated with a 30% mortality rate (Ludwig et al. 1997; Staatz et al. 2002; Davis et al. 2018). However, this prognosis is greatly affected by the underlying condition causing the peritonitis. Septic bile peritonitis carries a worse prognosis, with a mortality rate as high as 73% mortality, and the utilization of an open abdomen did not improve outcome (Ludwig et al. 1997).

References

Adams, R.J. et al. (2014). Closed suction drainage for treatment of septic peritonitis of confirmed gastrointestinal origin in 20 dogs. *Vet. Surg.* 43 (7): 843–851.

Bonczynski, J.J. et al. (2003). Comparison of peritoneal fluid and peripheral blood pH, bicarbonate, glucose, and lactate concentration as a diagnostic tool for septic peritonitis in dogs and cats. *Vet. Surg.* 32 (2): 161–166.

Buote, N.J. and Havig, M.E. (2012). The use of vacuum-assisted closure in the management of septic peritonitis in six dogs. *J. Am. Anim. Hosp. Assoc.* 48 (3): 164–171.

Cioffi, K.M. et al. (2012). Retrospective evaluation of vacuum-assisted peritoneal drainage for the treatment of septic peritonitis in dogs and cats: 8 cases (2003–2010). *J. Vet. Emerg. Crit. Care* 22 (5): 601–609.

Davis, D.J. et al. (2018). Influence of preoperative septic peritonitis and anastomotic technique on the dehiscence of enterectomy sites in dogs: a retrospective review of 210 anastomoses. *Vet. Surg.* 47 (1): 125–129.

D'Hondt, M. et al. (2007). Systemic peritoneal cavity lavage: a new strategy for treatment of the open septic abdomen. *Acta Chir. Belg.* 107 (5): 583–587.

Diebel, L.N. et al. (1992). Effect of increased intra-abdominal pressure on hepatic arterial, portal venous, and hepatic microcirculatory blood flow. *J. Trauma* 33 (2): 279–282; discussion 282–273.

Hondt, M. et al. (2011). Can vacuum-assisted closure and instillation therapy (vac-instill therapy) play a role in the treatment of the infected open abdomen? *Tech. Coloproctol.* 15 (1): 75–77.

Hosgood, G. (1990). The history of surgical drainage. *J. Am. Vet. Med. Assoc.* 196 (1): 42–44.

Hosgood, G. et al. (1989). Intraperitoneal circulation and drainage in the dog. *Vet. Surg.* 18 (4): 261–268.

Hosgood, G. et al. (1991). Open peritoneal drainage versus sump-penrose drainage: Clinicopathological effects in normal dogs. *J. Am. Anim. Assoc.* 27: 115–121.

Ivatury, R.R. et al. (2001). Abdominal compartment syndrome: recognition and management. *Adv. Surg.* 35: 251–269.

Ludwig, L.L. et al. (1997). Surgical treatment of bile peritonitis in 24 dogs and 2 cats: a retrospective study (1987–1994). *Vet. Surg.* 26 (2): 90–98.

Madback, F.G. and Dangleben, D.A. (2015). *Options in the Management of the Open Abdomen*. New York: Springer.

Salisbury, S.K. and Hosgood, G.L. (1989). Management of the patient with generalized peritonitis. *Problems in Vet. Med.* 1 (2): 168–182.

Schein, M. (2002). Surgical management of intra-abdominal infection: is there any evidence? *Langenbecks Arch. Surg.* 387 (1): 1–7.

Schein, M. et al. (1995). The abdominal compartment syndrome: the physiological and clinical consequences of elevated intra-abdominal pressure. *J. Am. Coll. Surg.* 180 (6): 745–753.

Spillebeen, A.L. et al. (2017). Negative pressure therapy versus passive open abdominal drainage for the treatment of septic peritonitis in dogs: a randomized, prospective study. *Vet. Surg.* 46 (8): 1086–1097.

Staatz, A.J. et al. (2002). Open peritoneal drainage versus primary closure for the treatment of septic peritonitis in dogs and cats: 42 cases (1993–1999). *Vet. Surg.* 31 (2): 174–180.

Szabo, S.D. et al. (2011). Evaluation of postceliotomy peritoneal drain fluid volume, cytology, and blood-to-peritoneal fluid lactate and glucose differences in normal dogs. *Vet. Surg.* 40 (4): 444–449.

Way, L.I. and Monnet, E. (2014). Determination and validation of volume to be instilled for standardized intra-abdominal pressure measurement in dogs. *J. Vet. Emerg. Crit. Care* 24 (4): 403–407.

Section II

Oral Cavity

6

Maxillectomy and Mandibulectomy

Bernard Séguin

Department of Clinical Sciences, College of Veterinary Medicine and Biomedical Sciences, Colorado State University, Fort Collins, CO, USA

6.1 Indications

The most common indication for maxillectomy or mandibulectomy is excision of a tumor. Other indications are a fracture where repair is or has been problematic, non-responding osteomyelitis, and osteonecrosis. Other indications for mandibulectomy are luxation of the temporomandibular joint (TMJ) and trismus. For a temporomandibular luxation, the TMJ is sacrificed by removing the condyloid process of the mandible. For trismus, a short segmental mandibulectomy of the caudal aspect of the body of the mandible is performed on the ipsilateral side of the lesion causing the trismus.

6.2 Surgical Techniques

The type and extent of maxillectomy or mandibulectomy performed depends on the location and size of the tumor or traumatized bone to be removed (Figures 6.1 and 6.2, Table 6.1). Although the width of the margins of normal tissue beyond the edge of the tumor necessary to achieve a complete excision has not been evaluated for malignant tumors of dogs and cats, a margin of 1–2 cm is typically recommended. A sterile skin marker and ruler can be used to appropriately measure the margins and draw the margins on the mucosa (Figure 6.3). Osteotomies have to be performed between two teeth and not through a tooth. These osteotomies are made in the interdental space away from the tumor beyond the proposed margin and not the interdental space toward the tumor. Complete excision of the tumor is the priority.

6.2.1 Maxillectomy

Hair is clipped from the superior lip and muzzle, particularly if the double approach will be used. For a segmental maxillectomy and subtotal and total maxillectomy (sometimes incorrectly referred to as hemimaxillectomy), the animal is positioned in lateral recumbency. For bilateral rostral premaxillectomy (incisivectomy), the animal is positioned in dorsal recumbency.

The mucosa is incised with a blade and scalpel handle all around the tumor. Typically, the incision will involve the buccal mucosa on the lateral aspect of the tumor and the oral mucosa of the hard palate on the medial aspect of the tumor, on the medial side of the dental arcade. The incision in the mucosa is made around the tumor (Figure 6.4). Cautery is avoided to incise the oral mucosa and submucosa tissues. Cautery can be used sparingly on the deeper tissues. If the incision on the medial side of the dental arcade in the hard palate needs to be performed more medially than the palatine artery, the transverse (medial to lateral) incisions in the mucosa of the palate are kept for toward the last steps of the dissection to avoid bleeding of the palatine artery while the rest of the surgery progresses. When the tumor is medial to the dental arcade and no mucosal margins are required on the lateral aspect of the maxilla, the incision is made just above the gingiva. When the tumor is lateral or has a lateral component to the dental arcade, the incision in the mucosa might have to be in the labial mucosa. Larger vessels, such as the infraorbital artery and vein, are isolated and ligated during the dissection when performed rostral to the

Gastrointestinal Surgical Techniques in Small Animals, First Edition. Edited by Eric Monnet and Daniel D. Smeak.
© 2020 John Wiley & Sons, Inc. Published 2020 by John Wiley & Sons, Inc.
Companion website: www.wiley.com/go/monnet/gastrointestinal

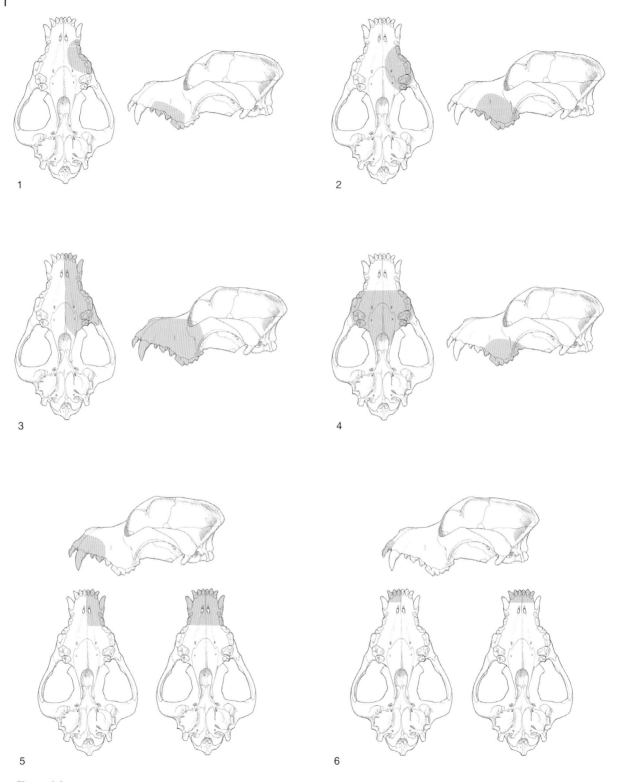

Figure 6.1

infraorbital foramen. The nerve can be injected with bupivacaine. For tumors that invade the lip, full-thickness segmental lip excision can be done en bloc with the maxillectomy. The incision is continued to the level

of the bone and the periosteum is elevated along the planned line of the osteotomy. Although an osteotome and mallet can be used, it is best to make the osteotomies with a power oscillating saw or burr. The osteotomies

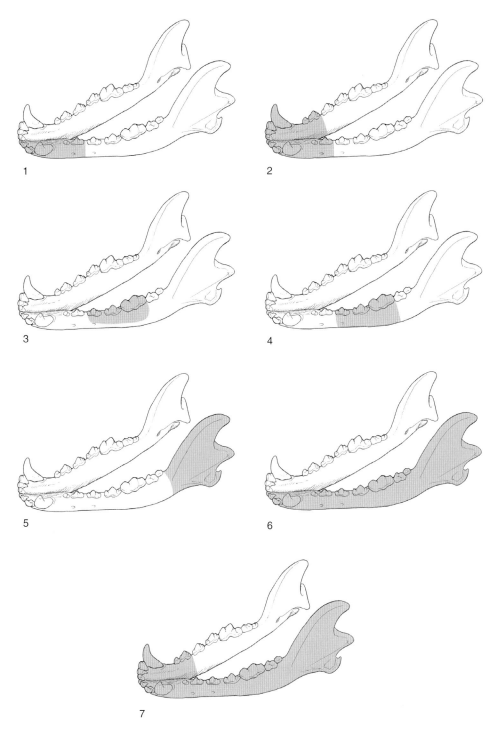

Figure 6.2

(lateral (dorsal to the dental arcade), medial to the dental arcade in the hard palate, and between the teeth (transversely connecting the lateral and medial osteotomies)) are performed. It is typically best to keep the caudal osteotomy for last, particularly when performing a caudal maxillectomy. Hemorrhage from the maxillary artery is the most common reason for significant blood loss. Ideally ligation of the maxillary artery is done before its transection, but exposure is limited and therefore not always possible. Therefore the caudal osteotomy is done last so the surgeon can readily and rapidly remove the maxillary bone segment and have access to the bleeding vessel and clamp it. Transection of the infraorbital artery is another source of blood loss

Table 6.1 Indications for and comments on the different types of mandibulectomies and maxillectomies.

Mandibulectomy procedures	Indications	Comments
Unilateral rostral	Lesions confined to rostral hemimandible Not crossing midline	Mandibular drift
Bilateral rostral	Bilateral rostral lesions crossing midline	Tongue "too long" Chelitis/ptyalism
Vertical ramus	Tumors confined to vertical ramus	Approach improved with cheilotomy
Complete unilateral	Lesions with extensive involvement of horizontal ramus and involvement of body or invasion or medullary canal	Mandibular drift, tongue hanging out of mouth
Segmental	Smaller tumors involving the mid portion of the body	No mandibular drift when canine preserved

Maxillectomy procedures	Indications	Comments
Unilateral rostral	Lesions confined to around teeth rostrally, one side	Ipsilateral mandibular canine can ulcerate skin of upper lip
Bilateral rostral	Lesions confined to incisive bone/rostral maxilla bilateral	Nose drops, can use cantilever suture to correct
Lateral/segmental	Laterally placed mid-maxillary lesions	Cosmetically will have a concave area in the muzzle
Bilateral	Palatine lesions that cross over midline	High rate of dehiscence, oronasal fistula

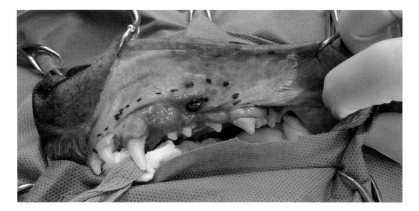

Figure 6.3

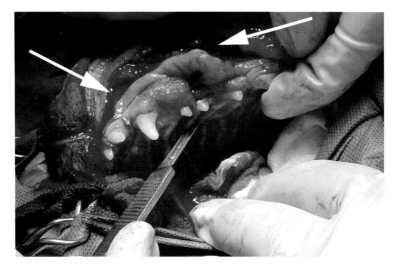

Figure 6.4

and having access to it will only be possible after removing the bone segment when it is transected caudal to the infraorbital foramen.

For tumors that have a significant dorsal component, a double approach can be necessary. The first approach is intra-oral as previously described. Additionally, a skin incision is done dorsally on the maxilla, at the dorsal aspect of the tumor (Figure 6.5.). The dorsal skin incision will allow the proper angle of the instrument (perpendicular to the bone surface) to perform the osteotomy. The subcutaneous tissues are incised all the way to periosteum and bone, where the osteotomy is required. The skin over the tumor is elevated, keeping a cuff of tissue on top of the tumor to serve as a margin. This is done in such a way that the dorsal approach can be connected with the intra-oral approach. If the skin is not movable over the tumor, a section of skin will need to be removed en bloc with the tumor.

Closure should be tension-free. A lip margin-based flap is created by undermining the labial mucosa and submucosa using a combination on blunt and sharp dissection. The labial flap is sutured to the cut edge of the hard palate in two layers. Bone tunnels can be created with a k-wire. Sutures are placed in the submucosa in the labial flap and through the bone tunnels. Alternatively, instead of using bone tunnels, the deep sutures are placed as a horizontal mattress in the submucosa of the labial flap and "deeper" aspect of the mucosa. on the hard palate side. Then mucosal sutures are placed. This can be with a simple interrupted, cruciate, or simple continuous pattern (Figure 6.6). Absorbable suture material is used intra-orally. If an approach was done through the skin dorsally as well, this is closed routinely.

For the rostral bilateral maxillectomy (including incisivectomy), the incision in the mucosa is done as previously prescribed, encircling the tumor (Figure 6.7). The

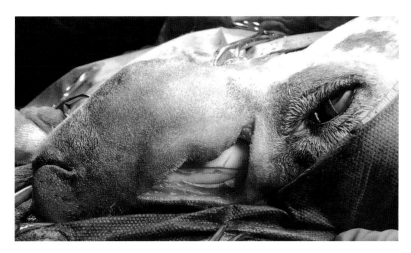

Figure 6.5

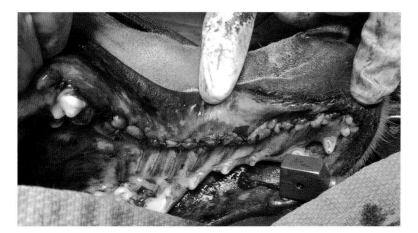

Figure 6.6

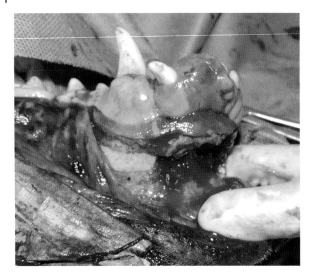

Figure 6.7

incision across the hard palate is kept for last, to avoid unnecessary bleeding from the palatine arteries until they can be occluded. For a small tumor located at the most rostral aspect of the incisive bone, a single osteotomy is made across the hard palate at the level between the most lateral incisor (103 and 203) and canine tooth. For larger tumors, the canine teeth are included in the excised segment. In this instance, dorsolaterally, osteotomies are made in a rostro-caudal direction from the rostral edge of the incisive bone for a short distance before engaging the maxilla. This is done on both sides. The osteotomies are joined with an osteotomy made across the hard palate (Figures 6.8 and 6.9). The attachments of the cartilages of the muzzle are cut from the maxilla and incisive bones. For the closure, bone tunnels can be created along the rostral edge of the hard palate. The defect is closed in two layers as previously described. The mucosa and submucosa in the rostral lips are elevated toward the mucocutaneous junction of the lips. The mucosa will be closed as a "T." The caudal aspect of the

labial mucosal/submucosal edge is sutured to the rostral cut edge of the hard palate until either side reaches midline. Then the labial mucosa from either side is sutured together (Figures 6.10 and 6.11). A cantilever suture can be placed to help with the nose dropping (see Section 6.4).

6.2.2 Mandible

Hair is clipped from the inferior lip including the cheek if a caudal mandibulectomy is performed, particularly when the ramus is removed. For segmental, unilateral subtotal, and total mandibulectomy, the animal is positioned in lateral recumbency. For bilateral rostral mandibulectomy, the animal is positioned in dorsal recumbency.

For tumors of the body of the mandible, the mucosa is incised with a blade and scalpel handle all around the tumor. Typically, the incision will involve the buccal mucosa on the lateral aspect of the tumor and the oral mucosa on the medical aspect of the tumor, on the medial side of the dental arcade. Cutting into the salivary duct ventral to the tongue is avoided if possible. Cautery is avoided to incise the oral mucosa and submucosa tissues. Cautery can be used sparingly on the deeper tissues to control bleeding. The incision is made as close to the gingiva when possible, when margins allow it. When the tumor is lateral or has a lateral component to the dental arcade, the incision in the mucosa might have to be in the labial mucosa. For tumors that invade the lip, full-thickness segmental lip excision can be done en bloc with the mandibulectomy. The incision is continued to the level of the bone and the periosteum is elevated along the planned line of the osteotomy. Dissection ventral to the mandibular segment to be removed is done such that the lateral and medial dissections connect. Although an osteotome and mallet can be used, it is best to make the osteotomies with a power oscillating saw or burr. Hemorrhage from the

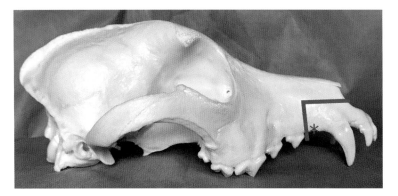

Figure 6.8

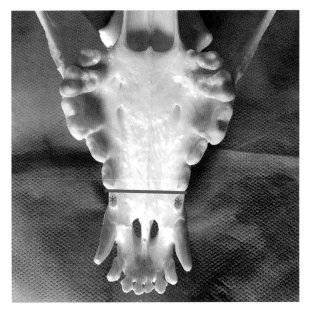

Figure 6.9

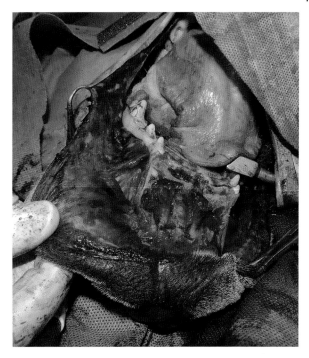

Figure 6.10

mandibular alveolar artery, which runs inside the mandibular canal with the corresponding vein, is addressed by grasping the vessel with small hemostat forceps and placing a small vascular clip if possible and available. Then the mandibular canal is packed with bone wax. If the vessel cannot be grasped or hemoclips are not available, the mandibular canal is simply packed with bone wax. If the segment of the mandible to be removed is caudal enough to be where the mandibular alveolar artery enters the mandible on the medial aspect through the mandibular foramen, the vessel is ligated before it enters the mandible. More rostrally, starting at the level of PM3 (teeth 307 and 407) the three mental branches exit the mandibular canal laterally through the caudal, middle, and rostral mental foramen.

A rim resection of the mandible can be done for small benign or small malignant tumor located at the edge of the gingiva and that do not show evidence of bone invasion on computed tomography. This is specifically for tumors of the body and not the ramus. With a rim resection, the ventral cortex of the mandible is preserved

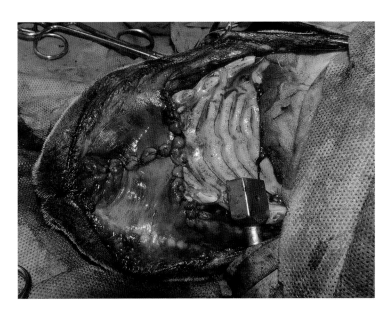

Figure 6.11

thereby preserving the structural unity of that mandible (Figure 6.12). The soft tissue dissection is similar other than there is no need to dissect ventrally and to connect the lateral and medial dissections. To perform the osteotomy, a biradial saw blade or burr can be used and the osteotomy is performed lateral to medial. Ideally, the osteotomy is made ventral to the roots of the teeth but if any roots were cut, the remnants are removed. The closure is similar where the labial mucosa is sutured to the oral mucosa ventral to the tongue covering the cut edges of the mandible at the osteotomy site.

For the rostral bilateral mandibulectomy, the incision in the mucosa is done as previously prescribed, encircling the tumor (Figure 6.13) similar to rostral maxillectomy but mandible. Depending on the margins required, if the caudal aspect of the mandibular symphysis (intermandibular suture) can be preserved, this will allow both the left and right mandibles to remain as one functional unit. But this should not be done at the expense of compromising margins. Once the soft tissues have been incised and elevated from the rostral mandible, the osteotomy is made across caudal to the canines or more caudal if indicated (Figure 6.14). For small tumors, particularly benign ones on midline in a larger dog, a wedge of bone preserving both canine teeth can be removed instead of performing a transverse osteotomy. It can be helpful to remove a wedge of the lower lip at its most rostral aspect when the osteotomy was across, caudal to the canine teeth. Without removing any lip, there can be excess lip and this can lead to dehiscence. Removing part of the lip becomes necessary if the tumor is invading the lip. For the clo-

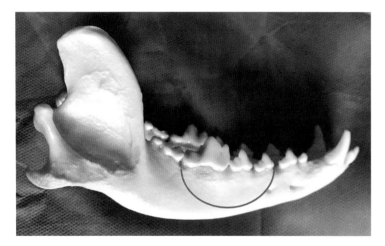

Figure 6.12

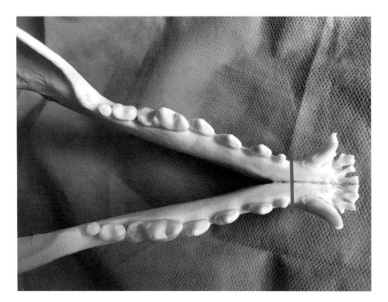

Figure 6.13

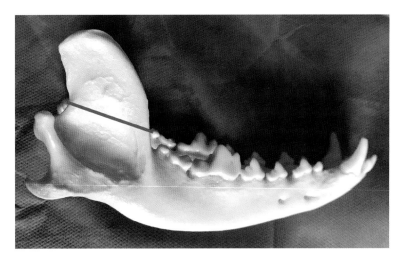

Figure 6.14

sure, bone tunnels can be created along the rostral edge if any of the symphysis was preserved. The defect is closed as previously described. The mucosa and sub-mucosa in the rostral lip are elevated toward the mucocutaneous junction of the lip. The mucosa will be closed as a "T." The caudal aspect of the labial mucosal edge is sutured to the gingiva of each mandible and to the oral mucosa ventral to the tongue, until either side reaches midline. Then the labial mucosa from either side is sutured together, similarly to a bilateral rostral maxillectomy.

The ramus or different sections thereof can be removed with or without parts of the body of the mandible. The ramus can be approached intra-orally when a segment of the body is removed as well en bloc with the ramus by incising the mucosa ventral to dorsal, starting caudal to the last mandibular molar tooth and going as far dorsal toward the palate. Alternatively, a skin incision can be made starting at the commissure of the lips and extending caudally full thickness into the cheek and over the ramus. If none of the body is removed and only the ramus or a part thereof, the skin incision is made over the ramus (caudal to the eye), ventral to the zygomatic arch. The TMJ can be preserved or involve removal of the condyloid process, thereby sacrificing the TMJ. When the coronoid process is part of the segment being removed, removing the part of the zygomatic arch right over it improves the approach and can make the dissection easier although it is not an absolute necessity. The muscles attached to the ramus are either elevated from the bone or cut to stay away from the tumor. The appropriate osteotomy is performed (Figures 6.14–6.16), preferably with an oscillating power saw.

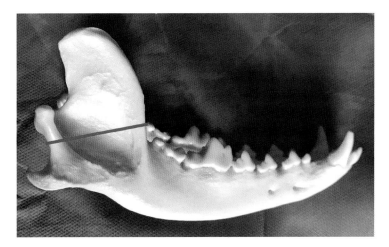

Figure 6.15

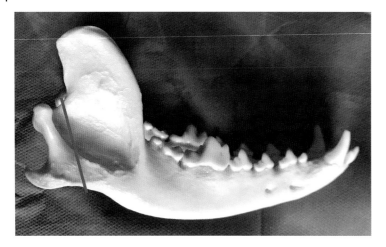

Figure 6.16

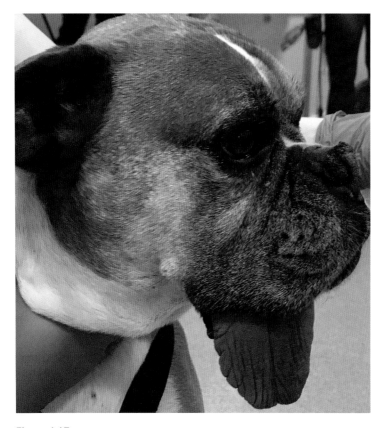

Figure 6.17

6.3 Tips

Changes to the cosmetic appearance will happen after maxillectomy and mandibulectomy. The severity of the change will depend on the location and extent of the excision. Client education is important to prepare them for the appearance of their pet. The appearance will be worse before it gets better, meaning the appearance right after surgery and upon discharge from the hospital will improve over time, particularly when the hair grows back. Having pictures of dogs and cats with a similar maxillectomy or mandibulectomy is very helpful for owners to be better prepared (Figure 6.17–6.20).

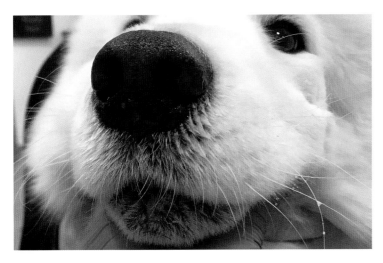

Figure 6.18

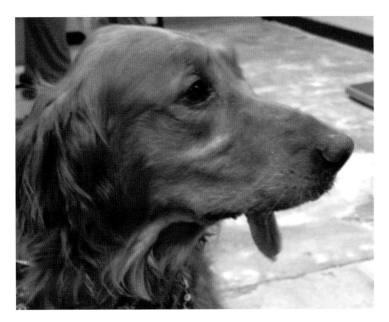

Figure 6.19

Before starting the incisions in the mouth, packing a gauze in the oropharynx in small dogs and cats and laparotomy sponge in large dogs is helpful to prevent blood from going down in the trachea or esophagus. Make sure to count the number of gauzes or laparotomy sponges that are packed so that at the end of surgery all of them are removed and accounted for. Use of a blade to cut mucosa but then cautery can be used for deeper tissue to control bleeding. Excessive use of cautery increases the risk of dehiscence.

Removal of any tooth roots left in the bone after the osteotomy. A classic example is when the osteotomy has been done caudal to the canine tooth across its root. The root is removed before closing to prevent the formation of an abscess and potentially be a source of pain. However, when cutting the root of the canine but the segment removed is the part caudal to the canine tooth, this author leaves the canine in place. Owners are warned about the possibility that the tooth may need to be removed at a later date but not necessarily and that preserving the canine in the situation of a mandibulectomy can help with mandibular drift by providing the "anchors" for jaw alignment through the locking mechanism of the upper and lower canine teeth. In the

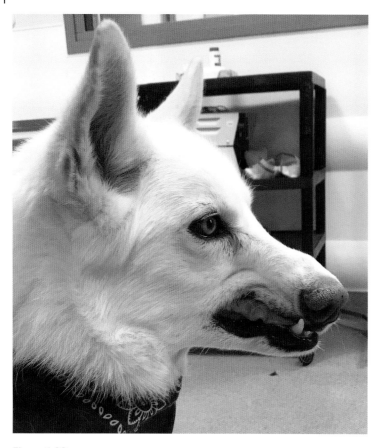

Figure 6.20

author's experience, these dogs will figure out how to play with their mandibles until the mandibular and maxillary canine teeth align properly. Dogs learn over time and the drift decreases.

When performing a mandibulectomy or maxillectomy that involves the caudal aspect, performing a full-thickness incision in the cheek from the commissure of the lips can be helpful for better exposure, particularly in dogs that do not have redundant tissue in that area.

Temporary occlusion of the carotid arteries can be done to decrease blood loss during surgery. This is more of a concern for caudal maxillectomies. This can be done in dogs but not in cats. Carotid artery occlusion in cats can be fatal.

It is recommended to place a feeding tube in all cats that undergo a mandibulectomy. Placing and feeding through a feeding tube for the first two weeks post-operatively in cases with an extensive maxillectomy, particularly those where the osteotomy medially will be at midline or beyond midline, might help prevent dehiscence.

6.4 Complications and Post-Operative Care

Immediately after surgery, the patient is maintained on IV fluids and given appropriate analgesia. Water can be offered when awake enough. Feedings can start the day after surgery. Soft food only is given for four weeks to promote proper healing in the mouth. Chew toys are removed for these four weeks. Oral medications can be given with soft food and is preferred over directly placing the medication in the mouth. If medications need to be given directly in the mouth, it is done away from the surgical site and sutures in the mouth. A recheck of the oral cavity is performed 2 weeks after surgery or sooner if signs of complications arise. Another examination is done at 4 weeks and every 3 months thereafter for 18 months if the neoplasm was malignant. Proper staging is also recommended at those visits.

6.4.1 Complications for Maxillectomy

Hemorrhage is more likely to occur when performing a caudal maxillectomy. Blood type and crossmatch the patient and have blood products available.

Infection is a very rare complication in spite of working in a contaminated area. The rich vascular supply in the oral cavity is believed to play a major role against infection.

Wound dehiscence, which leads to oronasal fistula, is one of the most common complications after maxillectomy. The risk may be as high as 33%, with caudal maxillectomies being at greater risk than rostral maxillectomies.

Ulcer formation of the upper lip is due to trauma by mandibular teeth. The most common culprit is the ipsilateral mandibular canine hitting the lip which has been drawn medially as a consequence of a rostral maxillectomy. Over time, the tissues can adapt and the ulcer heals. So no treatment is required in the majority of cases. For the more severe cases, the tooth or teeth can be removed or capped.

Eating difficulties are uncommon in dogs and cats after maxillectomy. More likely to see this complication after radical bilateral rostral maxillectomy. However, messy eating and drinking is not uncommon after maxillectomy. This is typically worse immediately after surgery and usually improves over several weeks.

Subcutaneous emphysema is rare despite the fact that the nasal passage often communicates with the subcutaneous area at the surgical site. Epistaxis after surgery is common and usually mild. It typically resolves within one week of surgery.

Stenosis of apertures of nasal passages can occur when a bilateral rostral maxillectomy (incisivectomy) is combined with nasal planectomy. Stenosis occurs in about 20% of the cases. Suturing techniques that create a closer apposition of skin to nasal mucosa should be favored over the purse-string suture.

Nose dropping occurs with incisivectomy (Figure 6.21). Cantilever suture can be placed, but in the author's opinion this technique does not fully elevate the nose to its normal position and instead pulls the planum caudally (Pavletic 2010).

6.4.2 Complications for Mandibulectomy

The majority of complications after mandibulectomy are minor and can be treated conservatively. Complication occurs more likely after total mandibulectomy. Thirty-eight percent of dogs treated with total mandibulectomy experience one or more complications. In cats, 95% had complications in the short term, and 76% in the long term. Nonetheless, 83% of cat

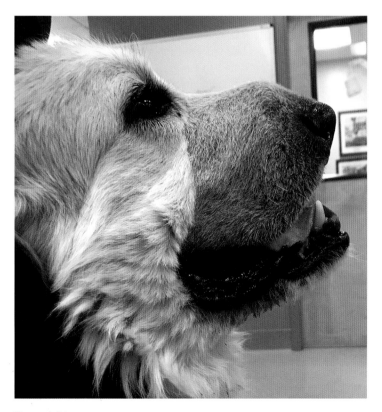

Figure 6.21

owners were satisfied with the outcome (Northrup et al. 2006).

Infection is very rare in spite of working in a contaminated area. The rich vascular supply in the oral cavity is believed to play a major role against infection.

Pseudo-ranula formation is a soft, fluctuant swelling ventral to the tongue, and along the frenulum which is more frequent after subtotal or total mandibulectomy. This swelling is rarely caused by accumulation of saliva such is the case with a true ranula but instead they are a hematoma or seroma/edema. They rarely need any treatment as they resolve on their own within 7–10 days after surgery.

Wound dehiscence has been seen in 8–33% of cases. Avoid tension at suture line and avoid using cautery to incise mucosa

The likelihood and severity of ptyalism/drooling is dependent on the location and extent of the mandibulectomy. Bilateral rostral mandibulectomy, total, or subtotal mandibulectomy, and large segmental mandibulectomy are likely to lead to significant drooling. It usually will be worse immediately post-operatively and improve, sometimes even resolve spontaneously after several weeks. Cheiloplasty can be helpful to decrease the severity if drooling.

Tongue protrusion (Figures 6.19 and 6.21) can happen after mandibulectomy. A cheiloplasty can be helpful in instances where a total mandibulectomy or significant segmental mandibulectomy was performed. When the tongue protrusion is a consequence of bilateral rostral mandibulectomy (Figure 6.21), no corrective measures are available.

Mandibular drift and malocclusion are more common after total or subtotal mandibulectomy or segmental mandibulectomy, particularly when the canine tooth is sacrificed as part of the mandibulectomy. In the author's experience, preserving both canines when performing a mandibulectomy helps prevent mandibular drift because of the interlocking of mandibular and maxillary canines when the jaw is closed. However, preserving a canine tooth should never been done at the risk of compromising surgical margins. Mandibular drift can lead to remaining canine creating an ulcer in hard palate. TMJ osteoarthritis has only been documented on histopathology (Umphlet et al. 1988). Replacement of the excised portion has been reported using 3D-printed implants (Bray et al. 2017). Reconstruction of the mandible has also been described using ulnar or rib autograft. Promotion of osseous ingrowth with use of rhBMP-2 has been reported (Spector et al. 2007). This is not currently recommended in cases where a malignant tumor was excised as there is not enough data to know the risk of promoting tumor recurrence. Elastic rubber chains can also be used to help maintain normal occlusion after segmental or subtotal or total mandibulectomy but 50% of dogs will develop mandibular drift once the orthodontic device is removed (Bar-Am and Verstraete 2010).

Almost every dog is eating voluntarily within three days of the surgery. Messy eating and drinking is not uncommon after mandibulectomy. This is typically worse immediately after surgery and usually improves over several weeks. Prehension difficulties are seen most commonly after bilateral rostral mandibulectomy, particularly with more aggressive surgeries such as when the osteotomy is done caudal to PM2. In cats, eating difficulties are more common. In one study, 42% of cats experienced eating difficulties in the long term, with 12% that never ate again (Northrup et al. 2006). But the author suspects this may be overestimated as we have also learned from the same study that some cats will take weeks to eat again and therefore will need a feeding tube. Having committed and patient owners is pivotal for a long-term positive outcome in cats.

Grooming difficulties are specific to cats. This is seen in 20% of cats after mandibulectomy but the risk varies with the type of mandibulectomy. Grooming difficulties appears to significantly negatively impact the quality of life for cats and owners should regularly groom their cat when this complication arises.

References

Bar-Am, Y. and Verstraete, F.J. (2010). Elastic training for the prevention of mandibular drift following mandibulectomy in dogs: 18 cases (2005–2008). *Vet. Surg.* 39 (5): 574–580.

Bray, J.P. et al. (2017). Clinical outcomes of patient-specific porous titanium endoprostheses in dogs with tumors of the mandible, radius, or tibia: 12 cases (2013–2016). *J. Am. Vet. Med. Assoc.* 251 (5): 566–579.

Northrup, N.C. et al. (2006). Outcomes of cats with oral tumors treated with mandibulectomy: 42 cases. *J. Am. Anim. Hosp. Assoc.* 42 (5): 350–360.

Pavletic, M.M. (2010). Nasal reconstruction techniques. In: *Atlas of Small Animal Reconstructive Surgery*, 3e (ed. M.M. Pavletic), 573–601. Ames: Wiley Blackwell.

Spector, D.I. et al. (2007). Immediate mandibular reconstruction of a 5 cm defect using rhBMP-2 after partial mandibulectomy in a dog. *Vet. Surg.* 36 (8): 752–759.

Umphlet, R.C. et al. (1988). The effect of partial rostral hemimandibulectomy on mandibular mobility and temporomandibular joint morphology in the dog. *Vet. Surg.* 17 (4): 186–193.

7

Glossectomy

Eric Monnet and Bernard Séguin

Department of Clinical Sciences, College of Veterinary Medicine and Biomedical Sciences, Colorado State University, Fort Collins, CO, USA

7.1 Indications

Glossectomy has been defined as partial (cranial to frenulum), subtotal (removal of the entire free segment of the tongue and a part of the genioglossus muscle caudal to frenulum), near-total (removal of 75% of the tongue) (Figure 7.1) and total glossectomy. Partial glossectomy is mostly performed for the surgical resection of tumor in the cranial part of tongue (Dvorak et al. 2004). Partial or subtotal glossectomy are most commonly performed in dogs however most of the tumors are located in the caudal part of the tongue and are bilateral in dogs making resection contraindicated (Beck et al 1986). Squamous cell carcinoma and melanoma are the two most common tumors diagnosed in dogs (Beck et al. 1986; Dvorak et al. 2004; Syrcle et al. 2008; Buelow and Manfra Marretta 2011; Culp et al. 2013). Median survival time has been reported at 216 and 241 days for squamous cell carcinoma and melanoma respectively. Tumors larger than 2 cm at the time of surgery had a more guarded prognosis (Culp et al. 2013). Rostral partial glossectomy can also be performed for the correction of trauma to the cranial part of the tongue.

Near-total glossectomy can be performed for tumor or trauma to the caudal part of the tongue or for tumor extending across midline caudal to the frenulum (Figure 7.2) (Dvorak et al. 2004; Syrcle et al. 2008; Buelow and Manfra Marretta 2011; Culp et al. 2013). However, after complete glossectomy feeding tubes have to be placed to support the patient in the long term (approximately one month). Most dogs eventually learn to eat and drink without assistance (Dvorak et al. 2004). Glossectomy may not be as well tolerated in cats and only 50% of the tongue can be amputated in this species.

7.2 Technique

After induction of general anesthesia, the dog or the cat is placed in sternal recumbency at the end of the table. The mouth is maintained open with a mouth gag.

For a partial rostral glossectomy, stay sutures are placed on the side of the tongue (Figure 7.3). A partial thickness incision is made on the dorsal surface of the tongue with a surgical blade. Hemostasis is performed with electrocautery. The dissection is extended ventrally until the lingual arteries and veins are identified and ligated. After transection of the lingual arteries and veins the resection is completed. The tongue is closed with a two-layer closure if possible (Figure 7.4). Monofilament absorbable suture size 4-0 is used for the closure. A simple continuous suture pattern is used to appose the ventral and the dorsal mucosa. The mucosa is made of a stratified epithelium on the dorsal side.

For a lateral resection, a Vshaped incision is performed on the margin of the tongue around the lesion to resect. Hemostasis is performed with electrocautery. Only one lingual artery and vein can be ligated. If both are ligated it will induce necrosis of the tip of the tongue The dorsal and ventral mucosa are then apposed with two layers of simple continuous sutures with 4-0 monofilament absorbable suture material.

7.3 Tips

Placement of an esophagostomy tube at the time of surgery is recommended to help support the patient in the post-operative period or even in the long term if a near-total glossectomy has been performed.

Gastrointestinal Surgical Techniques in Small Animals, First Edition. Edited by Eric Monnet and Daniel D. Smeak.
© 2020 John Wiley & Sons, Inc. Published 2020 by John Wiley & Sons, Inc.
Companion website: www.wiley.com/go/monnet/gastrointestinal

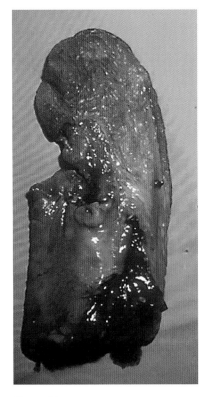

Figure 7.1

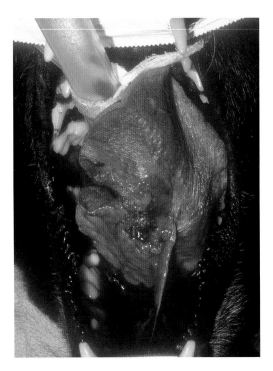

Figure 7.2

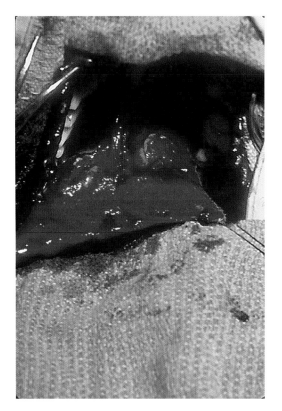

Figure 7.3

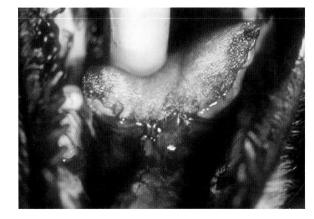

Figure 7.4

7.4 Complications

Complications of a glossectomy include hemorrhage (mostly during surgery), dehiscence, ptyalism, difficulty eating and drinking, necrosis of the cranial part of the tongue, and heat stroke if a large segment of the tongue has been removed (Beck et al. 1986; Dvorak et al. 2004; Syrcle et al. 2008). Dogs with near-total glossectomy are more at risk of heat stroke and activity should be limited when the outside temperature is elevated. Ptyalism is reported for near-total glossectomy and it can be controlled with resection of the mandibular and sublingual salivary glands.

Hemorrhage is usually well controlled during surgery with electrocautery, vessel sealant device or sutures. If the bleeding cannot be controlled, ligation of the carotid artery on the side of the bleeding is possible.

Dehiscence can happen in the post-operative period. A feeding tube should help prevent dehiscence. Usually if the dehiscence is minor it heals by second intention (Dvorak et al. 2004; Syrcle et al. 2008).

References

Beck, E.R. et al. (1986). Canine tongue tumors – a retrospective review of 57 cases. *J. Am. Anim. Hosp. Assoc.* 22 (4): 525–532.

Buelow, M.E. and Manfra Marretta, S. (2011). Major glossectomy in the dog. *J. Vet. Dent.* 28 (3): 210–214.

Culp, W.T. et al. (2013). Results of surgical excision and evaluation of factors associated with survival time in dogs with lingual neoplasia: 97 cases (1995–2008). *J. Am. Vet. Med. Assoc.* 242 (10): 1392–1397.

Dvorak, L.D. et al. (2004). Major glossectomy in dogs: a case series and proposed classification system. *J. Am. Anim. Hosp. Assoc.* 40 (4): 331–337.

Syrcle, J.A. et al. (2008). Retrospective evaluation of lingual tumors in 42 dogs: 1999–2005. *J. Am. Anim. Hosp. Assoc.* 44 (6): 308–319.

8

Tonsillectomy

Eric Monnet and Bernard Séguin

Department of Clinical Sciences, College of Veterinary Medicine and Biomedical Sciences, Colorado State University, Fort Collins, CO, USA

8.1 Indications

Tonsillectomy is mostly performed for the removal of neoplasia. Squamous cell carcinoma is commonly diagnosed in the tonsil in dogs. They have a tendency to metastasize rapidly to the local lymph nodes. Median survival with squamous cell carcinoma is two to four months after surgical excision. Metastasis has been diagnosed in 45% of the lymph nodes that seemed normal on palpation (Grant and North 2016). Computed tomography is recommended before surgery to evaluate the extent of the tumor (Figure 8.1) (Thierry et al. 2018). Surgery is mostly palliative for large tumors. The goal is to improve quality of life.

Tonsillectomy can also be performed for chronic tonsillitis. Tonsillectomy has also been performed for dogs with brachycephalic airway syndrome (Cook et al. 2015).

8.2 Technique

After induction of general anesthesia, the dogs are placed in ventral recumbency at the end of the table. The mouth is maintained open with a mouth gag to expose the back of the mouth and the tonsil. A temporary tracheostomy may be required if intubation is not possible because of the size of the tumor. Also a temporary tracheostomy might be helpful during surgery because it eliminates the endotracheal tube from the surgical field.

The oral mucosa is incised around the tonsil that is removed. Electrocautery is required to perform hemostasis. Placing stay sutures around the surgical incision helps with exposure of the surgical site and to minimize soft tissue trauma (Figures 8.2 and 8.3). The dissection is conducted 360° around the base of the tonsil. A vessel sealant device is recommended to perform the deeper dissection because it helps to maintain good hemostasis for good visualization (Cook et al. 2015; Belch et al. 2017). The hyoid apparatus should be preserved during dissection as well as the wall of the larynx.

After completion of the excision, a closed suction drain can be placed with an exit site on the side of the neck caudal to the vertical ramus of the mandible. The oral mucosa is then closed with a two-layer closure with monofilament absorbable suture. A simple continuous suture pattern is used (Figures 8.4 and 8.5).

8.3 Tips

Irrigating the surgical field with iced cold saline during the procedure can help minimize bleeding during the procedure.

An esophagostomy tube is placed at the end of the surgery to feed the patient and deliver medication while the oral mucosa is healing. This also might help decrease the risk of dehiscence.

8.4 Complications

The most common complications after tonsillectomy, especially if a large tumor was present, are hematoma formation, seroma, infection, and dehiscence. Local recurrence is also frequent after resection of a squamous cell carcinoma.

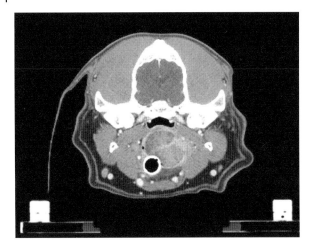

Figure 8.1

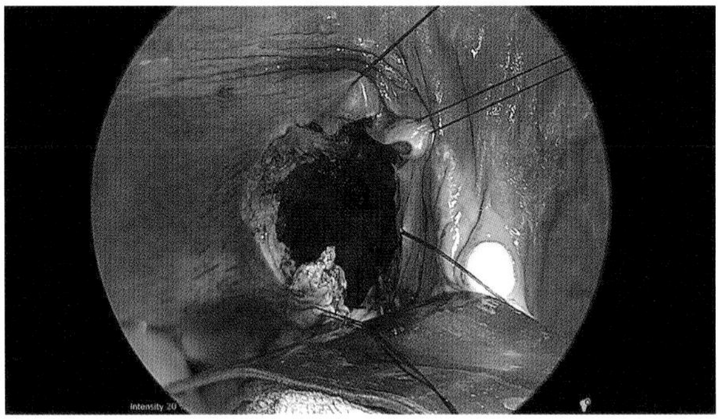

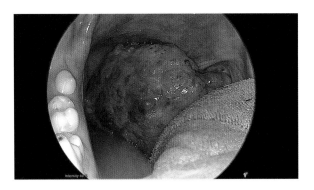

Figure 8.2

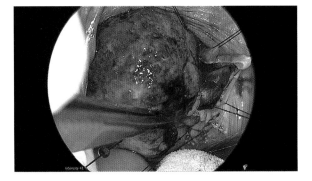

Figure 8.3

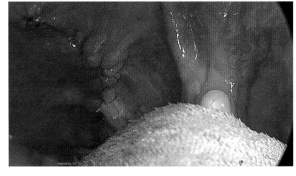

Figure 8.4

Figure 8.5

References

Belch, A. et al. (2017). Comparison of the use of LigaSure versus a standard technique for tonsillectomy in dogs. *Vet. Rec.* 180 (8): 196.

Cook, D.A. et al. (2015). Clinical effects of the use of a bipolar vessel sealing device for soft palate resection and tonsillectomy in dogs, with histological assessment of resected tonsillar tissue. *Aust. Vet. J.* 93 (12): 445–451.

Grant, J. and North, S. (2016). Evaluation of the factors contributing to long-term survival in canine tonsillar squamous cell carcinoma. *Aust. Vet. J.* 94 (6): 197–202.

Thierry, F. et al. (2018). Computed tomographic appearance of canine tonsillar neoplasia: 14 cases. *Vet. Radiol. Ultrasound* 59 (1): 54–63.

9

Palatal and Oronasal Defects
Chad Lothamer[1] and Jennifer Rawlinson[2]

[1] *Dentistry and Oral Surgery, College of Veterinary Medicine, University of Tennessee, Knoxville, TN, USA*
[2] *Department of Clinical Sciences, College of Veterinary Medicine and Biomedical Sciences, Colorado State University, Fort Collins, CO, USA*

9.1 Indications

Defects of the palate are generally divided into the categories of congenital malformations or acquired defects. Congenital defects are created by a failure of fusion of embryonic structures (Kelly and Bardach 2012). There are numerous classification systems for congenital palatal defects. Simply, defects are categorized as either primary cleft palates, secondary cleft palates, or a combination of the two, and also as unilateral or bilateral (Peralta et al. 2017). Primary cleft palate, also known as a cleft lip, involves failure of fusion between structures that will form the incisive bone, the upper lip, and the alveolar process. These paired embryonic structures include the nasal prominence and the maxillary prominence. Clinically this results in a defect that can be seen from the upper labia of the muzzle, extending into the nostril. The alveolar process may also be affected, creating a defect that may extend into the dental arch. Secondary cleft palates are defects of the hard and soft palate seen caudal to the palatine fissures. Secondary clefts form due to a failure of fusion between the paired palatine processes. These can range from small to large defects of both the hard and soft palate, to only small defects in the soft palate. Acquired defects can result as a consequence of trauma, a penetrating foreign body, electric cord injury, periodontal disease, neoplasia, radiation therapy, aggressive tooth extractions, or previous surgical dehiscence (Manfra Marretta 2012a, 2012b).

9.2 Surgical Techniques

The goal of repair of these defects is a separation of the oral and nasal cavities by continuous epithelized tissues. Flaps from local donor tissue sources are the primary means with which to close these defects. Ideally the flaps are well vascularized, tension-free, and when placed they are supported by underlying bone (Reiter and Holt 2012). The repair technique chosen should be the most simple with the highest chance of success (Zacher and Manfra Marretta 2013). Owners need to be made aware that overall the chance of a successful outcome for patients with a palatal defects is high. However, multiple procedures to salvage procedures may be required to achieve that successful outcome.

9.2.1 Repair of Congenital Clefts Palates

9.2.1.1 Primary Cleft Palate Correction Techniques
Closure of these defects involves treatment of malpositioned incisor teeth, separation of the nasal cavity from the oral cavity, and reconstruction of the cleft lip. Often times incisor teeth in the area of the cleft will impede the use of local tissues for various flap techniques, these teeth will need to be extracted and the surrounding tissues allowed to heal before definitive closure is attempted (Figure 9.1) (Fiani et al. 2016). Transposition flaps (see below) from the rostral palatal mucosa can be used to close the intra-oral defect. Grafts from alveolar

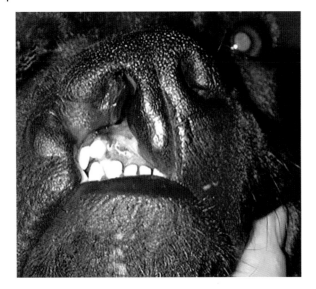

Figure 9.1

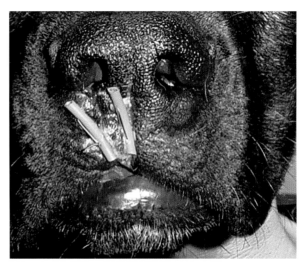

Figure 9.3

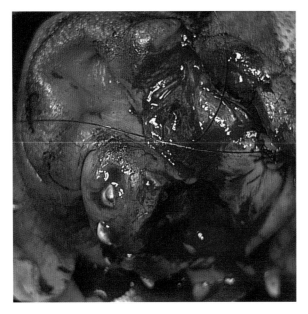

Figure 9.2

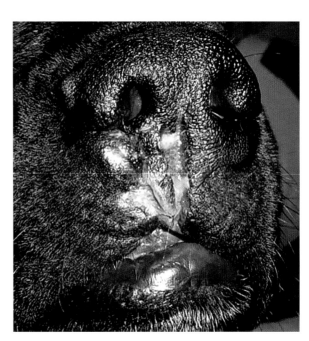

Figure 9.4

and nasal mucosal sources can be used to recreate a nasal floor (Figure 9.2) (Kirby et al. 1988). Closure of the cleft lip is performed by directly opposing labial, nasal planum, and mucosal tissues in the most aesthetic way possible; freshened edges are brought together and sutured in a simple interrupted pattern (Fiani et al. 2016). Suture material for all of these repairs is done with 4-0 or 5-0 absorbable monofilament material. Stents made out of Teflon or segment of red rubber tubing can be used to reinforce the suture across the nasal planum (Figure 9.3). The sutures are removed 10 days after surgery (Figure 9.4).

9.2.1.2 Secondary Cleft Palate Correction Techniques

9.2.1.2.1 *Von Langenbeck Technique* This technique is utilized for repair of narrow midline secondary cleft palates. It utilizes bilateral flaps, based on the greater palatine artery, which are repositioned medially to close the defect (Reiter and Smith 2005; Beckman 2011). The edges of the defect are cut to remove the intact epithelized tissue. Bilateral releasing incisions are made 2–3 mm palatal to the teeth to the caudal level of the defect on the hard palate. Periosteal elevators are used to lift the palatal mucosa on each side of the defect (Figure 9.5). The greater palatine artery exits its foramen

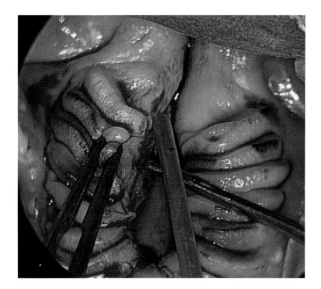

Figure 9.5

medial to the maxillary 4th premolar on each side, and care is taken not to damage the artery as it exits the foramen (Figure 9.6). The bilateral flaps are then repositioned medially covering the defect. The flaps are sutured together with absorbable monofilament in a simple interrupted pattern (Figure 9.7). The exposed maxillary bone in the areas of the releasing incisions are left to heal by second intention.

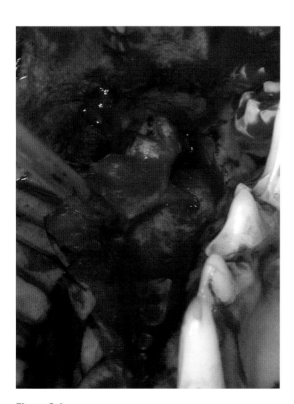

Figure 9.6

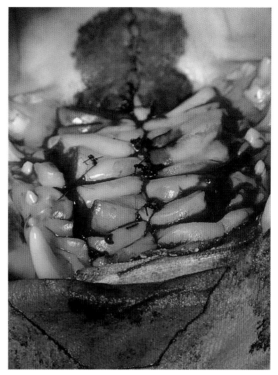

Figure 9.7

9.2.1.2.2 Overlapping Flap Technique This technique is utilized for repair of midline secondary cleft palates (Taney 2008). It utilizes tissue from one side of the defect that is elevated, flipped, and hinged at a point along the defect, the free end of the flap is then tucked under the mucosa on the contralateral side of the defect and sutured into place (Figure 9.8) (Taney 2008). This flap is created by making an incision on one side of the hard palate mucosa 2 mm palatal to the edge of the teeth. The length of the incision will run the length of the cleft. Incisions are made perpendicular to the rostral and caudal edges of the hard palate cleft (Figure 9.8a). The caudal incision needs to be placed far enough caudally to incorporate all of the greater palatine artery (Figure 9.8b), which exits its foramen medial to the maxillary 4th premolar, as well as far enough rostral to make the incision over bony support. Incising into the soft palate could create an iatrogenic oronasal fistula. The flap is then elevated from buccal to palatal, but not all the way to the medial edge of the defect (Figure 9.8c). Special attention is paid to the exit of the greater palatine artery, ensuring attachment of the artery to the flap. Attention will also need to be paid to the area of the palatine fissure more rostrally, and a partial thickness flap will be created over the fissure to prevent formation of an iatrogenic oronasal fistula. Once the flap has been elevated, the epithelial edge of the defect on the contralateral side is

(a)   (b)   (c)

(d)   (e)

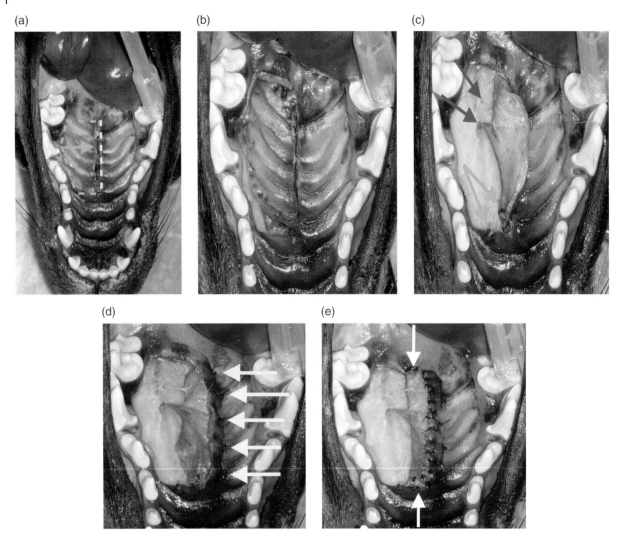

Figure 9.8

freshened and the soft tissue is elevated from the underlying bone, separating nasal and oral epithelium, again being careful to preserve the greater palatine artery (Figure 9.8d). The original flap is then hinged upon itself, and the free edge of the flap is tucked under the mucosa of the contralateral side so that the epithelium from the hinged flap is facing the nasal cavity. Absorbable monofilament sutures are placed in a horizontal or vertical mattress pattern from the hinged flap to the overlying mucosa of the contralateral side (Figure 9.8e). The bone exposed by the movement of the hinged flap is left to heal by second intention (Figure 9.9).

9.2.1.3   Soft Palate Repair Techniques
9.2.1.3.1   *Bilateral Medially Positioned Flaps*   This is a common technique for cleft soft palate repair (Sivacolundhu 2007). For this technique an incision is made from each edge of the soft palate defect from the caudal to midlevel of the pole of the tonsils to the rostral

aspect of the defect (Figures 9.10 and 9.11). Small blunt scissors are used to separate an epithelialized deep nasal layer from a more superficial oral layer. The left and right deep layer are then medially apposed and sutured together with an absorbable monofilament suture in a simple interrupted pattern, the suture should be tied so that the knots of this deep layer are tied on the nasal side of the defect (Figure 9.12). The more superficial oral layer is then closed in the same way except that the knots are tied facing the oral cavity. If any tension is present during the closure of the soft palate defect then partial thickness releasing incisions can be made in the caudal vestibular mucosa (Figure 9.13).

9.2.1.3.2   *Overlapping Flap Technique for Repair of the Soft Palate*   This technique for repair of soft palate defects has been described as difficult and usually unnecessary (Manfra Marretta 2012a, 2012b). A partial thickness hinged flap is created on each side of the soft

(a)　　　　　　　(b)　　　　　　　(c)

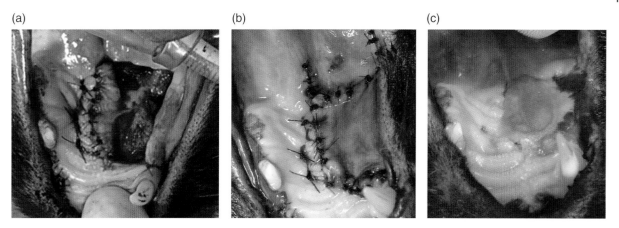

Figure 9.9

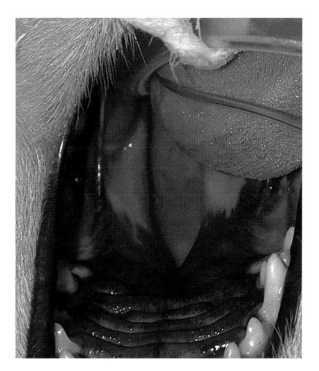

Figure 9.10

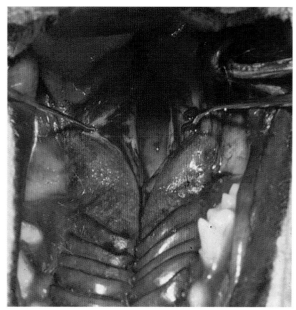

Figure 9.11

palate defect. One flap rotates epithelium from the oral cavity across the defect, and one flap rotates epithelium from the nasal cavity across the defect. The flaps are positioned so that the epithelium from the nasal cavity flap is facing the oral cavity and the epithelium from the oral cavity flap is facing into the nasal cavity. The flaps are sutured into place with absorbable monofilament material in a simple interrupted pattern.

9.2.2 Repair of Acquired Defects

9.2.2.1 Vestibular Mucoperiosteal Flaps
Vestibular mucoperiosteal flaps are flaps harvested from the buccal gingiva and vestibular mucosa, these are full-thickness pedicles flaps that receive blood supply from

the infraorbital artery and its branches (Manfra Marretta 2012a, 2012b; Manfra Marretta and Smith 2005). Vestibular mucoperiosteal flaps can be utilized to close defects along the alveolar crest often caused by loss of dentition with advanced periodontal disease, created when inappropriate or aggressive dental extractions have been performed, or used to close defects created with mass removal (Figure 9.14). These simple flaps when created appropriately and used in the correct locations have a high chance of success and should be the first type of closure attempted. Vestibular mucoperiosteal flaps can also be used as double flaps with hinged flaps from the palatal mucosa or epithelium from the fistula to create closures with epithelium on the nasal and oral side of defects (Wetering 2005). This technique is often used if a single-layer flap has previously failed to close the defect. Large vestibular mucoperiosteal flaps

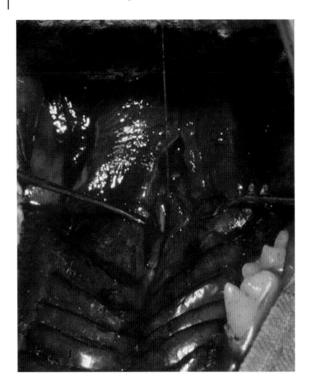

Figure 9.12

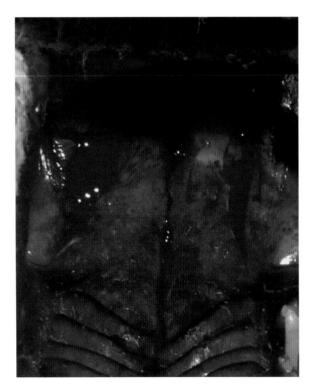

Figure 9.13

can be used to close more midline palatal defects, often extractions need to be performed six to eight weeks prior in order to harvest large enough flaps and to ensure the dentition does not get in the way of the flap. These large

flaps can be harvested from each side of the oral cavity and used as double overlapping flaps when two layers of tissue are desired. Before creation of the flap, defects should be debrided, removing 2–3 mm of mucosa surrounding the defect if it is chronic (Figure 9.14a). Ideally underlying bone will be exposed so that suture lines will be supported by this bone during closure. These flaps should be broad based ensuring good blood supply to the distal edge of the flap, ensuring an adequate amount of tissue to cover the defect, and to help to ensure that the flap will be tension-free at closure.

After freshening of the defect, vestibular mucoperiosteal flaps are created by making divergent incisions through the mucosa and periosteum to the bone at the mesial and distal aspect of the defect so that a trapezoidal flap is created (Figure 9.14). Periosteal elevators are used to elevate the flap from the underlying bone. It is important that divergent incisions extend past the gingiva into vestibular mucosa, as the vestibular mucosa has a much higher elastin content and is the tissue that will allow the flap to stretch over the defect without tension. The flap should be able to lay over the entire defect without retracting before closure is performed (Figure 9.14). Tension can be released by fenestrating the periosteum, which is the deepest layer of the flap, or by extending the divergent incisions into the vestibular mucosa. Care should be taken not to cut the infraorbital neurovascular bundle (white arrows) as it exits its foramen dorsal to the distal root of the maxillary third premolar, if incisions are made in this area (Figure 9.14c). Closure is performed with absorbable monofilament suture in a simple interrupted pattern with 2–3 mm between sutures. The first sutures placed are the free corners of the flap to the palatal mucosa, this helps to ensure that the flap does not get tacked down during closure, preventing the flap from covering the defect in a tension-free manner (Figure 9.14d–f).

Double-layer hinge flaps are often used to close defects in the area of the maxillary canine teeth when a single-layer flap has failed (Wetering 2005). This technique places a layer of epithelium facing both the nasal cavity, from the superficial layer of the palatal mucosa, and the oral cavity, from the superficial layer of the vestibular mucosa. The hinge flap is created by making a U-shaped incision from the edge of the defect into the palatal mucosa. Often a partial thickness flap is created to avoid uncovering the palatine fissures, which would only create another oronasal fistula. After elevation the U-shaped flap is folded over the defect, placing the epithelial layer into the nasal cavity side of the defect. The palatal mucosal flap is then sutured into place using absorbable monofilament suture in a simple

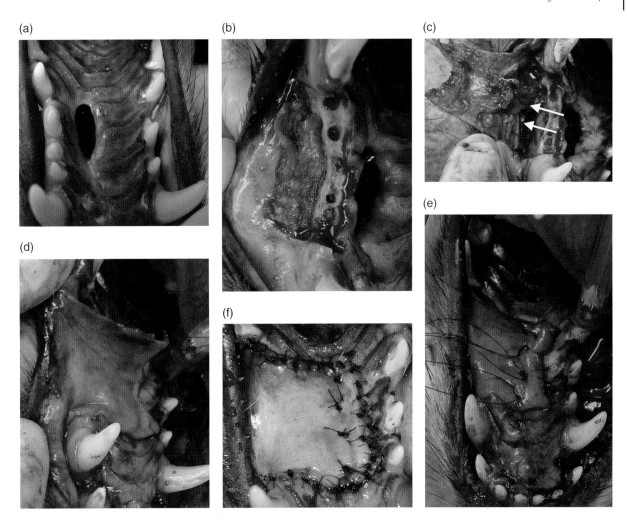

Figure 9.14

interrupted pattern. A buccal vestibular mucoperiosteal flap created as previously described is then placed over the U-shaped palatal flap and sutured into place. Any exposed bone or mucosa from the donor site of the palatal flap can be left to heal by second intention if the vestibular flap cannot cover it.

For defects of the hard palate than cannot be closed with palatal mucosa a technique has been described using large bilateral vestibular mucoperiosteal flaps (Zacher and Manfra Marretta 2013). Before flaps are created any teeth in the areas of the flap should be extracted and the extraction sites allowed to heal for six to eight weeks (Figure 9.15a). The repair is staged. The first surgery allowed for extraction of the right maxillary canine and premolar teeth. A palatal obturator was placed in the defect (pink) and secured in placed with dental composite to the left maxillary third and fourth premolar teeth (white) (Figure 9.15b). After eight weeks of healing, a second surgery was performed to close the defect. Three large vestibular mucoperiosteal flaps were utilized: a caudal right palatal-vestibular mucoperiosteal flap was transposed caudally (yellow), and two smaller vestibular mucoperiosteal flaps were harvested from the region of the canine teeth (blue and orange) (Figure 9.15c and d). Large vestibular flaps are created with an incision along the alveolar crest and then divergent incisions made to the labial mucocutaneous junction. Any palatal mucosa that will be covered by the flaps will need to have the superficial epithelial layer debrided to allow for the tissues to heal together, this is easily done with a diamond bur on a high-speed dental hand piece. One of the vestibular flaps will then be placed over the defect and sutured into place as described for the single-layer vestibular flap. The superficial epithelium of this deeper flap will need to be debrided before placing the second vestibular flap over the debrided deeper flap and suturing it into place.

(a)

(b)

(c)

(d)

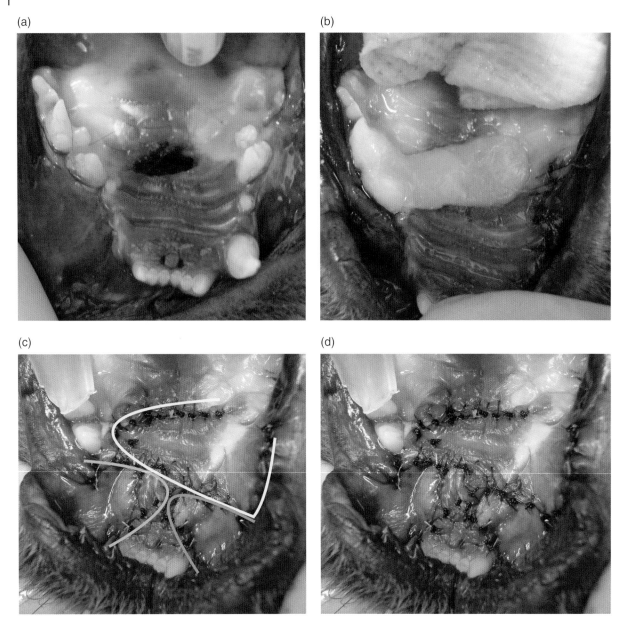

Figure 9.15

9.2.2.2 Palatal Mucoperiosteal Flaps

Closure of acquired palatal defects can be accomplished through the use of several palatal mucoperiosteal flaps whose blood supply is based on the left and right greater palatine arteries (Manfra Marretta 2012b). Each greater palatine artery exits from the greater palatine foramen, which is located medial to the distal aspect of the maxillary 4th premolar tooth, usually midway from the palatal aspect of the tooth to midline of the hard palate. The arteries course rostrally in a shallow groove toward the palatine fissures. The palatal mucoperiosteum behaves very similar to gingival mucosa in that it has a higher collagen content compared to elastin, making the tissue

tough, but it does not stretch in the way that vestibular mucosa does. This requires that the surgeon is careful in creating a flap large enough to easily cover the defect in a tension-free manner. Described palatal mucoperiosteal flaps include transposition flaps, advancement flaps, split palatal U-flaps, and rotating island flaps.

9.2.2.2.1 Transposition Flap The palatal mucoperiosteal transposition flap uses a U-shaped pedicle flap created in a distal to rostral orientation from one side of the palate to cover a small- to medium-sized off-midline defect in the contralateral hard palate rostral to the maxillary 4th premolar tooth to ensure that the greater palatine artery is incorporated into the flap (Figure 9.16a) (Manfra Marretta 2012a, 2012b). Two to three mm of palatal mucosa around the defect should be debrided, ideally uncovering a shelf of underlying healthy bone to support the suture lines of the flap closure (Figure 9.16b). A transposition flap that is at least 1.5–2 times the size of the defect is created (dashed blue lines), and the flap is elevated from the bone (Figure 9.16a). The base of the flap is located at the level of, or caudal to the foramen of the greater palatine artery (Figure 9.16c). Both the medial and lateral margins of the flap are partial thickness (yellow arrows), but the region by the greater palatine artery is full thickness. The greater palatine artery is preserved, and the rostral extent of the artery is ligated. The transposition flap is moved medially, and flap margins are trimmed to fit the surrounding tissue margins (Figure 9.16d). Distal to rostral incisions are made from 2 to 3 mm medial to the palatal aspect of the teeth and midline of the hard palate. The distal to rostral incision lines are connected rostrally by an incision perpendicular to the hard palate midline. The greater palatine artery will need to be ligated with this incision. Electrocautery and use of a laser for incisions should be avoided if possible to help ensure good healing of the donor and recipient tissues. Periosteal elevators are used to lift the U-shaped flap from the underlying bone, and care is taken not to damage the greater palatine

artery where it exits the bone from its foramen. The flap is then placed over the defect on the contralateral hard palate and sutured to the freshened recipient palatal mucosa with absorbable monofilament suture in a simple interrupted pattern (Figure 9.16d). The flap is secured with simple interrupted sutures where tissue margins abut and horizontal mattress sutures over the regions of partial thickness palatal tissue (black arrows). Creation and movement of the flap will create an area of exposed maxillary bone that will heal through second intention. If the clinician feels that the non-sutured side of the flap will not adequately lay against bone then holes can be created with K-pins or small cutting dental burs on a high-speed hand piece that can then be used to suture the flap to the underlying bone. The holes should be created so that flap covers the holes after suturing to prevent small fistula formation.

9.2.2.2.2 Split Palatal U-Flap The split palatal U-flap creates bilateral palatal transposition that are combined to cover midline palatal defects at the level of the maxillary 4th premolar teeth (Manfra Marretta 1991). Before creation of the flap, 2–3 mm of mucosa surrounding the defect should be debrided to ensure healthy freshened recipient tissue for the flap. Distal to rostral incisions are made bilaterally 2–3 mm palatal to the teeth and starting at the level or slightly rostral to

(a)   (b)   (d)

(c)

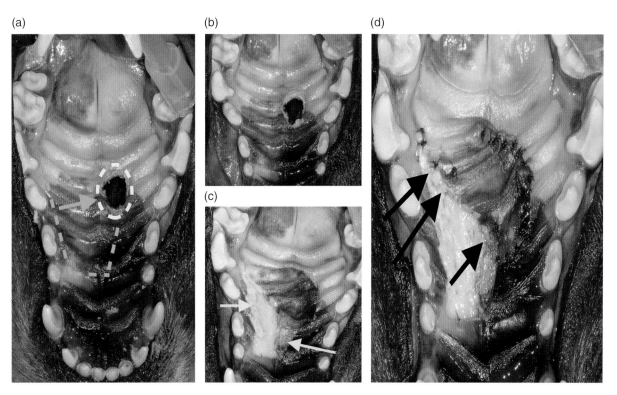

Figure 9.16

the defect. A U-shaped incision connects the distal to rostral incisions. Both of the greater palatine arteries will be encountered with this incision and will need to be ligated. An incision is made through the flap at midline, creating two separate flaps. The length of the flaps should be long enough so that when they are rotated they completely cover the palatal defect with the tips of the flaps supported by underlying bone. The flaps are carefully elevated from the underlying bone with periosteal elevators, making certain that the palatal artery is kept intact to ensure good blood supply to each flap. Once the flaps are elevated with periosteal elevators, one flap is rotated over the palatal defect and sutures to the freshened surrounding mucosa with absorbable monofilament in a simple interrupted pattern. The other flap is then rotated and sutured to the rostral aspect of the originally placed flap with the same suture technique. The bone exposed by the formation of the flap is left to heal by secondary intention. If the clinician feels that the rostral aspect of the second flap does not conform to the underlying bone well enough then holes can be made into the underlying bone with a K-pin or small cutting bur on a dental high-speed hand piece, the holes are then used to tack the flap down to the underlying bone with sutures. Care should be taken so that the holes in the bone are covered by the flap after suturing to prevent formation of small fistulas.

9.2.2.2.3 Rotating Palatal Island Flap The rotating island palatal flap is useful for caudal palatal defects in which rotation of the flap up to 180° will be needed to cover the defect (Figure 9.17) (Smith 2001; Woodward 2006). Two to three mm of tissue surrounding the defect (dashed yellow lines) should be debrided to create healthy freshened tissue (Figure 9.17a and b). This flap is created by making an oval-shaped incision. An island flap is at least 1.5–2 times the size of the defect (dashed blue lines). Two distal to rostral incisions of the palatal mucosa are made from the level of the distal aspect of the maxillary 1st molar tooth going rostral 2–3 mm palatal to the teeth and also at midline of the palate (Figure 9.17c). The distal to rostral incisions are connected both rostral to the incisions and distal to the incisions perpendicular to midline. The greater palatine artery will need to be ligated at the rostral incision (Figure 9.17d). The minor palatine artery may be encountered in the location of the distal incision, this small artery can be ligated if possible or incised with bleeding being controlled with application of pressure for several minutes. A periosteal elevator is used to elevate the flap while being careful to keep the major palatine artery intact and connected to the flap, while all of the palatal mucosa is elevated from the underlying bone. The flap can then be rotated up to 180°. However, less than that much rotation will ensure that the blood supply will remain intact to the flap. The size of the flap should completely cover the defect and be supporting by underlying bone around the defect. The flap should be sutured to the debrided tissue around the defect by absorbable monofilament suture by a simple interrupted pattern. The flap is secured with simple interrupted sutures where tissue margins abut and horizontal mattress sutures over the regions of partial thickness palatal tissue (white arrows) (Figure 9.17d and e). Exposed bone by the rotation of the creation of the palate will heal by secondary intention.

9.2.2.2.4 Palatal Advancement Flaps Advancement flaps are useful for repair of large caudal palatal defects (Rocha 2010). Before creation of the flap, 2–3 mm of tissue surrounding the defect should be debrided. A U-shaped flap is created distal to the defect. The created flap needs to extend to the soft palate mucosa as this mucosa has a higher elastin content and lower collagen content compared to the mucosa of the hard palate. This allows the tissue to be advanced over the defect without tension. This flap is usually created distal to the greater palatine arteries so that no major vessel is encountered with creation of this flap. The created flap is made full thickness through the hard palatal mucosa and can then be made partial thickness though the soft palatal mucosa. A periosteal elevator is used to elevate the mucosa overlying the bone of the hard palate and blunt tenotomy scissors can be used for dissection of the soft palatal mucosa in formation of the flap. Care needs to be taken with manipulation of the soft tissue mucosa as formation of any full-thickness defects of this tissue will result in formation of an oronasal fistula that will not heal by second intention and may also compromise blood flow to the rostral aspect of the flap. The flap is advanced in a rostral direction over the defect and sutured to the recipient soft tissue using absorbable monofilament suture in a simple interrupted technique.

9.2.2.3 Miscellaneous Palatal Repair and Salvage Techniques

9.2.2.3.1 Midline Palatal Fracture or Separation Midline palatal separation injuries are commonly seen in cats with falls from height or other traumas (Bonner et al. 2012). The repair can often be accomplished through reducing the injury with digital pressure and suturing of the soft tissue injury with absorbable monofilament suture in a simple interrupted pattern. For additional

(a)

(c)

(b)

(d)

(e)

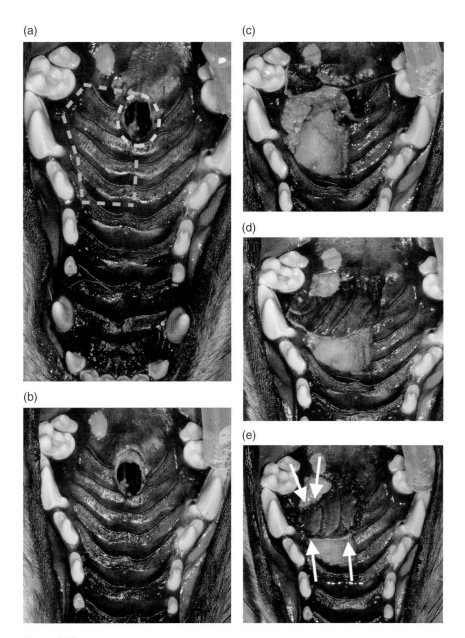

Figure 9.17

support a figure of eight cerclage wire can be placed around the maxillary canine teeth to resist tension at the fracture line. Care should be taken to not overtighten the wires, causing a malocclusion of the canine teeth.

9.2.2.3.2 Myoperitoneal Microvascular Free Flap This flap can be utilized when closure techniques utilizing local tissues have failed (Lanz 2001). Several sources of tissue and blood supply have been described to be harvested from the abdominal body wall. The infraorbital artery and superior labial vein are utilized to anastomose

the free tissue vasculature providing a robust tissue source for repair of oral defects.

9.2.2.3.3 Angularis Oris Mucosal Flap This flap has been described as a robust flap with a strong blood supply based on the Angularis Oris artery which is located in the caudal vestibular mucosa (Bryant et al. 2003). After harvesting this flap from the caudal vestibular mucosa the flap can be used to close defects to the level of the maxillary canine teeth. If the maxillary molar teeth are present, care needs to be taken to tunnel the flap through the mucosa caudal to the maxillary molar teeth to avoid trauma to the pedicle flap when the mouth is closed.

9.2.2.3.4 Obturators Various types and materials of obuturators have been described for use when other surgical options have failed or hold a poor prognosis (Smith and Rockhill 1996; Edstrom and Smith 2014). Obturators can be premade or manufactured in a lab specifically for an individual patient defect after an impression of the defect has been made with an appropriate material (Figures 9.18 and 9.19). Periodically obturators will need to be checked to ensure an adequate fit and to be cleaned.

9.2.2.3.5 Bone and Cartilage Grafts for the Support of Pedicle Grafts Both various autografts and allografts have been described for the use of closure of oral defects (Soukup et al. 2009; Lorrain and Legendre 2012). These grafts can be used alone as a scaffold material to allow the overgrowth of soft tissues, minimizing or closing a defect. Graft materials can also be used to provide additional support for pedicles or free grafts while they are healing to their recipient sites. After a defect has been debrided a bone or cartilage graft can be placed between the oral mucosa and bone, either being sutured to the underlying periosteum or to the overlying soft tissue. For defects less than 1 cm, often the freshened edges of a defect will have enough support from the graft to allow for reepithelization across the defect (Cox

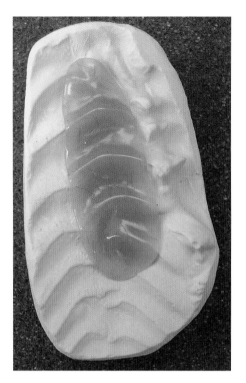

Figure 9.19

et al. 2007). If the bone or cartilage graft is placed to support an overlying mucosal graft then the bone or cartilaginous graft should be sutured into place far enough away from the edge of the defect as to not interfere with the suturing of the mucosal graft.

9.3 Tips

The timing of closure of defects is important for all types of defects. For congenital clefts, ideally the surgery is not performed until the patient is at least three to four months of age (Manfra Marretta 2012a). This is so that there are adequate amounts of tissue to work with and also so that any scar tissue that forms as a result of the surgery does not impede growth of the skull (Dremenak et al. 1970). Specifically for primary clefts, it is recommended to wait until six months of age as eruption of the permanent incisors can affect treatment plans (Fiani et al. 2016). For acquired defects, the health of the donor and recipient tissues needs to be taken into account as well as the underlying cause of the injury. If closing a defect created by a failed previous surgery then four to six weeks should be given for inflammation to subside and to allow adequate tissue healing before manipulation is attempted again (Hedlund 2002). Biopsies should be obtained from any tissues suspected

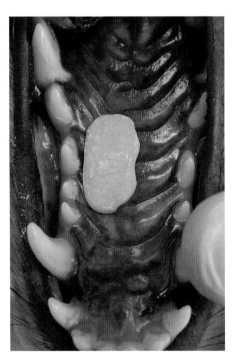

Figure 9.18

to have neoplasia or tissues that have unusual healing patterns (Manfra Marretta 2012b). For tissues previously treated with radiation therapy, the clinician and the owners need to be prepared for the unpredictable healing nature of this tissue. Wounds from electric cord injuries should be delayed until it is certain the patient is stable as pulmonary edema is a potential concurrent concern. Electric cord injuries also can take weeks to months to fully reveal the extent of the injury as osteonecrosis and sequestrum formation are not always evident acutely.

Diagnostic imaging is important for treatment planning for any category of defect. Due to superimposition of hard tissue structures, skull films can be confounding and give the least amount of usable data. For oronasal fistulas and defects in the alveolar bone, dental radiographs are useful and give adequate data without the superimposition of contralateral bones or teeth. Computed tomography has been shown to provide the most information concerning injuries of the skull when compared to radiographs (Bar-Am et al. 2008). Computed tomography has also revealed that soft tissue defects under-represent bony defects associated with congenital defects (Nemec et al. 2015). 3-D renderings generated from computed tomography are useful for both treatment planning and explanations of defects to owners.

9.4 Complications

Post-operative recommendations to minimize complications are based on the complexity of the defect and repair technique chosen. For repair of small and simple defects with a high chance of success recommendations include: appropriate pain management, a soft or gruel consistency diet for two weeks, and restriction of chew toys and activities that may damage the oral tissues for two weeks (Zacher and Manfra Marretta 2013). More complex repairs or those with a higher chance of failure or complication have recommendations that build upon

the previous recommendations and also include: use of a broad-spectrum antibiotic for 10–14 days, intravenous fluids and hospital support until the patient is comfortable and drinking on its own, and the use of a esophagostomy or gastrostomy tube to help with nutritional support and minimize oral tissue trauma from mastication during the initial healing period (Zacher and Manfra Marretta 2013).

The primary complication will be dehiscence of the flap. This occurs when there is tension on the flap, poor vascular supply, a lack of support at the suture lines, or a high bacterial load of the tissues. These etiologies can be minimized with proper technique. Tension is relieved with flaps of adequate size that have been properly undermined or released from the donor tissue. The flap should easily cover the defect without the need to be held in place or without the flap recoiling into its original position. To ensure good vascular supply, pedicle flaps should be wide-based. Proper planning and localization of vascular supply for axial flaps will help ensure success. A sterile marker can be used to help plan incisions before cutting. All tissues should be gently handled, stay sutures can be used rather than thumb forceps to minimize tissue handling and capillary bed damage. Proper knowledge of underlying bone support from diagnostic imaging with good surgical planning will help ensure the suture lines are supported with bone. While oral surgery is not a sterile procedure, a surgical technique of being as aseptic as possible will minimize post-operative complication associated with bacterial infections.

When failure of a flap does occur then an adequate amount of time needs to pass to allow for as much healing, angiogenesis, and minimization of local inflammation to occur before another attempt is made. Generally four to six weeks should be waited. Due to a change in the vascular supply and inherent fibrosis of repaired tissues, each subsequent attempted repair will have a decreased chance of success. This can be minimized by using the simplest technique with the highest chance for success as the first repair technique.

References

Bar-Am, Y., Pollard, R., and Verstraete, F. (2008). The diagnostic yield of conventional radiographs and computed tomography in dogs and cats with maxillofacial trauma. *Veterinary Surgery* 37 (3): 294–299.

Beckman, B. (2011). Repair of secondary cleft palate in the dog. *Journal of Veterinary Dentistry* 28 (1): 58–62.

Bonner, S., Reiter, A. et al. (2012). Orofacial manifestations of high-rise syndrome in cats: a retrospective study of 84 cases. *Journal of Veterinary Dentistry* 29 (1): 10–18.

Bryant, K., Moore, K. et al. (2003). Angularis oris axial pattern buccal flap for reconstruction of recurrent fistulae of the palate. *Veterinary Surgery* 32 (2): 113–119.

Cox, C., Hunt, G. et al. (2007). Repair of oronasal fistulae using auricular cartilage grafts in five cats. *Veterinary Surgery* 36 (2): 164–169.

Dremenak, C.R., Huffman, W.C., and Olin, W.H. (1970). Growth of maxillae in dogs after palatal surgery 2. *Cleft Palate Journal* 7 (3): 719–736.

Edstrom, E. and Smith, M. (2014). Prosthetic appliance for oronasal communication in a dog. *Journal of Veterinary Dentistry* 31 (2): 108–112.

Fiani, N., Verstraete, F., and Arzi, B. (2016). Reconstruction of congenital nose, cleft primary palate, and lip disorders. *Veterinary Clinics of North America* 46: 663–675.

Hedlund, C. (2002). Surgery of the oral cavity. In: *Small Animal Surgery*, vol. 21 (ed. T. Fossum), 274–306. St. Louis: Mosby.

Kelly K. and Bardach J. (2012). Biologic basis of cleft palate and palatal surgery. InL *Oral and Maxillofacial Surgery in Dogs and Cats* (ed. F. Verstraete and M. Lommer), 343–350. St. Louis: Elsevier. 35.

Kirby, B.M., Bjorling, D.E., and Mixter, R.C. (1988). Surgical repair of a cleft lip in a dog. *Journal of the American Animal Hospital Association* 24: 683.

Lanz, O. (2001). Free tissue transfer of the rectus abdominis myoperitoneal flap for oral reconstruction in a dog. *Journal of Veterinary Dentistry* 18 (4): 187–192.

Lorrain, R. and Legendre, L. (2012). Oronasal fistula repair using auricular cartilage. *Journal of Veterinary Dentistry* 29 (3): 172–175.

Manfra Marretta, S. (1991). Split palatal U-flap: a new technique for repair of caudal hard palate defects. *Journal of Veterinary Dentistry* 8 (1): 5–8.

Manfra Marretta, S. (2012a). Cleft palate repair techniques. In: *Oral and Maxillofacial Surgery in Dogs and Cats*, vol. 36 (eds. F. Verstraete and M. Lommer), 351–361. St. Louis: Elsevier.

Manfra Marretta, S. (2012b). Repair of acquired palatal defects. In: *Oral and Maxillofacial Surgery in Dogs and Cats*, vol. 37 (eds. F. Verstraete and M. Lommer), 363–372. St. Louis: Elsevier.

Manfra Marretta, S. and Smith, M. (2005). Single mucoperiosteal flap for oronasal fistula repair. *Journal of Veterinary Dentistry* 22 (3): 200–205.

Nemec, A., Daniaux, L., Johnson, E. et al. (2015). Craniomaxillofacial abnormalities in dogs with congenital palatal defects: computed tomographic findings. *Veterinary Surgery* 44 (4): 417–422.

Peralta, S., Fiani, N., Kan-Rohrer, K. et al. (2017). Morphological evaluation of clefts of the lip, palate, or both in dogs. *Journal of the American Veterinary Medical Association* 78 (8): 926–933.

Reiter, A. and Holt, D. (2012). Palate. In: *Veterinary Surgery Small Animal*, vol. 100 (eds. K. Tobias and S. Johnson), 1707–1717. St. Louis: Elsevier.

Reiter, A. and Smith, M. (2005). The oral cavity and oropharynx. In: *BSAVA Manual of Canine and Feline Head, Neck and Thoracic Surgery*, vol. 3 (eds. D. Brockman and D. Holt), 25. Gloucester: BSAVA.

Rocha, L. (2010). Soft palate advancement flap for palatal oronasal fistulae. *Journal of Veterinary Dentistry* 27 (2): 132–133.

Sivacolundhu, R. (2007). Use of local and axial pattern flaps for reconstruction of the hard and soft palate. *Clinical Techniques in Small Animal Practice* 22 (2): 61–69.

Smith, M. (2001). Island palatal mucoperiosteal flap for repair of oronasal fistula in a dog. *Journal of Veterinary Dentistry* 18 (3): 127–129.

Smith, M. and Rockhill, A. (1996). Prosthodontic appliance for repair of an oronasal fistula in a cat. *Journal of the American Veterinary Medical Association* 208 (9): 1410–1412.

Soukup, J., Snyder, C. et al. (2009). Free auricular cartilage autograft for repair of an oronasal fistula in a dog. *Journal of Veterinary Dentistry* 26 (2): 86–95.

Taney, K. (2008). Secondary cleft palate repair. *Journal of Veterinary Dentistry* 25 (2): 150–153.

Wetering, A. (2005). Repair of an oronasal fistula using a double flap technique. *Journal of Veterinary Dentistry* 22 (4): 243–245.

Woodward, T. (2006). Greater palatine island axial pattern flap for repair of oronasal fistula related to eosinophilic granuloma. *Journal of Veterinary Dentistry* 23 (3): 161–166.

Zacher, A. and Manfra Marretta, S. (2013). Oral and maxillofacial surgery in dogs and cats. *Veterinary Clinics of North America* 43: 609–649.

10

Salivary Gland Surgery

Daniel D. Smeak

Department of Clinical Sciences, College of Veterinary Medicine and Biomedical Sciences, Colorado State University, Fort Collins, CO, USA

10.1 Indications

Conditions involving the salivary glands and their respective ducts include trauma, a number of poorly understood inflammatory diseases, calculus formation, neoplasia, and rupture of salivary glands or ducts. With the exception of salivary gland abscessation, the majority of inflammatory diseases affecting these glands are best treated with medical therapy (Smith 1985; Boydell et al. 2000). Salivary gland abscesses are usually drained initially but excision of the affected gland may be recommended if it recurs.

Sialolithiasis is uncommon in cats and dogs, and most are found in the parotid duct, although the sublingual duct may also be affected (Harvey 1969; Knecht and Phares 1971; Schroeder and Berry 1988; Ryan et al. 2008). These calculi are usually radio-opaque, single, and the majority can be identified on plain skull radiographs or CT imaging (Smith 1985). Calculi may obstruct salivary ducts causing pain and swelling of the gland, but some eventually erode through the duct wall, causing a mucocele or fistula (Harvey 1977).

Salivary gland neoplasia is rare and most have been documented as adenocarcinomas of the mandibular or parotid glands (Withrow 2007). Other neoplasms of the salivary glands include squamous cell carcinoma, basal cell carcinoma, osteosarcoma, malignant fibrous histiocytoma, and mast cell tumor (Carberry et al. 1988). Male Siamese cats are over-represented, but no breed predilection in dogs has been reported (Withrow 2007). In general, wide excision of the salivary mass with local lymphadenectomy is recommended with or without adjunctive radiation therapy. Distant metastasis has been reported but may be slow to develop. Median survival times for dogs and cats with salivary gland neoplasms after aggressive resection ± local radiation range from 74 to over 500 days, depending mostly on the extensiveness of the tumor and stage of the disease on presentation (Hammer et al. 2001; Faustino and Dias Pereira 2007).

By far the most common surgical disease of the salivary glands is mucocele (or sialocele) formation, which is essentially a collection of saliva within the subcutaneous tissues. The most common source of leakage is from the mandibular and sublingual glands/ducts, and less often from the zygomatic and parotid glands (Schmidt and Betts 1978; Bellenger and Simpson 1992; Ritter et al. 2006). Just recently salivary mucocele formation has been documented in the nasopharygeal area in brachycephalic dogs (De Lorenzi et al. 2018). A case report has been reported of a mucocele originating from a minor sublingual salivary gland located in the soft palate which was successfully managed with complete excision (Watanabe et al. 2012). Poodles, German Shepherd dogs, silky terriers, and dachshunds may be over-represented, but no sex predilection has been documented. Mucoceles are uncommon in cats. Salivary mucoceles may be caused by trauma, migrating foreign bodies, calculi, following surgery for teeth extraction and hemimandibulectomy, and infiltrating neoplasia (Waldron and Smith 1991). For most the cause cannot be found, so the majority of mucoceles are considered spontaneous. However, it is still prudent to rule out these aforementioned primary causes before attempting surgical treatment because these causes could affect patient outcome, and likelihood of recurrence. It should be emphasized that mucoceles are not true cysts since the lining surrounding accumulated saliva is not secretory in nature. The inflammatory connective tissue lining, therefore, generally does not require excision. The primary goal of surgical therapy for

Gastrointestinal Surgical Techniques in Small Animals, First Edition. Edited by Eric Monnet and Daniel D. Smeak.
© 2020 John Wiley & Sons, Inc. Published 2020 by John Wiley & Sons, Inc.
Companion website: www.wiley.com/go/monnet/gastrointestinal

mucoceles is preventing further saliva leakage via complete excision of the respective "feeding" gland(s) (Waldron and Smith 1991).

Mucoceles generally present as slow-growing, painless, and soft fluctuant oral, perioral, or submandibular masses. The location of the mass and presenting complaint often points the clinician to the responsible gland. Patients can present with exophthalmos (zygomatic mucocele), labored breathing or dysphagia (pharyngeal mucocele, ranula), and most often with an intermandibular or rostral cervical swelling (cervical mucocele).

Diagnosis of uncomplicated (nonseptic, non-neoplastic) mucoceles is made by historical and physical examination findings including sampling the fluid-filled mass via fine needle aspiration. The aspiration should be performed under aseptic conditions to reduce contaminating the salivary pocket which could cause secondary infection. Fluid within mucoceles is typically viscous and clear- to "honey"-colored. Abscesses and neoplasia can also appear as swelling in these specific areas so a complete workup of patients with suspected mucoceles is necessary. Cytology should be obtained to help rule out these conditions. Uncomplicated mucoceles typically contain a moderate amount of nondegenerate nucleated cells and macrophages with a diffuse background of light violet-staining mucin. Staining a smear of the fluid with a mucin-specific stain such as periodic acid-Schiff can also help confirm that it is saliva.

When large ranulas or pharyngeal mucoceles cause significant respiratory compromise (Figure 10.1), emergency decompression of the swelling with a large-bore needle or #11 BP blade may be necessary to stabilize the patient before definitive surgery is planned (Weber et al. 1986). Most other types of mucoceles can be surgically treated on an elective basis.

10.2 Techniques

10.2.1 Anatomical Considerations

Four main pairs of salivary glands can be found in dogs and cats: the mandibular, sublingual, parotid, and zygomatic. The conjoined mandibular and sublingual glands are the source of most mucoceles in dogs and cats (Evans 1993). There are also numerous other small (minor) salivary glands located throughout the lining of the oral cavity, and paired molar glands found in the lower lip at the angle of the mouth in cats. Due to overabundance of salivary tissue in dogs and cats, ample salivary secretion can be expected even after bilateral removal of major salivary glands.

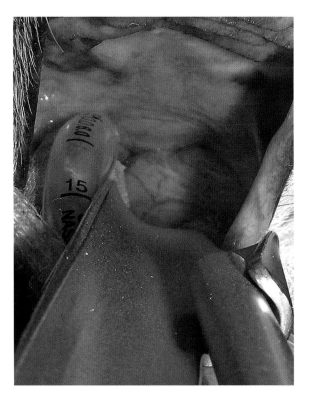

Figure 10.1

The mandibular gland is located between the branching maxillary and lingual facial veins, and within the same fibrous capsule on the rostral aspect, the monostomatic portion of the sublingual gland can be found. Both the mandibular and sublingual gland ducts course rostrally, tunneling between the masseter muscle, the mandible laterally, and the digastricus muscle medially. This limited duct path can create some difficulty for the surgeon when attempting exposure of the more rostral portions of this salivary complex via the lateral approach. This can complicate complete removal of the distal portion of the sublingual glands and increase the risk of mucocele recurrence. The ducts of the mandibular and sublingual glands often join together as they course under the mucosa of the tongue. These ducts eventually open at the sublingual papilla just lateral to the lingual frenulum. Clumps of sublingual salivary gland tissue, termed the polystomatic portion, can be found rostral to the monostomatic portion along the path of the sublingual duct. Ducts from the most terminal clumps of the polystomatic sublingual gland secrete directly into the oral cavity under the tongue (Cooke and Guilford 1992).

The triangle-shaped parotid gland is tightly adhered to the surrounding vertical ear canal. Multiple smaller ducts arising from the rostral portion of the parotid gland coalesce to form the major parotid duct which runs on the lateral surface of the masseter muscle. This ill-defined gland is covered by a thin capsule and is contiguous with deeper structures such as the facial nerve and regional major blood vessels. The duct opens within the oral cavity at the level of the fourth maxillary premolar.

The zygomatic gland is located in the periorbital region, rostromedial, and deep to the zygomatic arch, just rostral and ventrolateral to the globe, and dorsolateral to the pterygoid muscle. One or more ducts open at the deep caudolateral aspect of the oral cavity at the level of the last upper molar about 1 cm caudal to the parotid papilla. Duct anatomy is important for the surgeon to know, particularly during dissection or tumor removal in the maxillary region, to avoid inadvertent damage to the duct and iatrogenic mucocele formation (Clarke and L'Eplattenier 2010).

10.2.2 Removal of Sialoliths

A variety of surgical treatments for sialoliths have been described depending on the location of the calculus, presence of infection, ease of removing the affected gland, and likelihood of recurrence or stricture of the duct. Successful surgical treatments include removal of the stone within the duct followed by duct lavage ± repair, simple duct ligation, marsupialization of the duct within the oral cavity, or excision of the affected salivary gland(s) (Harvey 1969; Glen 1972). When the stone is near the papilla and the duct is dilated, the stone can be readily retrieved with an incision within the oral cavity. The duct incision can be marsupialized (sutured open to the oral mucosa) or left to heal by second intention. Multiple stone-like "pearls" located within a mucocele should not be confused with sialoliths. These structures are composed of proteinaceous material originating from mineralized folds within the mucocele lining (Imai 1976).

10.2.3 Cervical, Pharyngeal, Ranula Mucoceles (Mandibular and Sublingual Sialadenectomy)

Although most cervical, pharyngeal, and sublingual (ranula) mucoceles originate from the sublingual gland-duct complex alone, both the mandibular and sublingual glands are routinely removed due to the close anatomic association between the mandibular and sublingual glands and ducts. Some surgeons marsupialize pharyngeal and sublingual mucoceles (ranulas) in an effort to allow continuous drainage of the accumulated saliva, but without concurrent removal of the affected

glands, marsupialization alone often results in recurrence. If a cervical mucocele is very large and gravitates toward midline, determination of the affected side may be difficult.

Management of most sialoceles by simple incision or drainage is not recommended for definitive treatment due to a high risk of recurrence. The prognosis is excellent provided the entire affected salivary complex is surgically removed. Post-operative complications are mostly related to local wound issues, such as seroma, infection, recurrence, and bleeding. Placement of drains into a sialocele may not reduce the risk of seroma (Jeffreys et al. 1996).

10.2.3.1 Approaches to the Mandibular/Sublingual Salivary Complex

Two main approaches for mandibular and sublingual sialadenectomy have been described, a lateral or horizontal approach caudal to the angle of the mandible, and a ventral approach. The less invasive lateral approach provides less exposure to the rostral portion of the sublingual gland and requires rather aggressive retraction and deep dissection between the digastricus muscle and ventromedial mandible.

10.2.3.1.1 Lateral (or Horizontal) Approach The patient is positioned with the affected side up in lateral recumbency with a rolled towel situated under the neck (Figure 10.2) (Waldron and Smith 1991; Marsh and Adin 2013). The lateral aspect of the face from mid mandible to mid cervical regions is prepared for aseptic surgery. The skin and subcutaneous tissue and platysma muscle are incised horizontally from the caudal angle of the mandible to the junction of the linguofacial and maxillary veins (Figure 10.2). Dissection is continued more deeply with sharp dissection to expose the off-white fibrous capsule of the "disk-shaped" lobulated oval mandibular gland (Figure 10.3a). The mandibular lymph nodes must not be mistaken for the mandibular salivary gland. The mandibular lymph nodes are situated more rostroventral and are smaller and not lobulated. A horizontal incision is made through the fibrous capsule throughout the entire length of the gland (Figure 10.3b). The gland is grasped with Allis tissue forceps and the gland is bluntly dissected from the surrounding capsule of the conjoined mandibular and sublingual glands (Figure 10.3c). The gland's principal blood supply on the deeper medial side of the gland is electrocoagulated or ligated. Blunt dissection is continued in a rostral direction along the polystomatic portion of the sublingual gland and between the digastricus muscle and medial aspect of the mandible

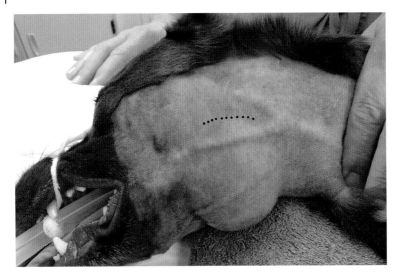

Figure 10.2

(a)

(b)

(c)

(d)

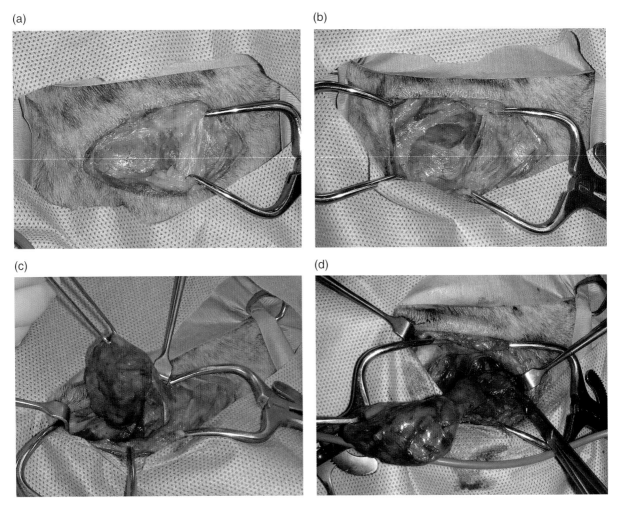

Figure 10.3

while the mandibular gland is held under tension (Figure 10.3d). A white linear lingual nerve should be identified coursing over the sublingual duct in the deep rostral aspect of the dissection plane. Hemostatic clips are used to "ligate" the sublingual duct just caudal to the nerve.

A tunneling technique has been described to improve rostral exposure and achieve increased length of the salivary gland excision (resulting in more complete salivary gland removal) when combined with the conventional lateral approach (Marsh and Adin 2013). Following mobilization of the sublingual and mandibular salivary gland complex, dissection is continued rostrally along the mandibular duct and associated sublingual gland extending between the digastricus muscle and mandible. A hemostat is applied to the duct rostral to the monostomatic portion of the gland complex, and the distal gland complex is removed caudal to the clamp. Blunt dissection is performed along the ventral aspect of the digastricus muscle and medially between the mandible and digastricus muscle to fully free it from surrounding tissue. The skin incision and subcutaneous tissue dissection is extended rostroventrally to allow for passage of curved Carmalt hemostatic forceps medial to the digastricus muscle up through the original tunnel (between the mandible and digastricus muscle) in a ventral to caudodorsal direction. The previously clamped stump remaining after removal of the mandibular and sublingual glands is transferred to the tunneled Carmalt forceps, and they are subsequently pulled medial and ventral to the digastricus muscle. Dissection is carried more rostrally and the remaining portion of the gland and duct are more easily excised while protecting the nearby lingual nerve.

Any saliva is suctioned from the mucocele pocket. Placement of a drain is at the discretion of the surgeon. Subcutaneous tissues, platysma muscle, and skin are closed routinely. If a drain is used, a bandage is placed around the cervical area until drain removal.

10.2.3.1.2 Ventral Approach

The patient is positioned in dorsal recumbency for the ventral approach (Ritter et al. 2006). The ventral cervical and intermandibular regions are prepared routinely for aseptic surgery. A skin incision is created starting from a point 5 cm caudal to the angle of the mandible on the affected side extending rostrally along and just medial to the mandible, to end at the rostral one-third of the mandible. If bilateral gland removal is planned, the skin incision can be made directly on ventral midline and each gland complex is removed by undermining and dissecting to each side. The subcutaneous tissue and platysma muscle

are incised along the skin incision line. The mandibular/sublingual gland complex is exposed and dissected from surrounding tissues as described for the lateral approach. Using caudal retraction on the mandibular gland, the sublingual gland is dissected dorsal to the digastricus muscle. A hemostatic forceps is tunneled under the digastricus muscle in a rostral to caudal direction and the forceps are spread to widen the "tunnel" and free the underlying portion of the sublingual gland. The freed portion of the polystomatic gland and duct are clamped and the distal large monostomatic sublingual and mandibular gland complex are excised (Figure 10.4). In the figure, the mandibular and monostomatic portion of the sublingual salivary glands have been excised and it is to the left in forceps. A Carmalt forceps is shown inserted under the digastricus muscle from the rostral aspect) and the tips of the forceps grasp the margin of the remaining sublingual gland stump (Figure 10.5). The clamped gland/duct stump is pulled rostrally under the digastricus muscle. For pharyngeal and cervical mucoceles, glandular tissue is ligated and resected to the level of the lingual nerve. In the figure the stump of the sublingual complex has been pulled through the tunnel under the digastricus muscle, and is dissected free. A yellow vessel loop encircles and helps retract the lingual nerve during rostral dissection (Figure 10.5).

The thin mylohyoideus muscle is incised in a line parallel and medial to the mandible to expose and allow further dissection of the rostral polystomatic portion of the gland up to the rostral portion of the tongue base. The duct is dissected and ligated as close to the sublingual caruncle as possible. The remaining gland/duct is removed, and the wound is lavaged and suctioned. If a ranula is present, the thin walled sac is generally readily dissected out and removed at its connection with the

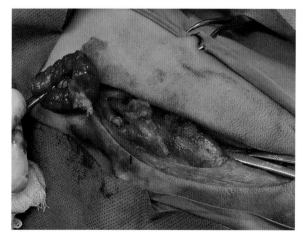

Figure 10.4

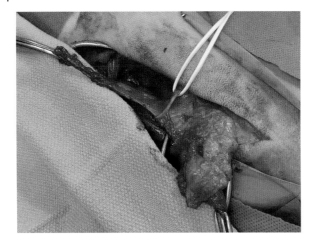

Figure 10.5

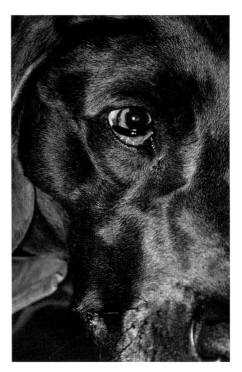

Figure 10.6

rostral portion of the sublingual gland/duct. In the figure the polystomatic portion has been dissected free. It will then be transferred underneath and rostral to the lingual nerve (yellow vessel loop) (Figure 10.5). The terminal ranula has been dissected from the base of the tongue (mass of tissue to the right held with Allis tissue forceps). The mylohyoideus muscle is closed first, then the subcutaneous tissue and skin are closed routinely. Resection of a cervical or pharyngeal mucocele is not generally necessary, and the wound can be drained with a passive or active drain system at the surgeon's discretion.

10.2.3.1.3 Marsupialization of Pharyngeal Mucoceles and Ranulas The sublingual swelling is incised with a #11 BP blade and a large elliptical portion of the overlying redundant sublingual or pharyngeal mucosa and underlying pseudocapsule of the mucocele is resected while avoiding important vascular structures in the region. The ill-defined fibrous pseudocapsule of the mucocele is identified and isolated. Cut edges of the mucosa are apposed with fine suture to the adjacent mucocele pseudocapsule with a simple continuous or interrupted pattern. The sutured opening is designed to keep the salivary pocket patent within the oral cavity to ensure adequate continuous drainage. This simple surgery may be considered as a temporary treatment when the patient has co-morbidities that limit a more extensive surgery (gland resection is the preferred treatment).

10.2.4 Zygomatic Salivary Mucocele

This uncommon mucocele should be suspected if the patient presents with exopthalmus, protrusion of the third eyelid, or a generally painless orbital or sub-zygomatic arch swelling (Figure 10.6). In some cases, a fluctuant

mass covered with normal-appearing mucosa is also evident in the region caudodorsal to the last maxillary molar. In straightforward cases the diagnosis can be confirmed with aspiration of saliva, but sialography, CT imaging, and biopsy may be indicated if neoplasia or other cause (foreign body) is suspected. Treatment consists of complete removal of the zygomatic gland.

10.2.4.1 Surgical Exposure (Approaches) for Zygomatic Sialadenectomy

A portion or all of the zygomatic arch is removed or reflected to gain access for zygomatic gland removal. With the patient in lateral recumbency, generously clip and aseptically prepare the skin centered over the zygomatic arch. Make an incision horizontally through the skin and subcutaneous tissue over the rostrodorsal aspect of the arch.

10.2.4.1.1 Zygomatic Arch Partial Excision (Limited Approach) The dorsal rim of the zygomatic arch is incised and dorsally reflected to expose the palpebral fascia and retractor anguli muscle. The periosteum is incised and ventrally reflected off the rostral half of the zygomatic arch. The dorsal half of the rostral zygomatic arch is removed with an oscillating saw or rongeurs (in small dogs) to expose the gland for removal. For closure, orbital fascia is sutured to the preserved periosteum. The subcutaneous tissue and skin are closed routinely.

10.2.4.1.2 Zygomatic Arch Osteotomy (for Maximum Exposure and Complete Periorbital Exploration) The masseter aponeurosis (leaving a small fringe of tissue for suture purchase later) is incised from the ventral rim of the rostral half of the zygomatic arch. The remaining soft tissue attachments are bluntly elevated with periosteal elevators. A tunnel is created with the elevators under the rostral zygomatic bone and under the mid zygomatic arch (just caudal to the orbital ligament). The periosteum on the zygomatic arch is vertically incised directly over the tunneled areas. The palpebral fascia at the dorsal aspect of the tunnels is incised and reflected. Bone holes (0.5 mm) are predrilled rostral and caudal to the periosteal incisions for future wire fixation. The arches are cut with an oscillating saw between the drill holes while carefully retracting and preserving structures deep to the cut, and the isolated arch is reflected dorsally. The rostroventral aspect of approach is explored to expose the zygomatic gland and mucocele (Figure 10.7). In the figure the isolated zygomatic arch has been retracted dorsally, and the zygomatic gland has been isolated with a stay suture to aid surgical resection. For closure, orthopedic wire is fed between the holes of each osteotomy to stabilize the isolated bone segment (Figure 10.8). The masseter aponeurosis is closed to the fringe of tissue left attached to the isolated zygomatic arch. The subcutaneous tissue and skin are closed routinely.

10.2.4.1.3 Gland Excision Technique Once adequate exposure is made, periorbital fat is carefully dissected and reflected to expose the zygomatic gland. Expect that the lobulated gland will be very soft (it lacks a discrete capsule) and is somewhat gelatinous in character. The gland is located in the rostroventral aspect of the periorbital space just under the broad remaining rostral zygomatic arch. The globe is dorsally retracted, and the

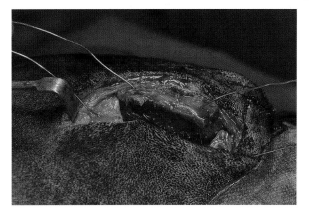

Figure 10.8

gland is bluntly and carefully dissected while avoiding the deep facial vein on the ventral aspect of the gland. The small malar artery is ligated or electrocoagulated on the ventral aspect of the gland. The site is lavaged with saline, and remaining free salivary fluid is suctioned. Drainage is generally not indicated.

10.2.5 Parotid Mucocele (Parotid Sialadenectomy)

Dog and cats with parotid mucoceles present with a nonpainful, fluctuant, soft tissue mass over the lateral aspect of the face in the region of the parotid gland. In about half of reported parotid mucoceles the cause remained undetermined, but these mucoceles can result from foreign body migration, sialolithiasis, neoplasia, and trauma (Guthrie and Hardie 2014). Recurrence is uncommon after complete parotidectomy and mucocele drainage (Proot et al. 2016). Facial nerve damage is a common complication during surgery (Carberry et al. 1988).

The anatomy surrounding the parotid gland is complex, so surgeons should dissect carefully with complete awareness of important anatomic structures in the region. In particular, the facial nerve courses directly medial and rostral to the parotid gland, so the facial nerve should be isolated and protected throughout the procedure.

A large area centered over the parotid gland extending to the rostral maxilla is prepared for aseptic surgery. With the patient in lateral recumbency, the skin and subcutaneous tissue are incised from the mid vertical ear canal to the caudal angle of the mandible. The platysma and parotidoauricularis muscles are incised and retracted to expose the parotid gland. The caudal auricular vein is ligated, and the parotid gland is bluntly dissected off the vertical ear canal in a caudal to rostral

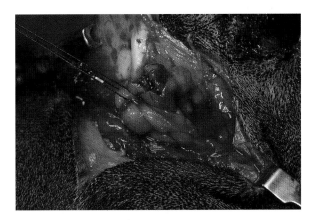

Figure 10.7

direction. The facial nerve is carefully isolated and protected as the gland is dissected from the ventral and deep aspect of the horizontal ear canal. The gland is meticulously dissected from surrounding tissues while maintaining hemostasis. Multiple small vessels that are encountered during dissection are electrocoagulated. The gland is dissected rostrally to the level of the affected duct where the duct is ligated and incised. Accessory glands (if present) are isolated and dissected free just dorsal to the parotid duct. Drainage is generally not indicated, and wound closure is routine.

10.3 Tips

If the history is inconsistent and the physical examination does not allow definitive identification of the affected side of a cervical mucocele, the author attempts to carefully squeeze the mandibular swelling while simultaneously observing the oral cavity for bulging on the affected side of the pharynx or sublingual areas. In addition, placing the patient on its back and observing if the swelling gravitates to one side may also indicate the side to operate. The author has some success first positioning the anesthetized patient in dorsal recumbency and preparing the ventral midline for aseptic surgery. A small incision directly into the cervical fluid pocket is created, and an index finger is inserted. The inserted finger is directed caudally along the submandibular space. The pocket generally extends further caudal on the affected gland complex side. Occasionally sialography or even CT imaging will help determine the affected side. Gland complexes on both sides can be removed without consequence if the affected side cannot be ascertained.

The author prefers the ventral approach overall for mandibular/sublingual gland excision, especially when treating sublingual mucoceles (ranulas) because it is easier to isolate and remove the entire sublingual gland complex to the frenulum of the tongue.

10.4 Complications and Outcome

The author does not recommend conservative management of mucoceles by simple incision and drainage, or periodic drainage with a large-bore needle, because of the high rate of recurrence and the risk of introducing infection. The prognosis is excellent provided the affected gland(s) is/are identified and removed entirely. Post-operative complications include bleeding, seroma, infection, and recurrence. Drain placement does not guarantee that a seroma will not occur. Recurrence rates of less than 5% have been reported for cervical mucoceles. Recurrence of a mucocele is usually due to incomplete removal of the affected gland or removal of the wrong side. If recurrence occurs, identify the remnant with sialography or CT imaging, and explore the region through the appropriate approach to help completely remove any remaining salivary tissue.

Bibliography

Bellenger, C.R. and Simpson, D.J. (1992). Canine sialocoeles – 60 clinical cases. *J. Small Anim. Pract.* 33: 376–380.

Boydell, P., Pike, R., Crossley, D. et al. (2000). Sialadenosis in dogs. *J. Am. Vet. Med. Assoc.* 16: 872–874.

Carberry, C.A., Flanders, J.A., Harvey, H.J. et al. (1988). Salivary gland tumors in dogs and cats: a literature and case review. *J. Am. Anim. Hosp. Assoc.* 24: 561–567.

Clarke, B.S. and L'Eplattenier, H.F. (2010). Zygomatic salivary mucocele as a postoperative complication following caudal hemimaxillectomy in a dog. *J. Small Anim. Pract.* 51: 495–498.

Cooke, M.M. and Guilford, W.G. (1992). Salivary gland necrosis in a wire-haired fox terrier. *N. Z. Vet. J.* 40: 69–72.

De Lorenzi, D., Bertoncello, D., Mantovani, C. et al. (2018). Nasopharyngeal sialoceles in 11 brachycephalic dogs. *Vet. Surg.* 47: 431–438.

Evans, E.H. (1993). *Miller's Anatomy of the Dog*, 3e. Philadelphia: Saunders.

Faustino, A.M. and Dias Pereira, P. (2007). A salivary malignant myoepithelioma in a dog. *Vet. J.* 173: 223–226.

Glen, J.B. (1972). Canine salivary mucoceles: results of sialographic examination and surgical treatment of fifty cases. *J. Small Anim. Pract.* 13: 515–526.

Guthrie, K.M. and Hardie, R.J. (2014). Surgical excision of the parotid gland for treatment of traumatic mucocele in a dog. *J. Am. Anim. Hosp. Assoc.* 50: 216–220.

Hammer, A., Getzy, D., Ogilvie, G. et al. (2001). Salivary gland neoplasia in the dog and cat: survival times and prognostic factors. *J. Am. Anim. Hosp. Assoc.* 37: 478–482.

Harvey, C.E. (1969). Canine salivary mucocele. *J. Am. Anim. Hosp. Assoc.* 5: 155–164.

Harvey, C.E. (1977). Parotid salivary duct rupture and fistula in the dog and cat. *J. Small Anim. Pract.* 18: 163–168.

Imai, Y. (1976). Physiology of salivary secretion. *Front. Oral Physiol.* 2: 184–206.

Jeffreys, D.A., Stasiw, A., and Dennis, R. (1996). Parotid sialolithiasis in a dog. *J. Small Anim. Pract.* 37: 296–297.

Knecht, C.D. and Phares, J. (1971). Characterization of dogs with salivary cyst. *J. Am. Vet. Med. Assoc.* 158: 612–613.

Marsh, A. and Adin, C. (2013). Tunneling under the digastricus muscle increases salivary duct exposure and completeness of excision in mandibular and sublingual sialoadenectomy in dogs. *Vet. Surg.* 42: 238–242.

Proot, J.L.J., Neilissen, P., Ladlow, J.F. et al. (2016). Parotidectomy for the treatment of parotid sialocoele in 14 dogs. *J. Small Anim. Pract.* 57: 79–83.

Ritter, M.J., von Pfeil, D.J.F., Stanley, B.J. et al. (2006). Mandibular and sublingual sialocoeles in the dog: a retrospective evaluation of 41 cases, using the ventral approach for treatment. *N. Z. Vet. J.* 54: 333–337.

Ryan, T., Welsh, E., McGorum, I., and Yool, D. (2008). Sublingual salivary gland sialolithiasis in a dog. *J. Small Anim. Pract.* 49: 254–256.

Schmidt, G.M. and Betts, C.W. (1978). Zygomatic salivary mucoceles in the dog. *J. Am. Vet. Med. Assoc.* 172: 940–942.

Schroeder, H. and Berry, W.L. (1988). Salivary gland necrosis in dogs: a retrospective study of 19 cases. *J. Small Anim. Pract.* 39: 121–125.

Smith, M.M. (1985). Surgery of the canine salivary system. *Compend. Contin. Educ. Pract. Vet.* 7: 457–464.

Waldron, D.R. and Smith, M.M. (1991). Salivary mucoceles. *Probl. Vet. Med.* 3: 270–276.

Watanabe, K., Miyawaki, S., Kanayama, M. et al. (2012). First case of salivary mucocele originating from the minor salivary gland of the soft palate in a dog. *J. Vet. Med. Sci.* 74: 71–74.

Weber, W.J., Hobson, H.P., and Wilson, S.R. (1986). Pharyngeal mucoceles in dogs. *Vet. Surg.* 15: 5–8.

Withrow, S.J. (2007). Cancer of the salivary glands. In: *Small Animal Clinical Oncology*, 4e (eds. S.J. Withrow and E.G. MacEwen), 47. Philadelphia: Saunders.

Section III

Esophagus

11

Esophagotomy

Eric Monnet

Department of Clinical Sciences, College of Veterinary Medicine and Biomedical Sciences, Colorado State University, Fort Collins, CO, USA

11.1 Indications

Esophagotomy is mostly performed to remove a foreign body wedged in the esophagus (Sutton et al. 2016). A foreign body can get wedged at the thoracic inlet, the base of the heart, or the lower esophageal sphincter. The foreign body should be removed first by endoscopy or pushed into the stomach with the endoscope to avoid an esophagotomy (Michels et al. 1994; Deroy et al. 2015). Every attempt should be made to avoid an esophagotomy because the risk of leakage and dehiscence with this procedure is very high (Pearlstein and Polk 1977). If a foreign body can be removed by endoscopy or pushed into the stomach, it is important to evaluate the integrity of the wall of the esophagus with either endoscopy or contrast study (Michels et al. 1994). Bronchoesphageal fistula is another indication of an esophagotomy (van Ee et al. 1986). Leiomyoma and leiomyosarcoma are tumors of the distal esophagus that only require an esophagotomy because the tumor is in the muscularis mucosa, muscularis propria, or the submucosa of the esophagus. Very often leiomyoma can be removed without entering the lumen of the esophagus. Interstitial cells of Cajal are thought to be the source of the leiomyoma. Those cells can differentiate in smooth muscle (leiomyoma), stromal (GIST), or neural sheath (schwanoma) (Beard and Reavis 2019). Leiomyosarcoma can also be resected with limited margins because those tumors are slow-growing (Farese et al. 2008; Ranen et al. 2008; Withrow 2013).

11.2 Technique

11.2.1 Surgical Approach of the Esophagus

The cervical esophagus is exposed with a ventral midline approach and separation of the sternohyoideus muscle cranially and sternothyroideus and sternocephalicus muscles caudally. After retraction of the trachea on one side, the esophagus is exposed.

The carotid artery, the vagus nerve and the recurrent laryngeal nerve are protected during the exposure of the esophagus. If needed, an osteotomy of the cranial part of the sternum is performed to extend the exposure into the cranial part of the thoracic cavity.

The thoracic esophagus is accessed through a right intercostal approach. A right intercostal approach in the third to the six intercostal space gives access to the esophagus in the cranial part of the thoracic cavity. The cranial vena cava has to be retracted ventrally to visualize the esophagus. The azygos vein is ligated to extend the exposure as it crosses over the esophagus at the base of the heart. A similar approach on the left side requires retraction of the brachiocephalic trunk to visualize the esophagus.

The caudal segment of the thoracic esophagus is reached with a left 8–10th intercostal thoracotomy to avoid the caudal vena cava. The vagus nerve is laying on the esophagus in a dorsal and ventral position. This approach can be extended through the diaphragm to reach the fundus and the body of the stomach (Taylor 1982). A gastrotomy is then performed to assist in

Gastrointestinal Surgical Techniques in Small Animals, First Edition. Edited by Eric Monnet and Daniel D. Smeak.
© 2020 John Wiley & Sons, Inc. Published 2020 by John Wiley & Sons, Inc.
Companion website: www.wiley.com/go/monnet/gastrointestinal

retrieving a foreign body wedged in the distal esophagus. The foreign body is grasped through the stomach and the lower esophageal sphincter. The forceps are guided by palpation of the distal esophagus. The foreign body can then be pulled and pushed at the same time. A radiograph is helpful to localize the site of the approach to treat the condition (Figure 11.1).

11.2.2 Esophagotomy

After exposure of the esophagus with the appropriate approach, stay sutures are placed on the wall of the esophagus (Figure 11.2a). In the caudal esophagus the vagus nerve is on the lateral side of the esophagus before dividing in a dorsal and a ventral trunk (Figure 11.2a and b). The vagal trunk present in the surgical field is retracted with suture after elevation from the wall of the esophagus. Stay sutures are then placed on each side of the future esophagotomy to help manipulate the wall of the esophagus. A #11 blade is used first to open the esophagus and Metzenbaum scissors are used to extend the incision to the appropriate length to remove the foreign body (Figure 11.2b). Suction should be ready to aspirate any fluid present in the esophagus at the time of the esophagotomy.

After removal of the foreign body the esophagotomy is closed with a one- or a two-layer closure (Oakes et al. 1993). If a two-layer closure is used the first layer includes the mucosa and submucosa with a simple continuous suture with 4-0 monofilament absorbable suture (Figure 11.3a). Knots are placed in the lumen of the esophagus. Simple interrupted sutures have also been used for the first layer. Then a second layer with a

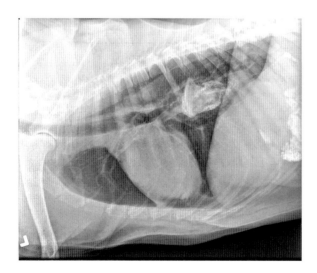

Figure 11.1

similar pattern and suture material is placed on the muscular layer and the adventitia (Figure 11.3b). Sutures are placed 2–3 mm from each other and 2 mm from the edges. It has been shown that one-layer closure is possible with a full-thickness simple continuous pattern. A 4-0 monofilament absorbable suture is used also (Oakes et al. 1993).

11.2.3 Patch

A patch of pericardium or muscle can be applied on the esophagotomy if the viability of the esophagus is questionable. Reinforcing the esophagotomy might help reduce the risk of leakage in the post-operative period. Muscle flaps have their own blood supply therefore it can unload the esophagotomy and improved its blood supply.

For the cervical esophagus the sternothyroideus muscle can be sutured over the esophagotomy with two simple continuous sutures (Figure 11.4) (Howard et al. 1975). A 4-0 monofilament absorbable suture is used. The sutures are placed partial thickness over the esophagus and 1–1.5 cm away from the incision.

For the thoracic esophagus, flaps of intercostal muscles have been described (Chernousov et al. 2009). Any intercostal space can be used. The choice of the space to use to create the flap depends on where the esophagotomy is located. It is important to prevent any tension on the flap. A flap is harvested maintaining its dorsal attachment with the intercostal artery and vein. The flap is then sutured to the esophagotomy as described above.

A flap of pericardium can also be used for the portion of the esophagus close to the base of the heart (Chernousov et al. 2009). After dissection of the phrenic nerve off the pericardium (Figure 11.5a), a flap based at the base of the heart and the great vessels is created with two parallel incisions toward the apex of the heart (Figure 11.5b). At the apex of the heart the two parallel incisions are connected and the flap can be rotated to cover the esophagotomy. The flap is sutured 360° around the esophagotomy with a 4-0 monofilament absorbable suture. Since the pericardium has been opened on the right side, the right atrium (RA) and the right ventricle (RV) are visible (Figure 11.6).

For the distal part of the esophagus a patch of diaphragm can be harvested with its base at the level of the esophageal hiatus (Figure 11.7a and b). The flap is 2 cm wide and it is sutured over the esophagotomy as described above. The liver (L) is then exposed after incision of the diaphragm (D) (Figure 11.8). For the distal esophagus the omentum can be pulled from the abdominal cavity through an incision in the diaphragm close

(a)

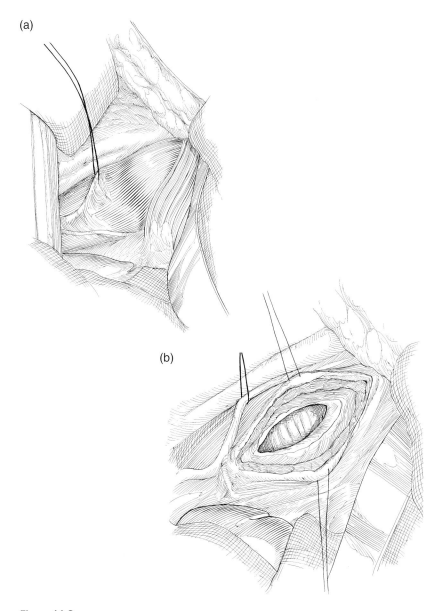

(b)

Figure 11.2

to the esophageal hiatus (Louie et al. 2019). The omentum is then wrapped around the distal esophagus (Chernousov et al. 2009).

If there is a defect in the wall of the esophagus after debridement of the necrotic part of the esophageal wall, the patch of muscle described above can be incorporated in the wall of the esophagus to prevent a stricture (Figure 11.8). The edges of the muscle flap are sutured to the edges of the esophagotomy (Figure 11.8). First interrupted mattress sutures are placed, followed by a simple continuous suture pattern on the edges. A 4-0 monofilament absorbable suture is used (Louie et al. 2019).

11.3 Tips

A one-layer closure of the esophagotomy with a simple continuous pattern has been associated with the weakest tensile strength and poor apposition (Oakes et al. 1993).

After induction of general anesthesia and before making an incision in the esophagus, it is important to advance a large-bore stomach tube in the proximal esophagus to empty as much as possible the cranial esophagus. It reduces the risk of contamination during surgery, especially when the surgery is performed in the thoracic cavity.

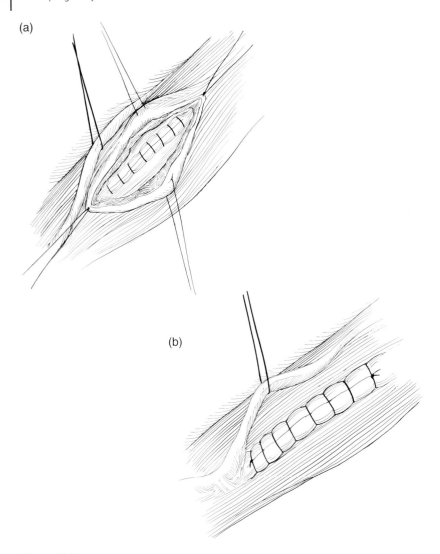

(a)

(b)

Figure 11.3

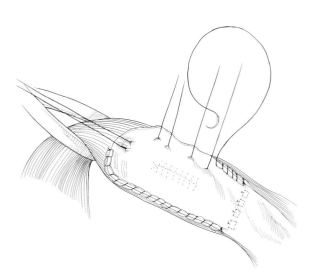

Figure 11.4

A gastrostomy tube is most likely indicated after any surgery on the esophagus. It allows feeding the patient without placing tension on the suture line (Pearlstein and Polk 1977). Because of its segmental blood supply and the lack of serosa, the esophagus is at higher risk of leakage and dehiscence. Esophagitis is also commonly associated with the presence of a foreign body and is another reason a gastrostomy tube is indicated.

Poor nutritional status is a risk factor for the development of leakage after surgery of the esophagus. Nutritional support should be instituted with a feeding tube prior to surgery to reduce the risk of dehiscence or leakage (Lerut et al. 2002; Lerut et al. 2009; Nobel et al. 2019).

The esophagus is the only segment of the gastrointestinal track to lack a serosal surface. The serosa typically helps to provide a seal after surgery and therefore the esophagus is at increased risk of leakage after esophagotomy (Nobel

(a)

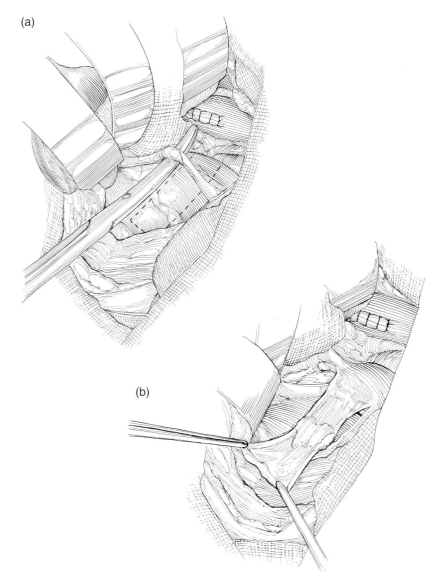

(b)

Figure 11.5

et al. 2019). Mobilizing the omentum in the pleural space and wrapping it around the esophagus can help provide a seal after surgery. However, the omentum does not have the tensile strength of a patch.

The esophagus has a segmental blood supply. Therefore, it is important to limit the dissection around the esophagus during surgery to minimize the risk of ischemia.

11.4 Complications

Leakage and dehiscence are two complications with very serious consequences for the patient when the esophagotomy was performed in the thoracic esopha-

gus. Leakage and dehiscence induce severe cellulitis in the subcutaneous tissue in the neck and a mediastinitis in the thoracic cavity. Thoracic radiographs show a dilation of the cranial mediastinum. Computed tomography scan with oral contrast is more sensitive than regular thoracic radiographs with contrast swallow (Nobel et al. 2019). Small leaks can be managed medically with antibiotic therapy and a gastrostomy tube. A thoracostomy tube should be placed if the small leakage is located in the thoracic esophagus. The thoracostomy tube can be used to lavage the pleural space (Nobel et al. 2019). If leakage is not responding to medical treatment or the leakage is large. Surgical exploration is required to patch the esophagotomy with either a muscle flap or the pericardium. Esophagectomy is attempted if the wall

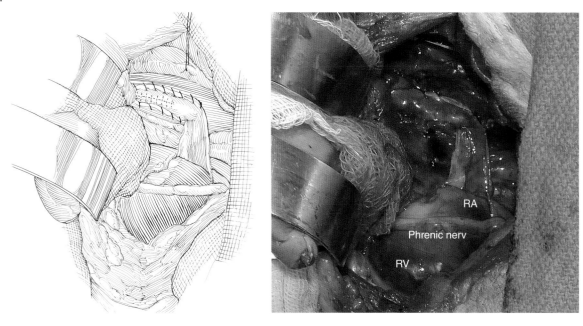

Figure 11.6

(a)

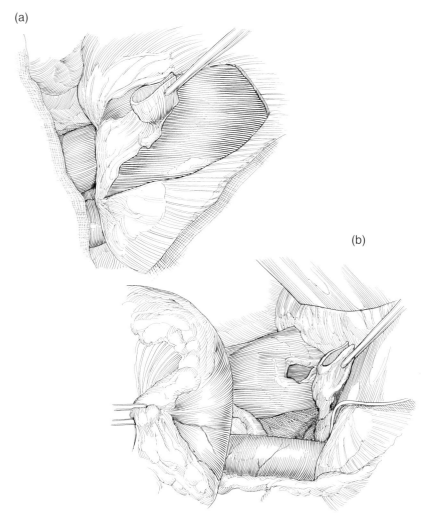

(b)

Figure 11.7

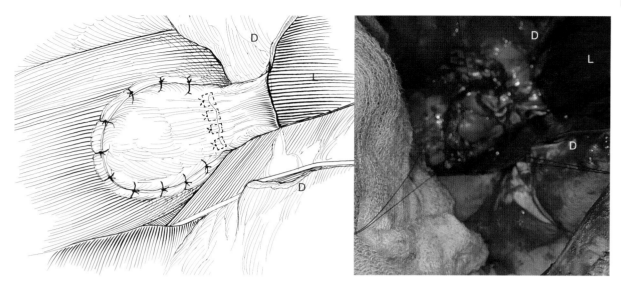

Figure 11.8

of the esophagus is not viable. If sepsis is present because of the leakage, surgical treatment should be attempted as soon as the patient is stabilized (Nobel et al. 2019).

Stricture can occur after an esophagotomy. It is very uncommon since the incision is longitudinal. It is usu-ally the result of the presence of foreign body and pressure necrosis of the mucosa. A stricture rate of 11% has been reported after foreign body retrieval from the esophagus with either endoscopy or surgery (Michels et al. 1995). Strictures can then be dilated with an endoscopic balloon.

References

Beard, K.W. and Reavis, K.M. (2019). Submucosal tumors of the esophagus and gastroesophageal junction. In: Shackelford's Surgery of the Alimentary Tract (eds. S.R. DeMeester et al.), 496–513. Philadelphia: Elsevier.

Chernousov, A.F. et al. (2009). Surgical treatment of esophageal fistula and perforation. In: Surgery of the Esophagus: Textbook and Atlas of Surgical Practice (eds. J.R. Izbicki et al.), 283–292. Berlin: Springer.

Deroy, C. et al. (2015). Removal of oesophageal foreign bodies: comparison between oesophagoscopy and oesophagotomy in 39 dogs. *J. Small Anim. Pract.* 56 (10): 613–617.

Farese, J.P. et al. (2008). Oesophageal leiomyosarcoma in dogs: surgical management and clinical outcome of four cases. *Vet. Comp. Oncol.* 6 (1): 31–38.

Howard, D.R. et al. (1975). Esophageal reinforcement with sternothyroideus muscle in the dog. *Canine Pract.* 2: 30–35.

Lerut, T. et al. (2002). Anastomotic complications after esophagectomy. *Dig. Surg.* 19 (2): 92–98.

Lerut, T. et al. (2009). Postoperative complications after transthoracic esophagectomy for cancer of the esophagus and gastroesophageal junction are correlated with early cancer recurrence: role of systematic grading of complications using the modified Clavien classification. *Ann. Surg.* 250 (5): 798–807.

Louie, B.E. et al. (2019). Surgical management of mid- and distal esophageal diverticula. In: Shackelford's Surgery of the Alimentary Tract (eds. S.R. Demeester et al.), 173–183. Philadelphia: Elsevier.

Michels, G.M. et al. (1994). Endoscopic retrieval of fish hooks in the stomach and esophagus in dogs and cats: a review of 62 cases. *Vet. Surg.* 23: 410.

Michels, G.M. et al. (1995). Endoscopic and surgical retrieval of fishhooks from the stomach and esophagus in dogs and cats: 75 cases (1977–1993). *J. Am. Vet. Med. Assoc.* 207: 1194–1197.

Nobel, T.B. et al. (2019). Anastomotic complications after esophagectomy: frequency, prevention and management. In: Shackelford's Surgery of the Alimentary Tract (eds. S.R. DeMeester et al.), 473–479. Philadelphia: Elsevier.

Oakes, M.G. et al. (1993). Esophagotomy closure in the dog: a comparison of a double-layer appositional and two single-layer appositional techniques. *Vet. Surg.* 22 (6): 451–456.

Pearlstein, L. and Polk, H.C. Jr. (1977). Esophageal anastomotic integrity. *Rev. Surg.* 34 (2): 137–140.

Ranen, E. et al. (2008). Oesophageal sarcomas in dogs: histological and clinical evaluation. *Vet. J.* 178 (1): 78–84.

Sutton, J.S. et al. (2016). Perioperative morbidity and outcome of esophageal surgery in dogs and cats: 72 cases (1993–2013). *J. Am. Vet. Med. Assoc.* 249 (7): 787–793.

Taylor, R.A. (1982). Transdiaphragmatic approach to distal esophageal foreign bodies. *J. Am. Anim. Hosp. Assoc.* 18 (5): 749–752.

van Ee, R.T. et al. (1986). Bronchoesophageal fistula and transient megaesophagus in a dog. *J. Am. Vet. Med. Assoc.* 188: 874–875.

Withrow, S.J. (2013). Esophageal cancer. In: Small Animal Clinical Oncology (eds. S.J. Withrow et al.), 399–401. St Louis: Elsevier Saunders.

12

Esophagectomy and Reconstruction

Eric Monnet

Department of Clinical Sciences, College of Veterinary Medicine and Biomedical Sciences, Colorado State University, Fort Collins, CO, USA

12.1 Indications

Esophagectomy is indicated for the resection of tumors, strictures, diverticulum, and non-viable segments of the esophagus after pressure necrosis from a foreign body (Kyles 2002; Hedlund 2007; Izbicki 2009; Thompson et al. 2012; Withrow 2013).

The most common types of neoplasia found in the esophagus are squamous cell carcinoma, leiomyosarcoma, fibrosarcoma, and osteosarcoma. Benign neoplasia like leiomyoma, adenomatous polyp, and plasmacytoma are rarely diagnosed and they may be encountered in the distal esophagus (Farese et al. 2008; Ranen et al. 2008; Withrow 2013).

The limiting factor for the resection of the esophagus is the amount of esophagus that can be resected. Since the esophagus is attached proximally to the pharynx and distally to the diaphragm and stomach it does not have much mobility. Therefore the amount of esophagus that can be safely resected is very limited.

12.2 Technique

The approaches to the cervical and thoracic esophagus are described in the chapter on esophagotomy.

12.2.1 Esophagectomy

The segment of esophagus to resect is dissected from the surrounding pleura and other tissue. The vagus nerves are preserved during the dissection. The dissection should not be extended more than 2 cm beyond the edges of the resection (Figure 12.1). Two stay sutures are first placed on each side of the esophagus beyond the edges of the resection. The edges of the resection are determined with palpation to localize the tumor or the stricture. A flexible endoscope can be used to confirm the location of the lesion to resect. If a stricture is present, passing a stomach tube helps determine the location of the stricture. The esophagus is incised with Metzenbaum scissors. A stomach tube can be introduced in the distal segment of the esophagus to prevent contamination (Figure 12.2).

Aspiration should be ready to collect any fluids leaking from the lumen of the esophagus. Usually Doyen clamps are not required to control reflux in the surgical field. However, Penrose drains or umbilical tape can be placed around the proximal and distal esophagus to facilitate manipulation and limit the amount of contamination.

The stay sutures are used to bring both ends of the esophagus close to each other to complete the anastomosis. The anastomosis is completed with either a one- or a two-layer closure. The anastomosis can be performed with simple interrupted or simple continuous suture pattern. A 4-0 monofilament absorbable suture should be used for the anastomosis (Oakes et al. 1993; Shamir et al. 1996; Shamir et al. 1999; Ranen et al. 2004; Hedlund 2007; Thompson et al. 2012; Sutton et al. 2016).

If a two-layer closure is used, the first layer includes the mucosa and submucosa. The submucosa is the holding layer of the esophagus. The knots are placed within the lumen of the esophagus to limit the amount of foreign materials in the wall of the esophagus. Then the second layer includes the muscularis and the adventitia. Placement of the second layer requires rotation of the esophagus to expose the back side of the wall of the esophagus. The same suture material is used for the

Gastrointestinal Surgical Techniques in Small Animals, First Edition. Edited by Eric Monnet and Daniel D. Smeak.
© 2020 John Wiley & Sons, Inc. Published 2020 by John Wiley & Sons, Inc.
Companion website: www.wiley.com/go/monnet/gastrointestinal

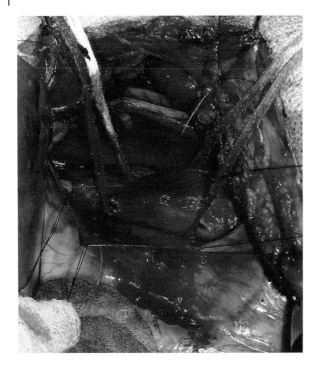

Figure 12.1

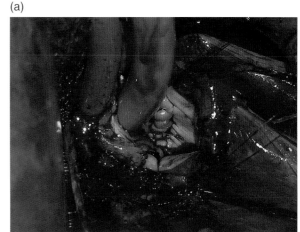

(a)

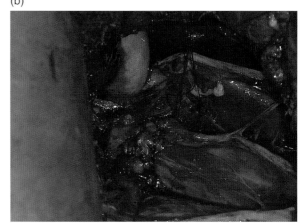

(b)

Figure 12.3

12.2.2 Dilation and Diverticulum of the Esophagus

Diverticulum is by definition the result of a bulging of the mucosa through the wall of the esophagus. It is usually the result of pressure applied from within the lumen of the esophagus by a foreign body. Pressure necrosis of the submucosa and muscularis results in the weakness of the wall of the esophagus. This type of diverticulum is called pulsion diverticulum. Usually these diverticula have a small entry site and accumulate lots of food and fluids. They need to be resected surgically (Chernousov et al. 2009; Louie et al. 2019).

With a persistent aortic arch, the entire wall of the esophagus is distended and a ventral dilation happens cranial to the base of the heart and also the cervical esophagus. It is a form of megaesophagus. It is not clear if those severe cases of distention should be resected or corrected surgically.

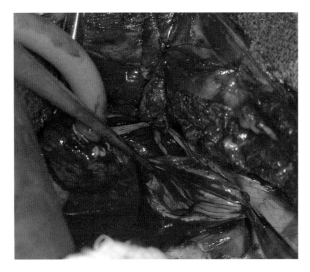

Figure 12.2

second layer. The knots are placed outside the wall of the esophagus. The suture should start on the back side of the anastomosis (Figure 12.3a). Then the front side is closed in a similar fashion (Figure 12.3b).

If a one-layer closure is used, a 4-0 monofilament is used to complete the anastomosis. A continuous or simple interrupted suture pattern with simple apposition can be used. A simple interrupted suture is less likely to interfere with dilation of the esophagus when a food bolus is going through.

12.2.2.1 Severe Dilation of the Esophagus
Due to a Persistent Aortic Arch

For a severe dilation of the cranial part of the thoracic esophagus related to a persistent aortic arch, the esophagus is approached through a left fourth intercostal thoracotomy. The ligamentum arteriosum compressing the esophagus is dissected, ligated, and transected.

The esophagus cranial to the ligamentum arteriosum is dissected ventrally. The vagus nerve is identified, dissected, and retracted dorsally or ventrally with sutures (Figure 12.4). Three or four stay sutures are then applied along the ventral border of the esophagus. A large stomach tube is introduced orally into the esophagus.

A thoraco-abdominal stapler is applied parallel to the axis of the esophagus across the diverticulum without compromising the lumen of the esophagus (Figure 12.4). A large gastrostomy tube can be placed in the esophagus to preserve the diameter of the lumen while applying the stapler. A 55 mm cartridge with 3.5 mm staples is used to resect the diverticulum. Two cartridges might be needed to go across the base of a large diverticulum. If two cartridges are needed they need to overlap over 1 cm to prevent any leakage. A 90 mm cartridge can be used but usually it is too long to be placed in the thoracic cavity. After firing the staples, a #15 blade is used to resect the diverticulum. The line of staples can be oversewn with a 4-0 monofilament absorbable suture.

12.2.2.2 Pulsion Diverticulum

A pulsion diverticulum is dissected from the surrounding tissue to isolate it from where it communicates with the lumen of the esophagus. Stay sutures are then placed in the wall of the esophagus at the base of the communication. The diverticulum is then resected with Metzenbaum scissors. The esophagus is then closed as an esophagotomy if it does not compromise the lumen of the esophagus. Staples can be placed at the base of the diverticulum and the muscularis layer is closed over the stapling line. If it does compromise the lumen of the esophagus, either an esophagectomy is performed or a muscular patch is applied in the defect and sutured to the edge of the defect as described in Chapter 11 (Chernousov et al. 2009; Zaninotto and Costantini 2019). Esophagectomy can be indicated if a severe stenosis is present.

12.2.3 Substitution

The distal esophagus can be replaced with a tube made from the stomach wall. After resection of the distal quarter of the esophagus, a reverse gastric tube is created along the greater curvature of the stomach keeping the base at the level of the fundus (Kyles 2002;

(a)

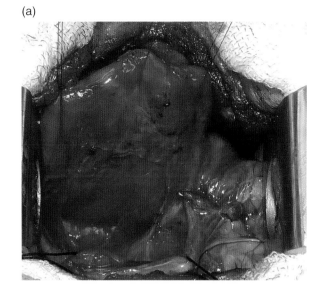

(b)

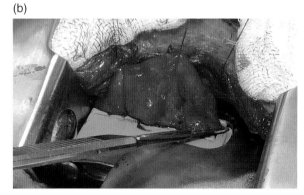

(c)

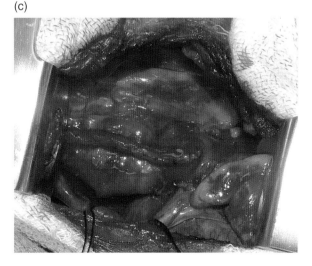

Figure 12.4

Hedlund 2007; Izbicki 2009; Depypere et al. 2019). The proximal esophagus has been replaced in dogs with a tube made from skin or skeletal muscle (Pavletic 1981; Straw et al. 1987). Esophageal replacement has been rarely performed in dogs because of the very high morbidity and mortality.

The right gastroepiploic artery and vein are ligated along the greater curvature of the stomach. Then a #11 blade is used to enter the stomach at the level of the ligature. The incision is extended dorsally and ventrally toward the lesser curvature over 3 cm on each side. Then the incision is extended dorsally and ventrally toward the fundus of the stomach staying parallel to the greater curvature. The stomach is then closed with a simple continuous suture pattern with 4-0 monofilament absorbable suture. The flap of the stomach wall based on the fundus is then closed as a tube with a simple continuous suture pattern with 4-0 monofilament absorbable suture. The tube can also be isolated with a gastrointestinal stapler. The utilization of the gastrointestinal stapler reduces the risk of contamination and it shortens the surgical time. One or two cartridges of staples are applied to create the tube starting from the suture applied around the right gastroepiploic artery and vein at the level of the pyloric antrum (Depypere et al. 2019).

The tube created from the stomach is then rotated and tunneled through the esophageal hiatus. It is then anastomosed to the proximal end of the esophagus.

Another alternative is to use a segment of jejunum or colon that is transposed in the thoracic cavity to replace the distal esophagus (Kuzma et al. 1989; Izbicki 2009). Pedicle segments of jejunum or colon can be used however their mobility reduces the amount of esophagus that can be replaced. Microvascular anastomosis have been tried with free segments of jejunum or colon with limited success in dogs because of leakage and thrombosis (Yasuda and Shiozaki 2011). Recently a pedicle of jejunum based on four arcades has been shown to be viable in dogs (Nucci and Monnet 2017). The pedicle of jejunum maintains its blood supply and the lower esophageal sphincter could be preserved to prevent gastroesophageal reflux in the post-operative period.

Skin has been used to replace the cervical esophagus in dogs. With a two-step procedure, a tube of skin is created by folding the skin on itself. The tube is left attached proximally and distally. The haired skin is inside the tube. Two weeks after creating the tube, it is transposed in the neck to replace the segment of esophagus with a proximal and distal anastomosis. The tube of skin does not have any peristalsis (Pavletic 1981).

12.3 Tips

The risk factors for leakage and dehiscence are the segmental blood supply, the lack of serosa, and the constant motion of the esophagus. The segmental blood supply of the esophagus places it at more risk for necrosis and dehiscence (Nobel et al. 2019). The esophagus cannot be placed at rest with a feeding tube since saliva is constantly traveling in the esophagus. However, it has been shown that placement of a gastrostomy tube after esophageal surgery can reduce the risk of dehiscence (Pearlstein and Polk 1977).

Poor nutritional status is a risk factor for the development of leakage after surgery of the esophagus. Nutritional support should be instituted with a feeding tube prior to surgery to reduce the risk of dehiscence or leakage (Nobel et al. 2019).

A simple continuous suture pattern with one layer was associated with the weakest tensile strength and was associated with poor apposition of the layers in the esophagus (Oakes et al. 1993).

12.4 Complications

Leakage and dehiscence are potential complications of esophagectomy because of the segmental blood supply of the esophagus. Also the esophagus does not have a serosal surface, which more likely increases the risk of leakage after surgery (Pearlstein and Polk 1977; Cassivi 2004; Nobel et al. 2019).

Leakage and dehiscence are two complications with very serious consequences for the patient when the esophagectomy is performed in the thoracic esophagus. Leakage and dehiscence induce severe cellulitis in the subcutaneous tissue in the neck and a mediastinitis in the thoracic cavity. Thoracic radiographs show a dilation of the cranial mediastinum.

Computed tomography scan with oral contrast is more sensitive than regular thoracic radiographs with contrast swallow (Nobel et al. 2019). Leakage has been classified with a grading scale from I–IV according to their severity and the presence or absence of clinical signs (Lerut et al. 2002; Cassivi 2004). Grade I is a leak that has been diagnosed on radiographs or CT scan but no clinical signs are present. Grade II is a leak that is associated with local inflammation (neck) or it is contained to the anastomosis on thoracic radiographs. Fever and leukocytosis are present. Grade III is associated with severe disruption of the anastomosis and sepsis. Grade IV is associated with necrosis of the anastomosis on endoscopy. Small leakage can be managed medically with antibiotic therapy and a gastrostomy tube. A thoracostomy tube should be placed if the small leakage is located in the thoracic esophagus. The thoracostomy tube can be used to lavage the pleural space (Nobel et al. 2019). If leakage is not responding to medical treatment or the leakage is large, surgical exploration is required to patch the esophagectomy with either a muscle flap or the pericardium. Esophagectomy is attempted if the wall of the esophagus is not viable. If sepsis is present because of the leakage, surgical treatment should be attempted as soon as the patient is stabilized (Nobel et al. 2019).

Stricture is another common complication of esophagectomy. It is important to have a good primary repair with apposition of each of the layers to minimize scar tissue formation. Two-layer closure may have a higher incidence of stricture than a one-layer closure (Nobel et al. 2019). Circular end-to-end stapling is associated with the highest rate of stricture after esophagectomy (Walther et al. 2003; Cassivi 2004).

In a study on 63 dogs and 9 cats, the immediate post-operative complication rate was 37% with aspiration pneumonia and respiratory distress being the most common complications (Sutton et al. 2016). Esophagectomy has been associated with an odds ratio of 11.25 for the risk of developing post-operative complications. Ninety percent of the patients were discharged from the hospital. Twenty-one percent of the dogs discharged from the hospital developed long-term complications: regurgitation, stricture, and dysphagia.

References

Cassivi, S.D. (2004). Leaks, strictures, and necrosis: a review of anastomotic complications following esophagectomy. *Semin. Thorac. Cardiovasc. Surg.* 16 (2): 124–132.

Chernousov, A.F. et al. (2009). Conventional resection of esophageal diverticula. In: Surgery of the Esophagus: Textbook and Atlas of Surgical Practice (eds. J.R. Izbicki et al.), 275–280. Berlin: Springer.

Depypere, L. et al. (2019). Options for esophageal replacement. In: Shackelford's Surgery of the Alimentary Tract (eds. S.R. DeMeester et al.), 438–466. Philadelphia: Elsevier.

Farese, J.P. et al. (2008). Oesophageal leiomyosarcoma in dogs: surgical management and clinical outcome of four cases. *Vet. Comp. Oncol.* 6 (1): 31–38.

Hedlund, C.S. (2007). Surgery of the esophagus. In: Small Animal Surgery (ed. T.W. Fossum), 372–409. St Louis: Mosby Elsevier.

Izbicki, J.R. (2009). Surgery of the Esophagus Textbook and Atlas of Surgical Practice (eds. J.R. Izbicki et al.), 386. Darmstadt: Springer.

Kuzma, A.B. et al. (1989). Esophageal replacement in the dog by microvascular colon transfer. *Vet. Surg.* 18 (6): 439–445.

Kyles, A.E. (2002). Esophagus. In: Textbook of Small Animal Surgery (ed. D. Slatter), 573–592. Philadelphia: Saunders.

Lerut, T. et al. (2002). Anastomotic complications after esophagectomy. *Dig. Surg.* 19 (2): 92–98.

Louie, B.E. et al. (2019). Surgical management of mid- and distal esophageal diverticula. In: Shackelford's Surgery of the Alimentary Tract (eds. S.R. Demeester et al.), 173–183. Philadelphia: Elsevier.

Nobel, T.B. et al. (2019). Anastomotic complications after esophagectomy: frequency, prevention and management. In: Shackelford's Surgery of the Alimentary Tract (eds. S.R. DeMeester et al.), 473–479. Philadelphia: Elsevier.

Nucci, D.J. and Monnet, E. (2017). Tissue blood flow to a pedicled jejunal autograft in the dog: a pilot study. *Vet. Surg.* 46 (6): 838–842.

Oakes, M.G. et al. (1993). Esophagotomy closure in the dog: a comparison of a double-layer appositional and two single-layer appositional techniques. *Vet. Surg.* 22 (6): 451–456.

Pavletic, M.M. (1981). Reconstructive esophageal surgery in the dog – a literature review and case report. *J. Am. Anim. Hosp. Assoc.* 17 (3): 435–444.

Pearlstein, L. and Polk, H.C. Jr. (1977). Esophageal anastomotic integrity. *Rev. Surg.* 34 (2): 137–140.

Ranen, E. et al. (2004). Partial esophagectomy with single layer closure for treatment of esophageal sarcomas in 6 dogs. *Vet. Surg.* 33: 428–434.

Ranen, E. et al. (2008). Oesophageal sarcomas in dogs: histological and clinical evaluation. *Vet. J.* 178 (1): 78–84.

Shamir, M.H. et al. (1996). Clinical evaluation of one-layer closure of esophageal incision utilizing the submucosa as the holding layer. *Vet. Surg.* 25 (3): 261–261.

Shamir, M.H. et al. (1999). Approaches to esophageal sutures. *Compend. Contin. Educ. Pract. Vet.* 21 (5): 414–421.

Straw, R.C. et al. (1987). Use of a vascular skeletal muscle graft for canine esophageal reconstruction. *Vet. Surg.* 16 (2): 155–163.

Sutton, J.S. et al. (2016). Perioperative morbidity and outcome of esophageal surgery in dogs and cats: 72 cases (1993–2013). *J. Am. Vet. Med. Assoc.* 249 (7): 787–793.

Thompson, H.C. et al. (2012). Esophageal foreign bodies in dogs: 34 cases (2004–2009). *J. Vet. Emerg. Crit. Care* 22 (2): 253–261.

Walther, B. et al. (2003). Cervical or thoracic anastomosis after esophageal resection and gastric tube reconstruction: a prospective randomized trial comparing sutured neck anastomosis with stapled intrathoracic anastomosis. *Ann. Surg.* 238 (6): 803–812; discussion 812–804.

Withrow, S.J. (2013). Esophageal cancer. In: Small Animal Clinical Oncology (eds. S.J. Withrow et al.), 399–401. St Louis: Elsevier Saunders.

Yasuda, T. and Shiozaki, H. (2011). Esophageal reconstruction using a pedicled jejunum with microvascular augmentation. *Ann. Thorac. Cardiovasc. Surg.* 17 (2): 103–109.

Zaninotto, G. and Costantini, M. (2019). Cricopharyngeal dysfunction and Zenker diverticulum. In: Shackelford's Surgery of the Alimentary Tract (eds. S.R. Demeester et al.), 157–172. Philadelphia: Elsevier.

13

Cricopharyngeal Myotomy and Heller Myotomy

Eric Monnet

Department of Clinical Sciences, College of Veterinary Medicine and Biomedical Sciences, Colorado State University, Fort Collins, CO, USA

13.1 Indications

Oropharyngeal dysphagia can result from abnormal prehension of food or abnormal swallowing disorders. Abnormal prehension can result from mechanical difficulty opening the mouth, oral mass, or pain on opening the mouth. Difficulty swallowing can be the result of pharyngeal dysphagia or cricopharyngeal dysphagia (Knecht and Eaddy 1959; Clifford et al. 1972, 1973, 1976; Allen 1991; Kyles 2002; Pfeifer 2003; Pollard et al. 2007; Langlois et al. 2014; Levine et al. 2014; Pollard et al. 2017; Zaninotto and Costantini 2019).

Pharyngeal dysphagia is most commonly associated with myasthenia gravis, polymyositis, polyneuropathy, brainstem disorders, or myoneural junction disorders. Cricopharyngeal dysphagia is the result of either weak pharyngeal constrictor muscles resulting in an inability to move the food bolus in the proximal esophagus, loss of coordination between the pharynx and the proximal esophagus, or cricopharyngeal dysphagia. Physical examination, neurological examination, thoracic radiographs and esophagram with visualization of the food bolus in the pharynx are important for the diagnosis of dysphagia.

Cricopharyngeal achalasia is diagnosed in young dogs and is associated with normal prehension of food and a normal gag reflex. The animal regurgitates the food almost immediately. During the esophagram a failure of opening of the upper esophageal sphincter is observed (Knecht and Eaddy 1959; Clifford et al. 1972, 1973; Allen 1991; Kyles 2002; Pfeifer 2003; Pollard et al. 2007, 2017; Pollard 2012; Langlois et al. 2014; Levine et al. 2014).

Cricopharyngeal myotomy is most commonly performed for the correction of cricopharyngeal achalasia (Allen 1991; Niles et al. 2001; Warnock et al. 2003; Papazoglou et al. 2006; Langlois et al. 2014; Zaninotto and Costantini 2019).

Heller myotomy is indicated for achalasia of the distal esophagus (Soffer 2019). This is a rare condition. Innervation to the esophagus has been damaged and the esophagus cannot contract appropriately to move the food bolus aborally, while the lower esophageal sphincter does not relax enough to allow the passage of the food bolus in the stomach. In one case report in a dog, achlasia of the distal esophagus was associated with a megaesophagus. Peristaltic waves were still present in this case (Boria et al. 2003).

13.2 Technique

13.2.1 Cricopharyngeal Myotomy

The cricopharyngeal muscle is a single striated muscle which makes up a part of the upper esophageal sphincter. It merges caudally with the muscle layers of the esophagus and it is bordered cranially by the thyropharyngeal muscle and the pharyngeal constrictor muscles (the palatopharyngeal muscle, the pterygopharyngeal muscle, and the hyopharyngeal muscle). There is a median raphe dorsal to the esophagus that blends caudally with the wall of the esophagus. The cricopharyngeal muscle is innervated by the vagus nerve via branches of the pharyngeal plexus and the laryngeal recurrent nerve.

The patient is placed in lateral recumbency with a roll under the neck (Figure 13.1). The surgery can be performed on the left or the right side. The larynx is

Gastrointestinal Surgical Techniques in Small Animals, First Edition. Edited by Eric Monnet and Daniel D. Smeak.
© 2020 John Wiley & Sons, Inc. Published 2020 by John Wiley & Sons, Inc.
Companion website: www.wiley.com/go/monnet/gastrointestinal

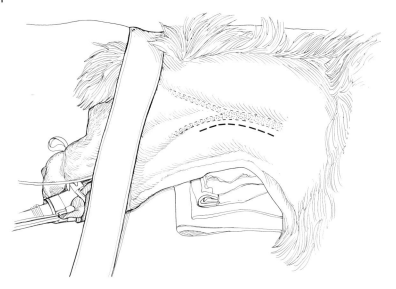

Figure 13.1

palpated and the jugular vein is visualized prior to make the skin incision.

A skin incision is made ventral to the jugular vein at the level of the bifurcation (Figure 13.1). After dissection through the platysma muscle, the jugular vein is retracted dorsally with a small Gelpy retractor (Figure 13.2a). The parotidoauricularis muscle is transected or retracted dorsally. The dissection is continued toward the dorsal border of the larynx. The cricopharyngeal muscle is identified immediately caudal to the thyropharyngeal muscle (Figure 13.2b). The cricopharyngeal muscle is transected and a segment resected if a myectomy is performed (Figure 13.3). It is important not to damage the wall of the esophagus during the dissection. An orogastric tube can be placed at the time of surgery to help identify the wall of the esophagus.

13.2.2 Heller's Myotomy

Heller's myotomy is indicated for achalasia of the distal esophagus (Colavita and Swanstrom 2019).

After a midline incision is performed to enter the abdominal cavity, the left lateral liver lobe is retracted following incision of the triangular ligament. The body of the stomach is retracted caudally and toward the right to visualize the esophageal hiatus (Figure 13.4a). The distal esophagus is then exposed. A partial thickness incision is performed in the ventral part of the esophagus (Figure 13.4b). The muscularis layer is cut from the most distal 2 cm of the esophagus to 2 cm over the stomach. The diaphragm should not be opened during the procedure.

13.3 Tips

13.3.1 Cricopharyngeal Myotomy

The procedure can be performed in dorsal or lateral recumbency. If the procedure is performed in dorsal recumbency it requires a 180° rotation of the larynx to visualize the cricopharyngeal muscle which can make the surgery more difficult. However, the ventral approach allows for a bilateral myotomy or myectomy.

A bilateral surgery is not performed routinely. It has been shown to be beneficial in one case after a unilateral myotomy was not successful in an eight-month-old Golden retriever (Langlois et al. 2014).

A myotomy of the thyropharyngeal muscle has also been performed at the time of a cricopharyngeal myotomy (Goring and Kagan 1982; Allen 1991).

It is important to dissect and transect all the muscle fibers. An orogastric tube helps identify the wall of the esophagus to prevent iatrogenic perforation of the esophageal wall while all the fibers are transected.

13.3.2 Heller's Myotomy

Heller myotomy has been performed with laparotomy, laparoscopy, or endoscopy in human patients. The laparotomy and the laparoscopic approaches are associated with a high rate of gastroesophageal reflux and a Nissen's fundoplication is routinely performed. The endoscopic approach is not associated with a high incidence of gastroesophageal reflux

(a)

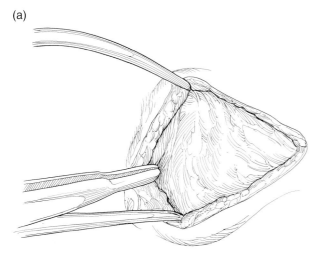

(b)

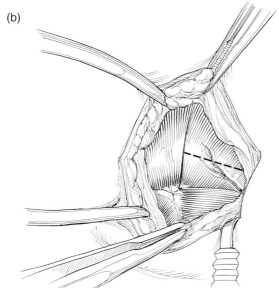

Figure 13.2

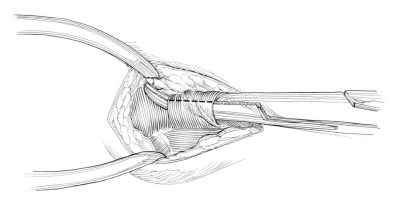

Figure 13.3

(a)

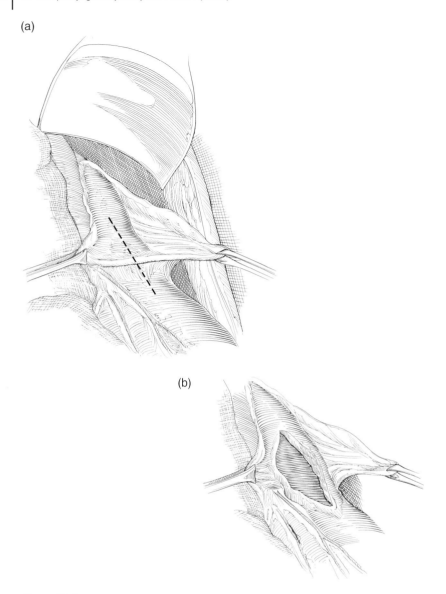

(b)

Figure 13.4

13.4 Complications

The prognosis after cricopharyngeal myotomy is considered good. Generally, the clinical condition of the patients is significantly improved. Some dogs may still cough intermittently. However, most of the documented studies have a short follow-up time of approximately seven weeks (Allen 1991). In a study with a longer follow-up time the outcome was less favorable, with 6 of 14 dogs showing no improvement after surgery (Warnock et al. 2003). The two years survival rate was 55%. Fibrosis of the surgical site has been a cause of recurrence in some cases. In another study with two to eight years of follow-up, five of six dogs had complete resolution of clinical signs with no recurrence (Niles et al. 2001). A myectomy was performed in those six dogs.

Cricopharyngeal myotomy may not improve, or may even exacerbate clinical signs if pharyngeal dysfunction is present. Video fluoroscopy is paramount to evaluate the synchronization between the contraction of the pharynx and the relaxation of the cricopharyngeal muscle and to subsequently achieve an accurate diagnosis prior to surgery (Pollard et al. 2007, 2017).

The long-term outcome and prognosis of dogs with esophageal achalasia and Heller's myotomy is not known. In one case report of true esophageal achalasia has been published (Boria et al. 2003). That case did well long term and the esophagus regained normal size 11 days after surgery. In other cases, the surgery was successful but the esophagus did not regain function after surgery (Clifford et al. 1967, 1972). The Heller's myotomy is associated with an excellent outcome in humans.

References

Allen, S.W. (1991). Surgical management of pharyngeal disorders in the dog and cat. *Prob. Vet. Med.* 3 (2): 290–297.

Boria, P.A. et al. (2003). Esophageal achalasia and secondary megaesophagus in a dog. *Can. Vet. J.* 44 (3): 232–234.

Clifford, D.H. et al. (1967). Esophagomyotomy (Heller's) for relief of esophageal achalasia in three dogs. *J. Am. Vet. Med. Assoc.* 151 (9): 1190–1201.

Clifford, D.H. et al. (1972). Management of esophageal achalasia in miniature schnauzers. *J. Am. Vet. Med. Assoc.* 161 (9): 1012–1021.

Clifford, D.H. et al. (1973). Comparison of motor nuclei of the vagus nerve in dogs with and without esophageal achalasia. *Proc. Soc. Exp. Biol. Med.* 142 (3): 878–882.

Clifford, D.H. et al. (1976). Classification of congenital neuromuscular dysfunction of the canine esophagus. *Vet. Radiol. Ultrasound* 17: 98–100.

Colavita, P.D. and Swanstrom, L.L. (2019). Endoscopic and surgical therapies for achalasia. In: Shackelford's Surgery of the Alimentary Tract (eds. S.R. Demeester et al.), 189–196. Philadelphia: Elsevier.

Goring, R.L. and Kagan, K.G. (1982). Cricopharyngeal achalasia in the dog: radiographic evaluation and surgical management. *Compend. Contin. Educ. Vet.* 5: 438–444.

Knecht, C.D. and Eaddy, J.A. (1959). Canine esophageal achalasia corrected by retrograde dilatation – a case report. *J. Am. Vet. Med. Assoc.* 135: 554–555.

Kyles, A.E. (2002). Esophagus. In: Textbook of Small Animal Surgery (ed. D. Slatter), 573–592. Philadelphia: Saunders.

Langlois, D.K. et al. (2014). Successful treatment of cricopharyngeal dysphagia with bilateral myectomy in a dog. *Can. Vet. J.* 55 (12): 1167–1172.

Levine, J.S. et al. (2014). Contrast videofluoroscopic assessment of dysphagic cats. *Vet. Radiol. Ultrasound* 55 (5): 465–471.

Niles, J.D. et al. (2001). Resolution of dysphagia following cricopharyngeal myectomy in six young dogs. *J. Small Anim. Pract.* 42 (1): 32–35.

Papazoglou, L.G. et al. (2006). Cricopharyngeal dysphagia in dogs: the lateral approach for surgical management. *Compend. Contin. Educ. Vet.* 28: 696–704.

Pfeifer, R.M. (2003). Cricopharyngeal achalasia in a dog. *Can. Vet. J.* 44 (12): 993–995.

Pollard, R.E. (2012). Imaging evaluation of dogs and cats with dysphagia. *ISRN Vet. Sci.* 2012: 15.

Pollard, R.E. et al. (2007). Preliminary evaluation of the pharyngeal constriction ratio (pcr) for fluoroscopic determination of pharyngeal constriction in dysphagic dogs. *Vet. Radiol. Ultrasound* 48 (3): 221–226.

Pollard, R.E. et al. (2017). Diagnostic outcome of contrast videofluoroscopic swallowing studies in 216 dysphagic dogs. *Vet. Radiol. Ultrasound* 58 (4): 373–380.

Soffer, E. (2019). Epidemiology, diagnosis, and medical management of achalasia. In: Shackelford's Surgery of the Alimentary Tract (eds. S.R. Demeester et al.), 184–196. Philadelphia: Elsevier.

Warnock, J.J. et al. (2003). Surgical management of cricopharyngeal dysphagia in dogs: 14 cases (1989–2001). *J. Am. Vet. Med. Assoc.* 223 (10): 1462–1468.

Zaninotto, G. and Costantini, M. (2019). Cricopharyngeal dysfunction and Zenker diverticulum. In: Shackelford's Surgery of the Alimentary Tract (eds. S.R. Demeester et al.), 157–172. Philadelphia: Elsevier.

14

Vascular Ring Anomaly

Eric Monnet

Department of Clinical Sciences, College of Veterinary Medicine and Biomedical Sciences, Colorado State University, Fort Collins, CO, USA

14.1   Indications

Vascular ring anomalies are congenital abnormalities resulting in compression of the esophagus. They are the result of the abnormal development of the aortic arches during embryological development.

During normal embryological development, the six aortic arches undergo remodeling to result in one aortic arch on the left side, a brachycephalic trunk, a left and right subclavian artery and a pulmonary artery. The ligamentum arteriosum that is connecting the aorta and the pulmonary artery as the ductus arteriosus does not compress the esophagus in the fetus.

Vascular ring anomalies have been listed as: a persistent right aortic arch with a left ligamentum arteriosum, a persistent right aortic arch with a left ligamentum arteriosum and an aberrant left subclavian artery, a double aortic arch, a left aortic arch with right ligamentum arteriosum, and a left aortic arch with right ligamentum arteriosum and right aberrant subclavian artery (Muldoon et al. 1997; Holt et al. 2000; MacPhail et al. 2001; Buchanan 2004; Krebs et al. 2014). The aforementioned vascular ring anomalies result in compression of the esophagus because the ligamentum arteriosum is encircling the esophagus and/or the aberrant subclavian artery is compressing the esophagus or because of a double aortic arch.

Approximately ninety percent of the clinical cases are the result of a right aortic arch with left ligamentum arteriosum plus or minus an aberrant left subclavian artery (Muldoon et al. 1997; Krebs et al. 2014; Townsend et al. 2016). Double aortic arches have been reported as case reports in dogs and cats (Martin et al. 1983; Ferrigno et al. 2001; Buchanan 2004; Du Plessis et al. 2006). Finally, left aortic arches with right ligamentum

arteriosum have been reported in German Shepherds (Hurley et al. 1993; Holt et al. 2000).

Dogs and cats with vascular ring anomalies present for regurgitation that most commonly develops at the time of switching from a liquid to a more solid diet. Very often, dogs and cats present with dilation in the neck that disappears after regurgitation. A continuous murmur can be auscultated if the ductus arteriosus is still patent at the time of diagnosis.

All vascular ring anomalies result in compression of the esophagus at the base of the heart with a cranial megaesophagus. An aberrant subclavian artery can result in an obstruction cranial to the base of the heart.

Beside the clinical signs, diagnosis of vascular ring anomalies includes thoracic radiographs with an esophagram (Figure 14.1). The esophagram reveals a dilation of the esophagus cranial to the base of the heart that can occupy most of the cranial mediastinum and a narrowing of the esophagus at the base of the heart. Usually the caudal esophagus is normal size with normal function. On thoracic radiographs, signs of aspiration pneumonia may be visualized . In the case of double aortic arches, computed tomography may be required to determine which aortic arch is predominant. A persistent left cranial vena cava can be seen in some cases. Flexible endoscopy of the esophagus is very valuable to determine the side of the aortic arch and determine the surgical approach (Figure 14.2) (Townsend et al. 2016). During endoscopy, pulsations against the wall of the esophagus are visible on the side of the aortic arch. If pulsations are visible on the right side of the esophagus, the aortic arch is on the right side of the esophagus and a left intercostal approach is warranted to correct the

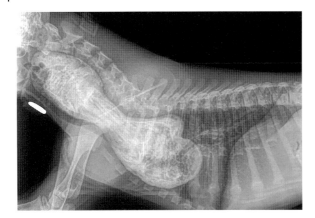

Figure 14.1

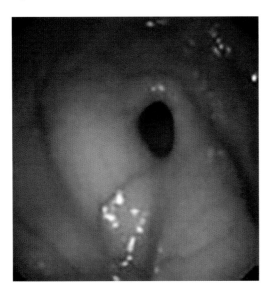

Figure 14.2

obstruction. If the pulsations are on the left side of the esophagus, the aortic arch is on the left side and a right intercostal approach is indicated. If pulsations are visible on both sides of the esophagus a double aortic arch is present and a CT scan or a MRI is indicated to determine the approach. The dominant aortic arch is preserved, therefore the approach is performed on the side of the smallest aortic arch, which is ligated.

14.2 Techniques

Correction of the esophageal obstruction requires either ligation and division of the ligamentum arteriosum or, in the case of a double aortic arch, ligation and division of the smallest aortic arch. Rarely, an aberrant subclavian contributes to an obstruction of the esophagus. The aberrant subclavian artery can be ligated and divided.

The surgery can be performed with an intercostal thoracotomy or with thoracoscopy (Muldoon et al. 1997; Holt et al. 2000; MacPhail et al. 2001; Krebs et al. 2014; Townsend et al. 2016). Thoracoscopy is only possible for the ligation and division of a ligamentum arteriosum and has only been reported for treatment of a persistent right aortic arch (MacPhail et al. 2001; Krebs et al. 2014; Townsend et al. 2016; Nucci et al. 2018).

14.2.1 Intercostal Thoracotomy

A left or a right fourth intercostal thoracotomy is performed to expose the ligamentum arteriosum and/or the subclavian artery. If a patent ductus arteriosus (PDA) is present, it has to be ligated at the time of surgery.

14.2.1.1 Ligamentum Arteriosum
The patient is placed in lateral recumbency. A skin incision is performed from dorsal to ventral at the level of the caudal border of the scapula. The subcutaneous tissues with the cutaneous trunci muscle are incised with electrocautery to minimize bleeding. The latissimus dorsalis muscle is then exposed and incised from ventral to dorsal with preferably electrocautery. After identifying the fourth intercostal space the bundles of the serratus dorsalis muscles are separated at the level of the fourth intercostal space. Ventrally the scalenus muscle is incised. The intercostal muscles are then incised in the fourth space. A Finochietto retractor is used to retract the ribs and expose the pleural space. The left or right cranial lung lobes are retracted caudally to expose the cranial mediastinum and the base of the heart. The ligamentum arteriosum is identified and dissected from the esophagus. The mediastinum covering the ligamentum arteriosum is incised first and then right-angle forceps are used to dissect the ligamentum arteriosum (Figure 14.3a). The vagus nerve and the laryngeal recurrent nerve should be identified before dissection and preserved. The ligamentum arteriosum is then double ligated with nonabsorbable suture and divided between the two sutures (Figure 14.3b). A large Foley catheter (20 F) is advanced in the esophagus from the mouth beyond the area of compression. The balloon is inflated and the catheter pulled back slowly. Fibers interfering with dilation of the esophagus should be divided. It is paramount not to damage the wall of the esophagus.

A thoracostomy tube is placed and the thoracotomy closed in a routine fashion.

14.2.1.2 Double Aortic Arch
If a double aortic is present, the dominant arch should be preserved. After performing a CT scan or an MRI

(a)

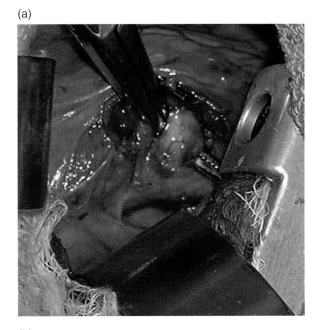

(b)

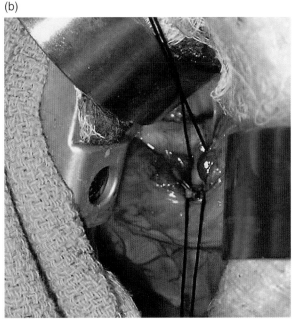

Figure 14.3

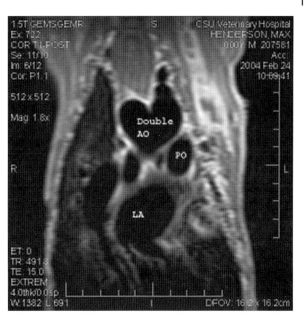

Figure 14.4

(Figure 14.4) to determine the major aortic arch, an intercostal thoracotomy in the left or right fourth intercostal space is performed to access the minor aortic arch. The aortic arch is exposed with caudal retraction of the left or right cranial lung lobe.

The aortic arch is dissected 360° with right-angle forceps (Figure 14.5a). The dissection should be large enough to be able to place two vascular clamps across the aortic arch. A red rubber feeding tube can be used as a guide to place the vascular clamp around the aortic arch (Figure 14.5b and c). Sufficient space must be left between the two forceps to be able to divide the aortic arch. After application of the vascular clamp the arterial pressure is monitored for five minutes to make sure it is not dropping, which would indicate that the remaining aortic arch does not provide adequate blood flow to perfuse the peripheral tissues. If the arterial pressure is decreased the clamps are removed and applied to the other aortic arch to evaluate its contribution to the blood flow. Exposure of the contralateral aortic arch is difficult. If the arterial pressure is equally affected by clamping of either aortic arch the ipsilateral aortic arch is clamped and divided.

After clamping the aortic arch, mattress sutures with pledgets made of Teflon are applied across the aortic arch on each side. Monofilament nonabsorbable suture size 4-0 is used. Then two simple continuous sutures with 4-0 monofilament nonabsorbable sutures are placed on each end of the aortic arch. The stitches should not be placed beyond the mattress sutures to reduce the risk of bleeding. The clamps are then removed. If some bleeding is present, mattress sutures with pledgets are added. The ligamentum arteriosum should be ligated and divided if the right aortic arch was preserved. If the ligamentum arteriosum is still patent, it should be clamped, divided, and sutured as described above for the aortic arch.

A thoracostomy tube is placed and the thoracotomy closed in a routine fashion.

(a)

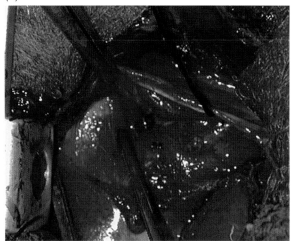

(b)

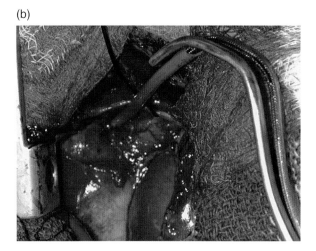

(c)

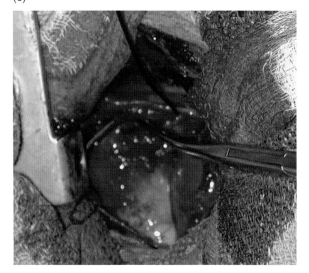

Figure 14.5

14.2.2 Thoracoscopy

The patient is placed in right lateral recumbency. The left cranial lung lobe is excluded by placing a bronchial blocker in the left cranial bronchi. A 5 Fr endobronchial blocker is placed under bronchoscopy.

An intercostal approach with three 5 mm cannulas is performed at the eighth or ninth intercostal space on the left side. The cannulas are all placed in the dorsal third of the same intercostal space. The vagus nerve is identified. A palpation probe is first used to palpate the ligamentum arteriosum (Figure 14.6). If the ligamentum arteriosum is not identified, a stomach tube is advanced in the esophagus to visualize the area of obstruction.

Fine-toothed grasping forceps are then used to elevate the ligamentum arteriosum into the pleural space. Dissection of the mediastinum covering the ligamentum is started with electrocautery with a J hook extension to the electrocautery pencil. Then right-angle forceps are used to complete the dissection 360° around the ligamentum arteriosum (Figure 14.7). Usually the wall of the esophagus is visible. Either hemoclips are applied to the ligamentum arteriosum before transection or a vessel sealant device is used (Figure 14.8).

After transection of the ligamentum arteriosum, the esophagus is well exposed with dissection of surrounding tissue and remaining fibers that could compress the esophagus.

A thoracostomy tube is then placed, the cannulas removed, and each cannula site closed routinely. A local block with a long-acting local anesthetic is performed in the intercostal space where the three cannulas were located and at the entrance of the thoracostomy tube.

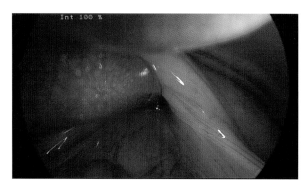

Figure 14.6

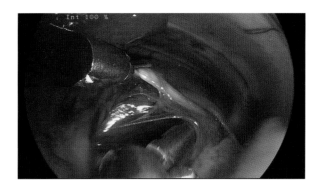

Figure 14.7

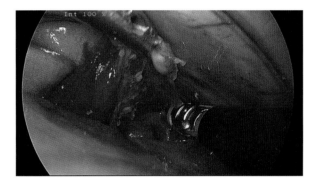

Figure 14.8

14.3 Tips

If a double aortic arch and a PDA are present, the PDA has to be dissected, clamped, divided, and sutured as described above for the aortic arch. The PDA has to be divided because it contributes to the compression of the esophagus after division of the left aortic arch.

An aberrant left cranial vena cava can be present also with a vascular ring anomaly. It covers the ligamentum arteriosum. The aberrant left cranial vena cava is dissected and retracted dorsally to expose the ligamentum arteriosum. If the retraction is difficult, the aberrant left cranial vena cava can be divided; usually the right cranial vena cava is present.

During thoracoscopy, the visualization of the ligamentum arteriosum is greatly improved if a stomach tube is placed in the esophagus.

One lung ventilation to exclude the left cranial lung lobe or the left cranial and caudal lung lobes greatly improves exposure. If one lung ventilation is not used, a fourth cannula is required to retract the left cranial lung lobe. A fan retractor or a palpation probe is used to retract the left cranial lung lobe.

During thoracoscopy placing the dog is a slight oblique position elevating the dorsal part of the thoracic cavity helps expose the ligamentum arteriosum. Utilization of a pediatric set (2.7 mm) can also prove advantageous during the dissection due to the limited available working space. A 5 mm vessel sealant device is required at the end to seal the ligamentum arteriosum.

The dilated cranial esophagus can be resected with a thoraco-abdominal stapler. The long-term benefit of the resection is not known (see Chapter 12).

14.4 Complications and Aftercare

Post-operatively the patients are monitored for signs of regurgitation. The thoracostomy tube is removed within 12 hours of surgery if the tube is not productive.

During surgery, it is important to identify the vagus and the recurrent laryngeal nerves. If the vagus nerve is damaged at the level of the ligamentum arteriosum it induces a megaesophagus in the distal esophagus with abnormal motility. Damage to the recurrent laryngeal nerve typically results in a unilateral laryngeal paralysis that should not be symptomatic.

After surgery, dogs are more likely to need to be maintained in a vertical position after eating to allow a food bolus to progress to the stomach. Since those dogs have a megaesophagus they are at higher risk for regurgitation and aspiration pneumonia. It is not known if the cranial esophagus regains some function after correction of the obstruction.

Thoracoscopic treatment of persistent aortic arch is an acceptable technique and it is not associated with higher morbidity or mortality when compared to treatment via thoracotomy (Nucci et al. 2018).

Generally, the quality of life of treated patients is greatly improved and owners are usually very satisfied with the outcome. However, the dogs still have to be fed in an elevated position for the rest of their life.

References

Buchanan, J.W. (2004). Tracheal signs and associated vascular anomalies in dogs with persistent right aortic arch. *J. Vet. Intern. Med.* 18 (4): 510–514.

Du Plessis, C.J. et al. (2006). Symmetrical double aortic arch in a beagle puppy. *J. Small Anim. Pract.* 47 (1): 31–34.

Ferrigno, C.R. et al. (2001). Double aortic arch in a dog (canis familiaris): a case report. *Anat. Histol. Embryol.* 30 (6): 379–381.

Holt, D. et al. (2000). Esophageal obstruction caused by a left aortic arch and an anomalous right patent ductus arteriosus in two German shepherd littermates. *Vet. Surg.* 29 (3): 264–270.

Hurley, K. et al. (1993). Left aortic arch and right ligamentum arteriosum causing esophageal obstruction in a dog. *J. Am. Vet. Med. Assoc.* 203 (3): 410–412.

Krebs, I.A. et al. (2014). Short- and long-term outcome of dogs following surgical correction of a persistent right aortic arch. *J. Am. Anim. Hosp. Assoc.* 50 (3): 181–186.

MacPhail, C.M. et al. (2001). Thoracoscopic correction of persistent right aortic arch in a dog. *J. Am. Anim. Hosp. Assoc.* 37 (6): 577–581.

Martin, D.G. et al. (1983). Double aortic arch in a dog. *J. Am. Vet. Med. Assoc.* 183 (6): 697–699.

Muldoon, M.M. et al. (1997). Long-term results of surgical correction of persistent right aortic arch in dogs: 25 cases (1980–1995). *J. Am. Vet. Med. Assoc.* 210 (12): 1761–1763.

Nucci, D.J. et al. (2018). Retrospective comparison of short-term outcomes following thoracoscopy versus thoracotomy for surgical correction of persistent right aortic arch in dogs. *J. Am. Vet. Med. Assoc.* 253 (4): 444–451.

Townsend, S. et al. (2016). Thoracoscopy with concurrent esophagoscopy for persistent right aortic arch in 9 dogs. *Vet. Surg.* 45 (S1): O111–O118.

15

Hiatal Hernia

Eric Monnet

Department of Clinical Sciences, College of Veterinary Medicine and Biomedical Sciences, Colorado State University, Fort Collins, CO, USA

15.1 Indications

Hiatal hernias are congenital or acquired in origin. Upper airway obstruction has been identified as a common cause of hiatal hernia in dogs (Ellison et al. 1987; Hardie et al. 1998; Holt et al. 1998; Lorinson and Bright 1998; Mackin 1998; Sivacolundhu et al. 2002; Mayhew et al. 2017). Chinese Sharpei and English Bulldogs are the two breeds most commonly reported with hiatal hernias. Brachycephalic dogs should be evaluated with chest radiographs during a work-up for a suspected hiatal hernia (Hardie et al. 1998; Broux et al. 2018).

Hiatal hernias are only surgically treated if they are inducing vomiting or regurgitation. If an underlying condition has been identified, it should be corrected first. Medical treatment with omeprazole, sucralfate, and cisapride should be initiated. If the patient is not improving then surgical treatment is indicated.

Thoracic radiographs with barium are sufficient to make the diagnosis of a sliding hiatal hernia. Sometimes several radiographs are required to visualize the stomach in the thoracic cavity through the esophageal hiatus (Figure 15.1). Flexible endoscopy of the upper gastrointestinal tract is recommended to confirm the diagnosis of a hiatal hernia and to evaluate the diameter of the esophageal hiatus before surgery. When the endoscopy is retroflexed in the stomach to look back at the cardia, the imprint of the diaphragm is visible on the stomach, delineated by the black arrows, (Figure 15.2) and the lower esophageal sphincter is not visible around the endoscope. The white arrows in Figure 15.2 are pointing to the lower esophageal sphincter (Figure 15.2). With flexible endoscopy the lower esophageal sphincter is visualized in the

thoracic cavity and it is open. The mucosa around the lower esophageal sphincter is usually inflamed because of chronic gastroesophageal reflux (Figure 15.3).

15.2 Techniques

Several techniques have been used to treat hiatal hernia in dogs and cats. Earlier techniques involved creating a plication of the fundus of the stomach around the lower esophageal sphincter as described in human patients (Sivacolundhu et al. 2002). This technique resulted in bloating of the stomach in several cases.

The current recommended surgical technique aims at stabilizing the lower esophageal sphincter in the peritoneal space (Ellison et al. 1987). The positive pressure of the abdominal cavity helps close the lower esophageal sphincter and prevent reflux in the lower esophagus.

15.2.1 Laparotomy

After a midline incision and abdominal exploration, the left lateral and middle liver lobes are retracted caudally with malleable retractors to expose the esophageal hiatus (Figure 15.4). The triangular ligaments are incised to help mobilize the liver lobes.

The hernia is then reduced by applying traction on the body and fundus of the stomach. If a liver lobe, a loop of intestines, or the spleen are in the hernia, the content of the hernia is reduced first. The esophageal hiatus is opened from ventral to dorsal. The phrenico-esophageal membrane is retracted with Allis tissue forceps or stay sutures and incised (Figure 15.5). This membrane

Gastrointestinal Surgical Techniques in Small Animals, First Edition. Edited by Eric Monnet and Daniel D. Smeak.
© 2020 John Wiley & Sons, Inc. Published 2020 by John Wiley & Sons, Inc.
Companion website: www.wiley.com/go/monnet/gastrointestinal

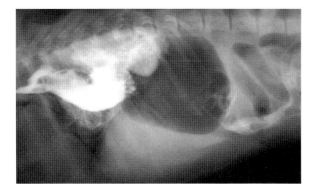

Figure 15.1

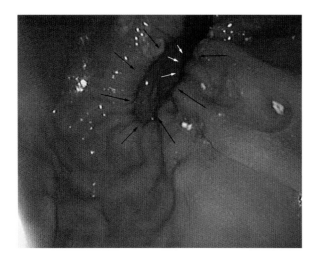

Figure 15.2

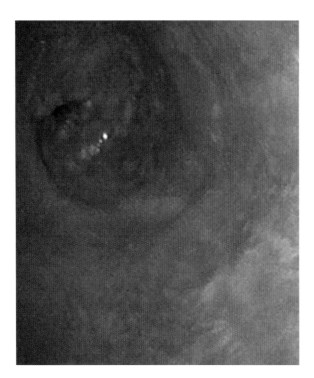

Figure 15.3

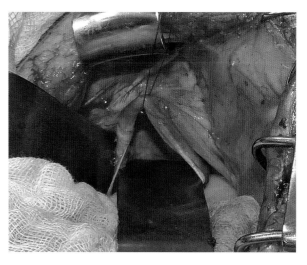

Figure 15.4

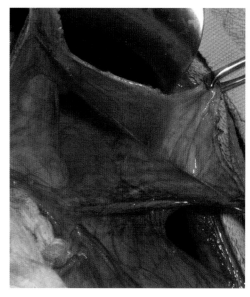

Figure 15.5

is usually very distended in dogs with a sliding hiatal hernia. The incision should be confined to the ventral half of the membrane because the vagus nerves run at the 3 and 9 o'clock position. At this point the pleural space is open and the patient should be on a ventilator.

After resection of the ventral part of the membrane, the esophageal hiatus is plicated with mattress sutures (Figure 15.6a). Nonabsorbable suture material size 2-0 or 3-0 is used for the plication. The esophageal hiatus is reduced to a smaller diameter without inducing a stenosis of the lower esophagus. Usually a large gastrostomy tube is advanced through the mouth into the stomach and the plication should be snugged around the esophagus but not tight. The author likes to be able to place a

(a)

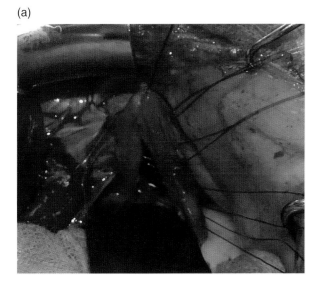

(b)

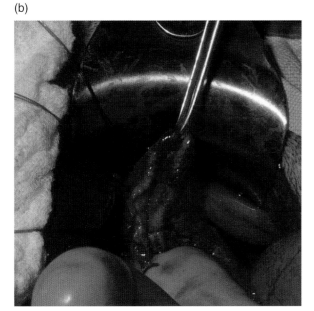

Figure 15.6

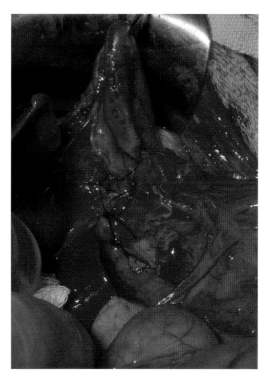

Figure 15.7

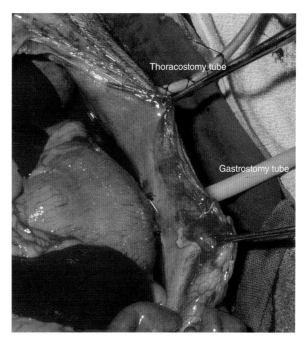

Figure 15.8

finger around the esophagus while the gastrostomy tube is in place (Figure 15.6b).

An esophagopexy is completed on each side of the esophagus (Figure 15.7). Nonabsorbable suture size 3-0 are used to pexy the lower esophagus to the esophageal hiatus. Usually one or two cruciate sutures are placed on each side of the esophageal hiatus to complete the esophagopexy.

Finally the body of the stomach or the fundus of the stomach is pexied to the left side to the abdominal cavity under moderate tension. Usually a tube gastropexy is placed (Chapter 4) (Figure 15.8). A 20 Fr Foley catheter is used. The gastrostomy tube can be used to feed the patient after surgery and to deliver medications while the esophagitis is resolving.

15.2.2 Laparoscopy

Hiatal hernias can be corrected with laparoscopy. The patient is placed in a dorsal oblique recumbency position. The patient is tilted 20° toward the right side to improve visualization of the esophageal hiatus on the left side.

Multiport or single-port access can be used to complete the surgery. If a single-port access system is used, it is recommended by the author to place it in the abdominal wall on the left side where the tube gastropexy will be placed at the end of surgery. When the single-port access system is removed the gastropexy can be performed through the incision used to place the single-port access system. If a single-port access system is used, an extra cannula is needed to provide retraction of the liver lobe.

If a multiport system is used, the first cannula is placed caudal to the umbilicus and the second cannula is placed cranial to the umbilicus. The first cannula is used to introduce the endoscope while the second cannula is used to introduce a retractor or a palpation probe to retract the liver lobes. The third cannula is placed in the middle third of the left side of the abdominal wall, 2–3 cm caudal to the last rib. The gastrostomy tube will be placed at that site.

The fourth cannula is placed in the abdominal wall on the left side between the first and the second cannula.

A fan retractor or a palpation probe is used to retract the left lateral liver lobe and expose the triangular ligament (white arrows) of the left lateral liver lobe (Figure 15.9). The triangular ligament is then incised with electrocautery. Fine-toothed grasping forceps are then used to expose the esophageal hiatus (Figure 15.10). The esophageal hiatus is grabbed ventrally and pulled toward the sternum. Another pair of fine-toothed grasping forceps are used to grab and pull the fundus of the stomach toward the caudal abdomen to reduce the hernia (Figure 15.11). Traction is applied until the distal esophagus is visible in the abdomen (white arrows).

The phrenico-esophageal membrane is then dissected with electrocautery or a vessel sealant device (white arrows) (Figure 15.12). The esophageal hiatus is then partially closed with a simple continuous suture. A 3-0 absorbable, barbed, unidirectional suture is used. The suture is used to lift the hiatus toward the sternum to better visualize the edges of the hiatus (Figure 15.13).

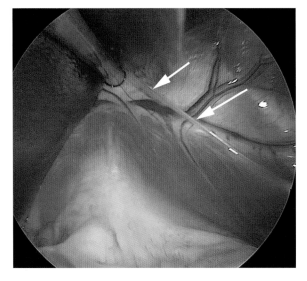

Figure 15.9

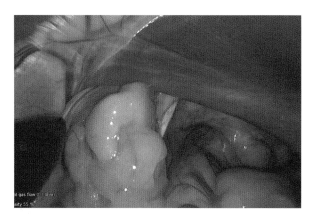

Figure 15.10

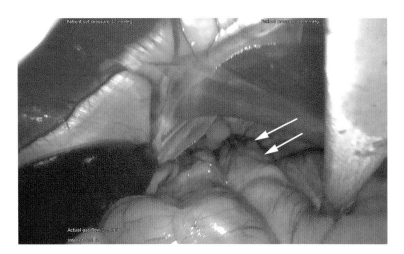

Figure 15.11

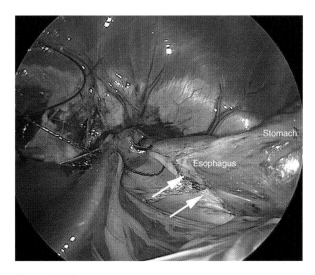

Figure 15.12

A gastrostomy tube can be placed in the esophagus to help determine how much of the hiatus needs to be closed. An esophagopexy is then completed with two cruciate sutures on the right and left side between the wall of the distal esophagus and the edges of the esophageal hiatus. Monofilament, absorbable suture size 3-0 is used for the esophagopexy. The unidirectional barbed suture can also be used to perform the esophagopexy by extending the suture used to close the hiatus along one side of the esophagus (Figure 15.14).

A tube gastropexy is then completed between the body of the stomach and the left abdominal wall. A 20 Fr Foley catheter is used. The gastropexy is completed at the level of the single-port access.

(a)

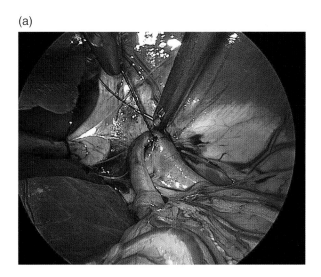

(b)

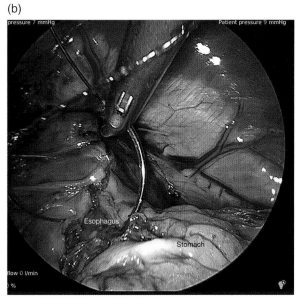

Figure 15.13

(a)

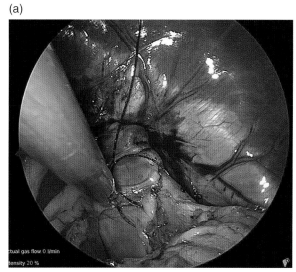

(b)

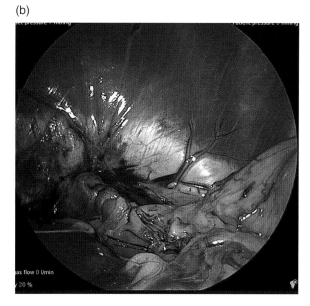

Figure 15.14

15.3 Tips

It is important to gain a good exposure of the esophageal hiatus for the procedure. Malleable retractors are very useful during laparotomy.

Dissection of the esophageal membrane is only performed on the ventral part to avoid damaging the vagus nerves. The vagus nerves travel at 3 and 9 o'clock along the esophagus.

15.4 Complications and Post-Operative Cares

A flexible endoscopic examination of the upper gastrointestinal tract can be performed after surgery to confirm the appropriate reduction of the hernia and the closure of the lower esophageal sphincter around the endoscope. The imprint of the esophageal hiatus should no longer be visible and the lower esophageal sphincter should be visualized in close contact with the endoscope (Figure 15.15).

Dogs and cats with hiatal hernias very often have esophagitis which needs to be treated. In the post-operative period, the patient is treated with pantoprazole and/or omeprazole, sucralfate, and cisapride. This treatment is maintained for two weeks (Ellison et al. 1987;

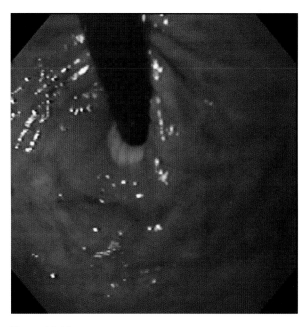

Figure 15.15

Sivacolundhu et al. 2002). The gastrostomy tube is removed one week after surgery.

If a megaesophagus was present before surgery, the dog or the cat will need to be monitored with repeated chest radiographs. The megaesophagus will hopefully improve while the esophagitis is getting under control.

References

Broux, O. et al. (2018). Effects of manipulations to detect sliding hiatal hernia in dogs with brachycephalic airway obstructive syndrome. *Vet. Surg.* 47 (2): 243–251.

Ellison, G.W. et al. (1987). Esophageal hiatal hernia in small animals: literature review and a modified surgical technique. *J. Am. Anim. Hosp. Assoc.* 23: 391–399.

Hardie, E.M. et al. (1998). Abnormalities of the thoracic bellows: stress fractures of the ribs and hiatal hernia. *J. Vet. Intern. Med.* 12 (4): 279–287.

Holt, D. et al. (1998). Medical treatment versus surgery for hiatal hernias. *J. Am. Vet. Med. Assoc.* 213 (6): 800.

Lorinson, D. and Bright, R.M. (1998). Long-term outcome of medical and surgical treatment of hiatal hernias in dogs and cats: 27 cases (1978–1996). *J. Am. Vet. Med. Assoc.* 213 (3): 381–384.

Mackin, A. (1998). Abnormalities of the thoracic bellows: stress fractures of the ribs and hiatal hernia. *J. Vet. Intern. Med.* 12 (6): 478–480.

Mayhew, P.D. et al. (2017). Prospective evaluation of surgical management of sliding hiatal hernia and gastroesophageal reflux in dogs. *Vet. Surg.* 46 (8): 1098–1109.

Sivacolundhu, R.K. et al. (2002). Hiatal hernia controversies – a review of pathophysiology and treatment options. *Aust. Vet. J.* 80 (1–2): 48–53.

Section IV

Stomach

16

Anatomy and Physiology of the Stomach

Eric Monnet

Department of Clinical Sciences, College of Veterinary Medicine and Biomedical Sciences, Colorado State University, Fort Collins, CO, USA

The anatomy and the physiology of the stomach need to be fully understood before performing surgery on the stomach, and especially if a major resection and reconstruction are planned. The physiology of the stomach, especially acid secretion, is profoundly affected by major reconstructive surgical procedures such as the Billroth II or the Roux-en-Y.

16.1 Anatomy

16.1.1 Divisions

The stomach is divided in five regions: the cardia, the fundus, the body, the pyloric antrum, and the pylorus. Proximal to the cardia is the lower esophagus, and the two blend together. The pylorus connects the stomach with the duodenum (Evans 1993).

16.1.2 Morphology and Glandular Organization

The wall of the stomach is covered by a peritoneal layer which forms the serosa. Underneath the serosa, three layers of smooth muscles make up the muscular layer or muscular propria. The middle, circular layer creates the pyloric sphincter. The outer layer is made of longitudinal muscle fibers. The longitudinal fibers along the greater curvature fuse with the esophagus and the duodenum. The longitudinal fibers on the dorsal and ventral aspect of the stomach stop at the level of the body of the stomach. The inner layer is made of oblique muscle fibers. Underneath the muscularis propria is the submucosa, a collagen rich layer of connective tissue. The submucosa includes a rich network of capillary, and

lymphatics. The mucosa is the inner layer of the stomach, comprised of a surface epithelium, lamina propria, and muscular mucosa (Evans 1993; Wilson and Stevenson 2019).

The gastric mucosa consists of columnar glandular epithelium. The composition of the glandular epithelium varies with the different regions of the stomach. In the cardia the epithelium mostly produces mucous via mucus producing cells. The body of the stomach contains most of the parietal cells and chief cells . Parietal cells mostly produce acid, ghrelin, and leptin. Chief cells produce pepsin and leptin. Enterochromaffin-like cells (ECL cells) which produce histamine are mostly in the body of the stomach while G cells which produce gastrin are in the antrum. D cells producing somatostatin are found both in the body and the antrum of the stomach (Wilson and Stevenson 2019).

16.1.3 Blood Supply

The stomach receives its blood supply from the celiac artery with the right and left gastric arteries supplying the lesser curvature, and the left and right gastroepiploic arteries supplying the greater curvature (Evans 1993).

16.1.4 Innervation

The stomach is innervated by the vagus nerve and the sympathetic system through the celiac plexus. Caudal to the hilus of the lungs the left and right vagus nerve separate into a dorsal and a ventral branch. The left and right dorsal branches fuse together to create the dorsal vagal trunk and left and right ventral branches fuse together to create the ventral vagal trunk. Both trunks supply branches to the esophagus before passing through the

Gastrointestinal Surgical Techniques in Small Animals, First Edition. Edited by Eric Monnet and Daniel D. Smeak.

diaphragm. The ventral trunk produces plexuses that innervate the stomach and the liver. Hepatic branches run in the lesser omentum. Other branches innervate the pylorus and the duodenum after following the right gastric artery and the pancreaticoduodenal artery (Stromberg 1993). The dorsal trunk supplies the cardia and the fundus of the stomach and forms a plexus in the dorsal surface of the stomach. The myenteric plexus (Auerback's plexus) is located between the different layers of muscle in the stomach wall while the Meissner's plexus is located in the submucosa of the stomach.

The sympathetic innervation arises from T5 to T10 and travels via the splanchnic nerve to the celiac ganglion. Post-ganglionic fibers travel within the celiac artery to the stomach.

Cholinergic, serotoninergic, and peptidergic neurons are present in the stomach with nonadrenergic noncholinergic pathway. Acetylcholine, serotonin, substance P, calcitonin, bombesin, cholecystokinin, and somatostatin are the neuropeptides present in the intrinsic gastric nervous system (Wilson and Stevenson 2019).

16.2 Physiology

16.2.1 Gastrin

Gastrin is produced by G cells in the pyloric antrum. It is synthesized as a pre-propeptide and it is processed into biologically active peptides (Figure 16.1). Three different types of gastrin have been identified: big, little, and mini gastrin. Little gastrin (G 17) represents 90% of the gastrin in the antrum while big gastrin (G 34) predominates in the systemic circulation because of its longer half-life.

Gastrin secretion is stimulated by protein and it is inhibited by presence of acid in the stomach. Somatostatin inhibits release of gastrin by the G cells. Gastrin stimulates the production of acid by the parietal cells, however it is likely that the greatest production of acid due to gastrin secretion is histamine mediated. Hypergastrinemia is associated with a trophic effect of the gastric mucosa, especially in ECL cells. Hypergastrinemia is induced by antisecreting agents, uremia, vagotomy, and retained gastric antrum, after gastrectomy (Wilson and Stevenson 2019).

16.2.2 Somatostatin

Somatostatin is produced by D cells in the fundus and the pyloric antrum (Figure 16.1). D cells exert a direct paracrine effect on parietal cells and G cells. Somatostatin

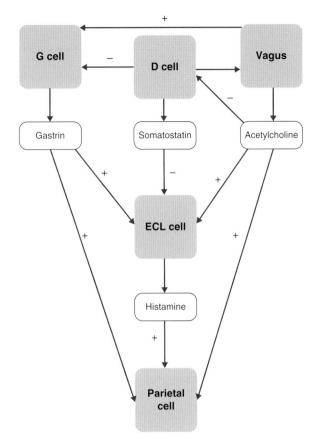

Figure 16.1

inhibits G cells, parietal cells, and ECL cells. Release of somatostatin by D cells results in inhibition of acid secretion. Acetylcholine inhibits the release of somatostatin.

16.2.3 Histamine

Histamine is stored in the ECL cells and the mast cells present in the stomach wall (Figure 16.1). ECL cells have receptors for gastrin, acetylcholine, and epinephrine, which stimulate histamine release. The somatostatin receptors on the ECL cells inhibit gastrin-induced histamine release.

16.2.4 Ghrelin and Leptin

Ghrelin is a peptide secreted by parietal cells in the fundus of the stomach. It is an appetite stimulant and it plays a role in energy metabolism (Jeusette et al. 2005, 2006). Ghrelin receptors in the hypothalamus appear to be responsible for increased food intake. Leptin is a peptide which is secreted by chief cells of the stomach. Leptin is also responsible for the regulation of metabolism and its effect on food intake is the opposite of the effect of ghrelin (Jeusette et al. 2005, 2006).

16.2.5 Other Gastric Secretory Products

Gastric juice is the result of secretion of the parietal cells, the chief cells, and the mucous cells in addition to saliva. The main electrolytes in the stomach fluid are sodium, potassium, and bicarbonate. Mucus and bicarbonate are secreted by the mucous cells and the neck cells. The mucus and the bicarbonate neutralize the gastric acid at the gastric mucosal surface.

An intrinsic factor produced by the parietal cells is important for the absorption of Vitamin B12. After gastrectomy, injection of Vitamin B12 is needed because of the reduction in production of the intrinsic factor.

Pepsinogen is produced by the chief cells and the mucous neck cells. It is a proteolytic enzyme. It is converted to pepsin by the acid present in the stomach.

16.2.6 Acid Secretion

Parietal cells produce acid under the influence of gastrin, histamine, and acetylcholine released from the vagus nerve (Figure 16.1).

The vagus nerve has a major influence on acid secretions in the stomach. The vagus nerve innervates the G cells and the ECL cells both of which stimulate acid secretion. Acetylcholine is the principle neurotransmitter modulating acid secretion in the stomach. Somatostatin produced by the D cells reduces the production of acid by inhibiting gastrin production by the G cells and histamine production by the ECL cells.

Parietal cells which produce acid have gastrin receptors, muscarinic receptors, histamine receptors, and somatostatin receptors on their cell membrane. Gastrin, produced by the G cells, has a direct effect on parietal cells to increase acid secretion. The production of gastrin is stimulated by proteins and histamine produced by the ECL cells. Acid in the lumen of the stomach inhibits production of gastrin. Somatostatin produced by D cells has a paracrine effect on the G cells and also inhibits the production of gastrin. The administration of H2 inhibitors blunts the effect of histamine on gastrin secretion.

Acid secretion is stimulated by the ingestion of food. There is a cephalic phase, a stomach phase, and an intestinal phase of acid secretion. The cephalic phase is mediated by the vagus nerve, which stimulates acid production by a direct action on parietal cells and enterochromaffin-like cells. The cephalic phase accounts for 20–30% of the total acid secreted. The gastric phase is stimulated by food entering the lumen of the stomach. Some nutrients (proteins and aromatic amino acids) have a direct effect on G cells to produce gastrin. Gastric distention by food entering the stomach induces a vagal response that triggers acid secretion by the parietal cells. The gastric phase counts for 60–70% of the acid secretion. The intestinal phase is not clearly understood. It is mediated by a distinct acid-stimulatory peptide hormone from the small bowel mucosa (Wilson and Stevenson 2019).

16.3 Acid Secretion and Gastrectomy

Acid secretion in the stomach is a major cause of complications after gastrectomy in dogs and cats. During gastrectomy (Billroth I or II, or a Roux-en-Y procedure) it is important to completely remove the pyloric antrum distally. If pyloric antrum is left on the pyloric/duodenal stump it is exposed to alkaline ph. This alkaline pH stimulates G cells to produce more gastrin which will induce gastritis. This process is termed "the retained antrum syndrome" and results in severe gastritis and ulceration (Lee et al. 1986; Gibril et al. 2001; Dumon and Dempsey 2019).

Vagotomy has been advocated to reduce the risk of gastritis after gastrectomy in human patients. During a Billroth II or a Roux-en-Y it is not unusual to perform a vagotomy. Vagotomy was initially recommended for the treatment of peptic gastric ulcers. Three different types of vagotomy have been described: truncal vagotomy, selective vagotomy, and proximal vagotomy. Truncal vagotomy consists of transecting the dorsal and the ventral vagal trunk as they cross the diaphragm. This technique is associated with hypomotility of the stomach, which is not a problem if a Billroth I or II has been performed, since the pylorus has been removed during those procedures. The gall bladder and the rest of the GI tract are affected by the vagotomy. It can result in cholelithiasis and diarrhea. The selective vagotomy is similar to the truncal vagotomy, but the hepatic and the celiac branches of the ventral and dorsal vagal trunks are preserved. Stomach hypomotility and post-operative diarrhea still generally occur. Finally, during the proximal vagotomy all the branches going to the lesser curvature are transected, preserving the branches going to the pylorus. There is no increased rate of diarrhea with this procedure and the pylorus, if present, is still functional (Broderick and Matthews 2007; Ali et al. 2019; Dumon and Dempsey 2019).

16.4 Stomach Motility and Gastrectomy

The enteric nervous system, including the parasympathetic and the sympathetic pathways as well as the intrinsic nervous system, control the gastric motor function. Depolarization of the smooth muscle generates myogenic activity in the wall of the stomach. The resting potential of the cell membrane of the smooth muscle is different between the pacemaker cells of Cajal and the pylorus. Pacemaker cells are located in the mid-body of the stomach along the greater curvature. The difference in potential might explain the reduced rate of contraction of the pylorus (Wilson and Stevenson 2019).

During a fasting state, the pacemaker cells generate slow waves of depolarization toward the pylorus. Those waves do not induce a contraction. A pattern of electrical activity named the myoelectric migrating complex (MMC) is generated during the fasting phase. Four phases have been identified. Phase I is the quiescent phase, with only slow waves maintaining a tone within the wall of the stomach. Phase II is associated with motor spikes, which generate contraction in the middle of the slow waves. Phase III is characterized by an increased number of motor spikes and gastric contractions are triggered every 15–20 seconds. This phase helps evacuate undigested large particles from the stomach. Phase IV is a period of recovery before phase I starts again. The MMC maintains clearance of the stomach.

After ingesting a meal there is a phase of relaxation that allows the stomach to stretch. This relaxation mostly occurs in the fundus of the stomach. This relaxation is mediated by the vagus nerve. Truncal vagotomy affects this relaxation phase and early emptying of the stomach occurs. The stomach is responsible for mixing and grinding ingested, solid food. Repetitive contraction of the antrum is responsible for this activity. Emptying of the stomach occurs under the influence of neural and hormonal mediators.

Vagotomy results in a lack of relaxation, bloating, accelerated emptying of liquid and delayed emptying of solids. Since the vagus nerve is responsible for contractions of the antrum and relaxation of the pylorus, if a truncal vagotomy is performed, the pylorus has to be removed or bypassed. However, the risk of "dumping syndrome," entry of unsuitable material into the duodenum and proximal jejunum, is increased by the Billroth I (Humphrey et al. 1972a,b; Dumon and Dempsey 2019).

References

Ali, A. et al. (2019). Surgery for peptic ulcer disease. In: Shackelford's Surgery of the Alimentary Tract (eds. C.J. Yeo et al.), 673–701. Philadelphia: Elsevier.

Broderick, T.J. and Matthews, J.B. (2007). Vagotomy and drainage. In: Shackelford's Surgery of the Alimentary Tract (eds. C.J. Yeo et al.), 811–830. Philadelphia: Elsevier Saunders.

Dumon, K. and Dempsey, D.T. (2019). Postgastrectomy syndromes. In: Shackelford's Surgery of the Alimentary Tract (eds. C.J. Yeo et al.), 719–734. Philadelphia: Elsevier.

Evans, H.E. (1993). The digestive apparatus and abdomen. In: Miller's Anatomy of the Dog (ed. H.E. Evans), 385–462. Philadelphia: W.B. Saunders Company.

Gibril, F. et al. (2001). Retained gastric antrum syndrome: a forgotten, treatable cause of refractory peptic ulcer disease. *Dig. Dis. Sci.* 46 (3): 610–617.

Humphrey, C.S. et al. (1972a). Incidence of dumping after truncal and selective vagotomy with pyloroplasty and highly selective vagotomy without drainage procedure. *Br. Med. J.* 3 (5830): 785–788.

Humphrey, C.S. et al. (1972b). Effect of truncal vagotomy (t.V.), selective vagotomy (s.V.) and pyloroplasty, and highly selective vagotomy (h.S.V.) without drainage on the response to meat extract in man. *Br. J. Surg.* 59 (11): 906.

Jeusette, I. et al. (2006). Effect of ovariectomy and ad libitum feeding on body composition, thyroid status, ghrelin and leptin plasma concentrations in female dogs. *J. Anim. Physiol. Anim. Nutr.* 90 (1–2): 12–18.

Jeusette, I.C. et al. (2005). Effects of chronic obesity and weight loss on plasma ghrelin and leptin concentrations in dogs. *Res. Vet. Sci.* 79 (2): 169–175.

Lee, C.H. et al. (1986). The clinical aspect of retained gastric antrum. *Arch. Surg.* 121 (10): 1181–1186.

Stromberg, M.W. (1993). The autonomic nervous system. In: Miller's Anatomy of the Dog (ed. H.E. Evans), 776–799. Philadelphia: W.B. Saunders.

Wilson, R.L. and Stevenson, C.E. (2019). Anatomy and physiology of the stomach. In: Shackelford's Surgery of the Alimentary Tract (eds. C.J. Yeo et al.), 634–646. Philadelphia: Elsevier.

17

Gastrotomy
Eric Monnet

Department of Clinical Sciences, College of Veterinary Medicine and Biomedical Sciences, Colorado State University, Fort Collins, CO, USA

17.1 Indications

A gastrotomy is most commonly performed in dogs and cats for retrieval of a foreign body lodged in the stomach or to release a linear foreign body anchored in the pylorus. Gastrotomies are also used to collected full-thickness gastric biopsies.

17.2 Techniques

After performing a midline laparotomy and exploration, the stomach is exposed in the cranial part of the abdominal cavity.

Stay sutures are placed midway between the lesser and the greater curvature in the body of the stomach (Figure 17.1). An incision is first made with a #11 blade and then extended with Metzembaum scissors (Figure 17.2). The wall of the stomach is well vascularized. Usually blood vessels bleeding in the wall of the stomach are ignored unless they persist after the incision is completed. The gastrotomy should be long enough to allow retrieval of the foreign body without tearing the wall of the stomach. The lumen of the stomach should be inspected to make sure that the entire foreign body has been removed. If a linear foreign body is present and it is entering the duodenum, inducing plication of the small intestine, only the part of the foreign body present in the stomach is removed after cutting the foreign body close to the pylorus. Usually, there is an anchoring point of the foreign body at the pylorus that prevents it from migrating into the small intestine.

After removing the foreign body or harvesting the full-thickness biopsy, the incision is closed with a simple continuous appositional pattern with 4-0 monofilament absorbable suture. The mucosa of the stomach has a tendency to evert in dogs and cats. The mucosa can be pushed back in the lumen of the stomach while the full-thickness sutures are placed.

The line of suture should be started before the beginning of the incision and continue past the end of the incision (Figure 17.3). The first and the last suture where the knots are placed do not provide a good seal. There is no need to perform a second layer closure with an inverting suture pattern after completing a simple continuous appositional closure (Figure 17.4).

Another option for the closure of the gastrotomy is to apply staples. A stay suture is added in the middle of the gastrotomy to elevate the two sides of the gastrotomy into the stapler. A TA 55 or 90 with 4.8 mm staples are used to complete the closure.

17.3 Tips

Traditionally, a two-layer closure has been described for closure of the stomach. However, it is the author's experience that one-layer closure with a simple continuous appositional suture pattern is safe in dogs and cats. When a simple continuous suture is used it is important to place the first and the last stitches with the knots outside the incision (Figures 17.3 and 17.4).

Stomach mucosa has a tendency to evert after a gastrotomy which might interfere at the time of closure. It is possible to push the mucosa inside the lumen of the stomach during closure of the gastrotomy to prevent eversion of the mucosa. A modified Gambee pattern is also useful for placing the mucosa inside the lumen of the stomach during closure. It is very important to make sure the submucosa is still engaged in the line of closure.

Gastrointestinal Surgical Techniques in Small Animals, First Edition. Edited by Eric Monnet and Daniel D. Smeak.
© 2020 John Wiley & Sons, Inc. Published 2020 by John Wiley & Sons, Inc.
Companion website: www.wiley.com/go/monnet/gastrointestinal

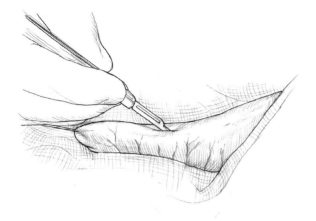

Figure 17.1

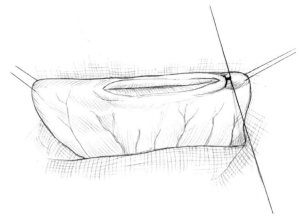

Figure 17.3

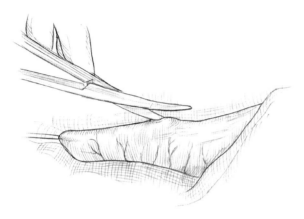

Figure 17.2

17.4 Complications and Post-Operative Cares

Post-operatively the patient is fed as soon as they are awake and able to swallow. Water is given first in small amount to make sure the patient is not regurgitating or vomiting.

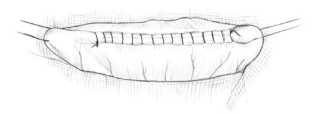

Figure 17.4

If the patient tolerates water, food is given at 1/4 maintenance of their resting energy requirement (RER).

Since the stomach has a very good blood supply dehiscence is very rare after a gastrotomy. However, the patient should be closely monitored for signs of septic peritonitis.

Antiemetic medications are recommended if the patient has been vomiting before surgery. Gastroprotectants are used if signs of gastritis were obvious during surgery or if the patient was vomiting a lot before surgery.

18

Gastrectomy

Eric Monnet

Department of Clinical Sciences, College of Veterinary Medicine and Biomedical Sciences, Colorado State University, Fort Collins, CO, USA

18.1 Indications

Neoplasia, ulceration with or without perforation, and necrosis of the stomach wall due to a gastric dilatation and volvulus are the most common indications for a gastrectomy in dogs and cats.

Adenocarcinoma is the most common gastric tumor in dogs. It represents 70–80% of all gastric tumors diagnosed in dogs. It is usually infiltrative and expansile with a central ulceration. Adenocarcinoma is very commonly located along the lesser curvature of the stomach (Swann and Holt 2002). Other tumors diagnosed in the stomach of dogs and cats include eiomyosarcoma, lymphoma, mast cell tumors, plasmacytoma, and fibrosarcoma (Swann and Holt 2002; Frost et al. 2003; Withrow 2013). Leiomyomas and gastrointestinal stromal tumors (GIST) have also been described in the stomach of dogs. GIST occurs equally in male and female dogs at a mean age of 11 years. Leiomyoma occurs most commonly in male dogs around 11 year of age. Leiomyoma typically do not metastasize while GIST can metastasize to the liver (Frost et al. 2003).

Ulceration of the stomach can be a simple epithelial erosion or a full thickness lesion through the submucosa with bleeding or perforation. Ulceration can be caused by physical trauma to the epithelium, acute or chronic gastritis, neoplasia of the stomach, Zollinger–Ellison syndrome, parasites (*Helicobacter* spp.), inflammatory bowel disease, gastric dilatation-volvulus (GDV), liver disease, uremia, and non-steroidal anti-inflammatory drug therapy (Mansfield and Abraham 2013).

Partial gastrectomy is also commonly performed during the surgical treatment of gastric dilatation and volvulus. The necrosis associated with a GDV most commonly occurs along the greater curvature of the body of the stomach (Matthiesen 1985; Clark and Pavletic 1991).

18.2 Technique

Gastrectomy is a well-tolerated surgery in dogs and cats. The entire stomach can be resected for the treatment of gastric carcinoma (Jeong et al. 2013). However, it is accepted that 60% of the stomach can be removed in dogs and cats without too many consequences on the gastrointestinal physiology of the patient.

It is important to preserve the cardia and the lower esophageal sphincter. If this is not done, a lot of gastroesophageal reflux can develop, which will induce esophagitis and affect the quality of life of the patient (Pavletic 1981).

The gastrectomy can be local or segmental depending on the amount of resection needed. Local gastrectomies are indicated for resection of an ischemic gastric wall during GDV, ulcers, and small tumors. Segmental gastrectomies are recommended for large tumors or infiltrative tumors like adenocarcinoma. A circular portion of the stomach is resected during a segmental gastrectomy.

18.2.1 Local Gastrectomy for Resection of Neoplasia or Ulcer

After an abdominal exploration the stomach is isolated from the rest of the abdominal cavity with laparotomy sponges and towels. Stay sutures are placed around the area to resect to limit the contamination of the abdominal cavity (Figure 18.1a).

Gastrointestinal Surgical Techniques in Small Animals, First Edition. Edited by Eric Monnet and Daniel D. Smeak.
© 2020 John Wiley & Sons, Inc. Published 2020 by John Wiley & Sons, Inc.
Companion website: www.wiley.com/go/monnet/gastrointestinal

(a)

(b)

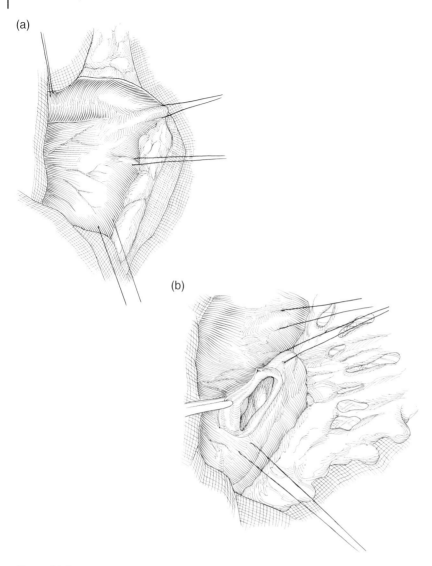

Figure 18.1

An incision is made in healthy tissue with a #11 blade. The incision is extended with Metzenbaum scissors around the area to resect (Figure 18.1b). Since the stomach wall is very vascular, bleeding occurs from blood vessels in the wall. Those bleeders are usually ignored as they will stop bleeding on their own. If the bleeding persists, a small suture can be placed around the vessel or electrocautery can be used to control the bleeding.

If the gastrectomy includes the lesser or greater curvature, the right gastric artery and vein or the left or right gastroepiploic artery and vein are ligated.

After completing the resection (Figure 18.2a) the stomach wall is closed with 4-0 monofilament absorbable suture with a continuous full-thickness pattern. A one-layer closure is sufficient to close the stomach (Figure 18.2b). It is not unusual to apply two or three lines of suture to be able to close the stomach.

18.2.2 Local Gastrectomy During a Gastric Dilatation-Volvulus

GDV is associated with necrosis of the greater curvature at the level of the body of the stomach and fundus.

Resection of the necrotic stomach wall during GDV surgery is better performed with staples, however it can be performed as described above with hand sutures. The utilization of a stapling device reduces both surgical time and the risk of contamination of the abdominal cavity (Clark and Pavletic 1991).

The viability of the stomach is mostly evaluated with subjective parameters: color, peristalsism, thickness, and bleeding on incision of the serosa (Matthiesen 1987).

After identifying how much stomach has to be resected a thoraco-abdominal (TA) stapler or a gastrointestinal anastomosis (GIA) stapler are used to com-

(a)

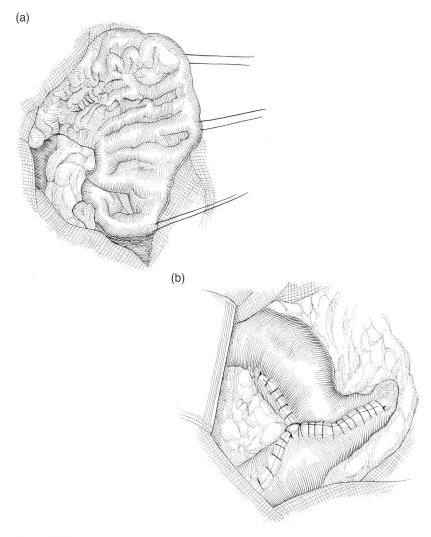

(b)

Figure 18.2

plete the gastrectomy. The TA stapler applies two rows of staples in the wall of the stomach. The GIA stapler applies six rows of staples in the wall of the stomach and a blade cuts between the six rows, leaving three rows in the patients and three rows with the segment of the stomach being removed. It therefore reduces the risk of contamination even more than the TA stapler. The stapler is applied in healthy tissue across the greater curvature of the stomach. A TA 55 mm or 90 mm long are used with 4.8 mm staples. If more than one cartridge of staples is required to complete the resection the two rows should overlap over 1 cm to make sure the gastrectomy is well sealed. The GIA stapler exists in 50, 60, 80, 90, and 100 mm long cartridges with 4.8 mm staples.

Stay sutures are placed along the greater curvature of the stomach to help manipulate the stomach within the stapler (Figure 18.3). After the staples are applied, the necrotic part of the stomach is removed. An oversew of the staple line is usually performed with 4-0 monofilament absorbable suture with an inverting Cushing pattern.

18.2.3 Segmental Gastrectomy

If the pathology requiring resection is located in the pyloric antrum or the pylorus, a segmental resection is performed. A Billroth I, II or a Roux-en-Y reconstruction is then required (Chapters 19, 20, and 22).

If the pathology requiring resection is located in the body of the stomach and/or the fundus and infiltrating more than 50% of the circumference of the wall of the stomach, a segmental resection of the body and/or fundus can be performed.

After placement of stay sutures in the stomach wall on each side of the planned segmental resection, the left and right gastric artery and vein and the left and right

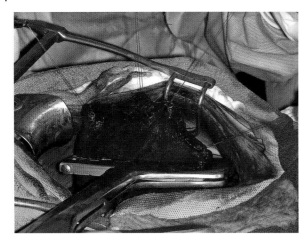

Figure 18.3

gastroepiploic artery and vein are ligated at the appropriate location. The greater and lesser omentum are dissected away from the greater and lesser curvature.

The wall of the stomach is incised in healthy tissue on each side of the planned resection with a #11 blade and the incisions are continued with Metzenbaum scissors 360° to completely resect the segment of stomach (Figure 18.4a).

The two extremities of the stomach are sutured together with two simple continuous apposition pattern with 4-0 monofilament absorbable sutures (Figure 18.4b). The dorsal side is sutured first within the lumen of the stomach. Then the ventral side is sutured in a similar fashion. It might be necessary to partially close the proximal end of the stomach since it might be of a larger diameter. Another option is to close the proximal part of the stomach with a thoraco-abdominal stapler and then perform an end-to-side

(a)

(b)

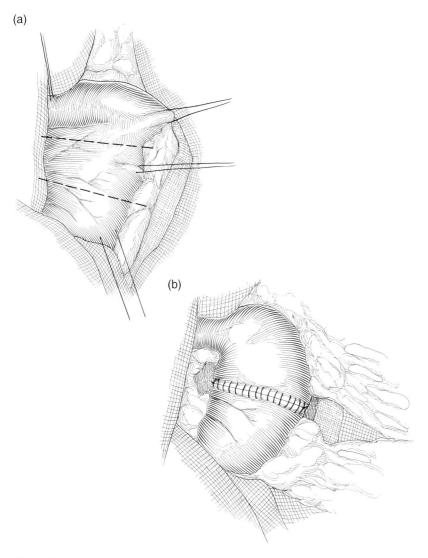

Figure 18.4

anastomosis of the distal end of the stomach on the dorsal side of the proximal stomach, like for a Billroth I.

18.3 Tips

A two-layer closure with a simple continuous, appositional pattern followed by a continuous inverting pattern has traditionally been recommended. However, the author has been using a simple continuous, full-thickness, appositional pattern without increased risk of complications.

The addition of a gastrostomy tube or J through G tube is helpful in the post-operative period. The jejunostomy tube can be used during the immediate post-operative period to start feeding the patient. Patients that require a gastrectomy have typically been anorexic and vomiting. The gastrostomy tube can be used to suction the stomach to reduce gastroesophageal reflux. The combination of a J through G tube allows both tubes to be placed through one surgical site.

If a gastrostomy tube cannot be placed because of the location of the closure of the gastrectomy, only a jejunostomy is placed.

If the gastrectomy is performed for the resection of an ulcer or neoplasia, it is paramount to biopsy the gastric lymph node (Withrow 2013).

18.4 Complications and Post-Operative Cares

After surgery, dogs and cats are monitored for signs of septic peritonitis. Leakage can occur within the first 24 hours after surgery and dehiscence of the stomach more likely occurs three to four days after surgery. The utilization of staples may reduce the risk of dehiscence and peritonitis.

Addition of a gastrostomy tube or J through G tube is recommend in order to provide adequate post-operative care. The gastrostomy tube is used primarily to suction the stomach to reduce the risk of regurgitation/vomiting and subsequent aspiration pneumonia. Aspirating the stomach might affect the electrolytes imbalance. Electrolytes have to be monitored and corrected accordingly. Also, the fluid rate has to be adjusted to compensate for the amount of fluid removed from the stomach. The jejunostomy tube is used to provide enteral feeding immediately after surgery.

Patients are maintained on pantoprazole and sucralfate in the post-operative period to treat the gastritis that is usually present in the dogs and cats that need a gastrectomy. Ondansetron is used to control vomiting for at least 24 or 48 hours.

If a large resection was performed, small meals several times a day should be offered to the patient. If less than 60% of the stomach has been resected, normal stomach function and physiology should resume.

References

Clark, G.N. and Pavletic, M.M. (1991). Partial gastrectomy with an automatic stapling instrument for treatment of gastric necrosis secondary to gastric dilatation-volvulus. *Vet. Surg.* 20 (1): 61–68.

Frost, D. et al. (2003). Gastrointestinal stromal tumors and leiomyomas in the dog: a histopathologic, immunohistochemical, and molecular genetic study of 50 cases. *Vet. Pathol.* 40 (1): 42–54.

Jeong, O. et al. (2013). Comparison of short-term surgical outcomes between laparoscopic and open total gastrectomy for gastric carcinoma: case-control study using propensity score matching method. *J. Am. Coll. Surg.* 216 (2): 184–191.

Mansfield, C.S. and Abraham, L.A. (2013). Stomach: ulcer. In: Canine and Feline Gastroenterology, 1e (eds. R.J. Washabau and M.J. Day), 637–650. St Louis: Elsevier Saunders.

Matthiesen, D.T. (1985). Partial gastrectomy as treatment of gastric volvulus: results in 30 dogs. *Vet. Surg.* 14 (3): 185–193.

Matthiesen, D.T. (1987). Indications and techniques of partial gastrectomy in the dog. *Semin. Vet. Med. Surg.* 2 (4): 248–256.

Pavletic, M.M. (1981). Reconstructive esophageal surgery in the dog – a literature review and case report. *J. Am. Anim. Hosp. Assoc.* 17 (3): 435–444.

Swann, H.M. and Holt, D.E. (2002). Canine gastric adenocarcinoma and leiomyosarcoma: a retrospective study of 21 cases (1986–1999) and literature review. *J. Am. Anim. Hosp. Assoc.* 38 (2): 157–164.

Withrow, S.J. (2013). Gastric cancer. In: Withrow and MacEwen's Small Animal Clinical Oncology, 5e (eds. S.J. Withrow et al.), 402–405. St Louis: Elsevier Saunders.

19

Billroth I

Eric Monnet

Department of Clinical Sciences, College of Veterinary Medicine and Biomedical Sciences, Colorado State University, Fort Collins, CO, USA

19.1 Indications

Billroth I is a surgical procedure used to reconstruct the upper gastrointestinal tract after partial gastrectomy. This procedure is indicated when the gastrectomy includes only the pyloric antrum and the proximal duodenum. The common bile duct remains intact. The remaining section of the duodenum and the body of the stomach can be brought together with minimal tension to perform a gastro-duodenostomy.

The most common indications for a Billroth I are pyloric obstruction due to neoplasia, resection of ulcer in the pyloric antrum, and correction of a severe pyloric obstruction or hypertrophy. If neoplasia is the underlying disease, a 1–2 cm margin should be taken for the gastrectomy. However, pyloric adenocarcinoma may not resected appropriately (Walter et al. 1985; Walter and Matthiesen 1989; Eisele et al. 2010; Ali et al. 2019).

19.2 Technique

After a midline laparotomy, the abdominal cavity is explored. The stomach and the proximal duodenum are exposed and isolated from the rest of the abdominal cavity.

To perform this surgery, the local anatomy should be well understood. The common bile duct, the pancreatic duct, the pancreatic-duodenal artery, the hepatic artery, the right gastroepiploic artery and the right gastric artery, and the portal vein are present in the surgical field. All those structures have to be identified and preserved.

Two stay sutures are placed on the pyloric antrum were the gastrectomy is going to be performed (Figure 19.1). The stay sutures help minimize contamination

from stomach contents. The right gastroepiploic artery is dissected from the greater curvature of the pyloric antrum (Figure 19.1). The right gastric artery is dissected from the lesser curvature without damaging the main hepatic artery and the portal vein dorsal to the right gastric artery (Figure 19.2). Hemostasis is performed for each branch penetrating the wall of the pyloric antrum with either sutures, electrocautery or a vessel sealant device (Figure 19.3). The dissection is extended over the duodenum with dissection of the pancreatic-duodenal artery. The common bile duct and the pancreatic duct have to be preserved.

Doyen clamps have to be placed across the duodenum to minimize contamination (Figure 19.4). The contents of the stomach should be suctioned when the stomach is open. Doyen clamps can also be placed across the stomach but they are not always very efficient because of the stomach wall thickness.

The pyloric antrum is resected first. It is easier to perform the gastrectomy with a thoraco-abdominal stapler with 4.8 mm staples (Figure 19.4). It reduces the risk of contamination of the peritoneal cavity. The distal segment of the stomach can be clamped with a crushing clamp or a Doyen clamp to reduce the risk of contamination. The resection is completed with a surgical blade. The pyloric antrum is then transected after placement of a Doyen clamp on the duodenum (Figure 19.4). If staples have been used the stump of the stomach is oversewn with a continuous inverting pattern with 4-0 monofilament absorbable suture.

The gastro-duodenal anastomosis is then completed on the dorsal side of the body of the stomach (Figure 19.5). Two stay sutures are placed to maintain the duodenum against the wall of the stomach. A #11 blade is used to perform a gastrotomy where the anastomosis is going to

Gastrointestinal Surgical Techniques in Small Animals, First Edition. Edited by Eric Monnet and Daniel D. Smeak.
© 2020 John Wiley & Sons, Inc. Published 2020 by John Wiley & Sons, Inc.
Companion website: www.wiley.com/go/monnet/gastrointestinal

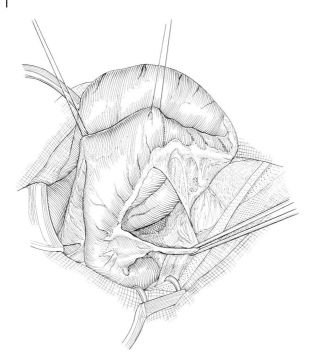

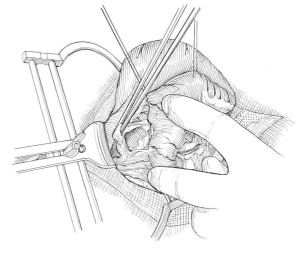

Figure 19.2

Figure 19.1

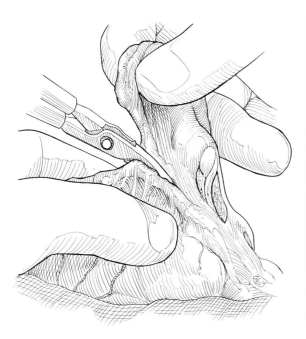

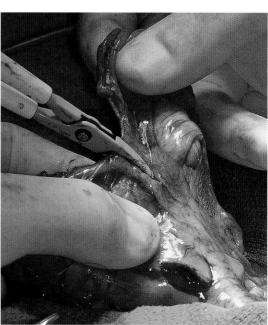

Figure 19.3

be performed. The length of the incision should match the diameter of the duodenum. One of the stay sutures is then used to start the anastomosis by suturing the back wall of the duodenum with the back wall of the stomach (Figure 19.6). A simple continuous suture pattern is used with 4-0 monofilament absorbable suture. The second stay suture is then used to complete the gastro-duodenal anastomosis of the proximal wall (Figure 19.7).

A gastrostomy and/or a jejunostomy tube can be placed at the end of the surgery. The gastrostomy tube can be used to decompress the stomach and minimize the risk of regurgitation and aspiration pneumonia. The jejunostomy tube will bypass the surgical site and help feed the patient if vomiting is still occurring. A gastrojejunostomy tube can also be placed at the time of surgery to facilitate post-operative care (Cavanaugh et al. 2008).

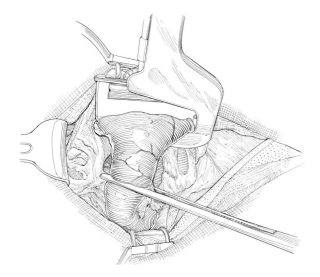

Figure 19.4

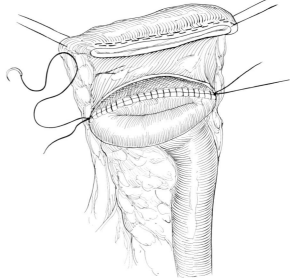

Figure 19.6

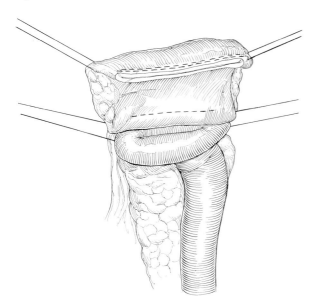

Figure 19.5

19.3 Tips

There has been lot of variation in the technique. The duodenogastric anastomosis can be performed end to end after reducing the diameter of the stomach to match the diameter of the duodenum, or end-to-side on the dorsal or the ventral part of the stomach. Also, an end-to-side on the duodenum has been described (Ali et al. 2019). Suturing the duodenum to the dorsal part of the stomach is more likely beneficial to slow down gastric emptying. Staplers can be used to complete the entire surgery. A thoraco-abdominal or a gastrointestinal stapler is used for the gastrectomy and an end-to-end anastomosis stapler is used for the duodenogastric anastomosis. The end-to-end anastomosis staplers are usually too large to be used in a dog because the diameter

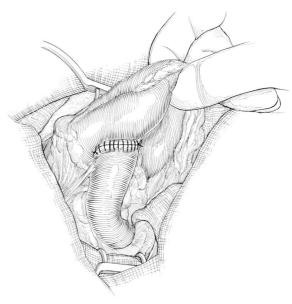

Figure 19.7

of the duodenum is not sufficient to introduce the distal anvil of the end-to-end anastomosis device.

A vagotomy at the time of surgery help increase the gastric emptying time. The vagotomy will also reduce acid secretion in the stomach from the parietal cells (Ali et al. 2019).

19.4 Complications

After surgery patients are monitored for the development of a septic peritonitis. Continuous electrocardiogram and pressure monitoring with measurement of blood glucose and lactate are strongly recommended in monitoring the patients. If septic peritonitis develops an abdominal exploration is required to inspect the surgical site.

Electrolytes should be monitored and corrected, especially if the stomach contents have been suctioned via the gastrostomy tube in the post-operative period.

Nausea can happen after a Billroth I and it is more likely related to the dumping syndrome (see Chapter 20). Dumping syndrome is not very common after Billroth I.

Vomiting can happen after a Billroth I. It is more likely due to biliary reflux in the gastric lumen. When bile reflux is present the gastric mucosa is very inflamed and friable on endoscopy with superficial erosion. Parietal and gastrin cells start to atrophy. Very often patients need ondansetron as needed after surgery and in the long term. Cisapride can also be used to reduce the risk of vomiting and improve gastrointestinal motility. If bile reflux is present, a surgery to divert the bile away from the stomach might be indicated, with interposition of a loop of bowel between the proximal duodenum and the stomach.

Stricture can develop at the level of the anastomosis. The surgical site should then be revised.

References

Ali, A. et al. (2019). Surgery for peptic ulcer disease. In: Shackelford's Surgery of the Alimentary Tract (eds. C.J. Yeo et al.), 673–701. Philadelphia: Elsevier.

Cavanaugh, R.P. et al. (2008). Evaluation of surgically placed gastrojejunostomy feeding tubes in critically ill dogs. *J. Am. Vet. Med. Assoc.* 232 (3): 380–388.

Eisele, J. et al. (2010). Evaluation of risk factors for morbidity and mortality after pylorectomy and gastroduodenostomy in dogs. *Vet. Surg.* 39 (2): 261–267.

Walter, M.C. and Matthiesen, D.T. (1989). Gastric outflow surgical problems. *Probl. Vet. Med.* 1 (2): 196–214.

Walter, M.C. et al. (1985). Pylorectomy and gastroduodenostomy in the dog: technique and clinical results in 28 cases. *J. Am. Vet. Med. Assoc.* 187 (9): 909–914.

20

Billroth II
Eric Monnet

Department of Clinical Sciences, College of Veterinary Medicine and Biomedical Sciences, Colorado State University, Fort Collins, CO, USA

20.1 Indications

Billroth II is one of the surgical procedures used to reconstruct the upper gastrointestinal tract in dogs and cats. It is indicated when the gastrectomy is removing the pylorus, the pyloric antrum, and part of the body of the stomach. Very often the proximal duodenum is resected, including the connection with the common bile duct. A Billroth II is indicated when the resection does not allow a gastro-duodenostomy because of tension.

It is recommended to remove the entire pyloric antrum during a Billroth II surgery to minimize gastrin production and acid secretion (Ali et al. 2019).

20.2 Technique

After a midline laparotomy, the abdominal cavity is explored. The stomach and the proximal duodenum are exposed and isolated from the rest of the abdominal cavity.

To perform this surgery, the local anatomy should be well understood. The common bile duct, the pancreatic duct, the pancreatic-duodenal artery, the hepatic artery, the right gastroepiploic artery and the right gastric artery, and the portal vein are present in the surgical field. All those structures have to be identified and preserved.

20.2.1 Gastrectomy

After identification of the margins for the resection the dissection is started along the lesser and greater curvature of the stomach. All the branches from the right gastroepiploic artery, and the right gastric artery are ligated as they penetrate the wall of the stomach (Figure 20.1). Utilization of a stapler device or a vessel sealant device greatly facilitates this part of the procedure.

Stay sutures are then placed on the body of the stomach along the lesser and greater curvature. It is recommended to use stapling equipment to perform a Billroth II. It more likely shortens the surgical time and reduces the risk of contamination of the peritoneal cavity.

If stapling equipment is not available the risk of contamination is higher. Doyen clamps can be used on the body of the stomach to try to minimize the risk of contamination. However, most of the time the gastric wall is too thick and the Doyen clamps are not efficient. Placement of the stay sutures and aspiration of the stomach contents are paramount to minimize contamination. Crushing clamps are placed on the wall of the stomach and the duodenum where the resections are going to be performed (Figure 20.2). The stomach is then incised along the crushing clamps on the distal segment of the stomach.

20.2.2 Dissection of the Duodenum

The dissection is then extended along the duodenum with dissection of the cranial duodeno-pancreatic artery. The common bile duct is identified and ligated. If staples are not available the distal duodenum is clamped with Doyen clamp distally without damaging the pancreas to prevent contamination. Crushing clamps are placed on the proximal section of the duodenum at the level of the resection. An incision is then made to resect the duodenum, the pylorus, and the section of the stomach that has been previously isolated (Figure 20.3).

Gastrointestinal Surgical Techniques in Small Animals, First Edition. Edited by Eric Monnet and Daniel D. Smeak.
© 2020 John Wiley & Sons, Inc. Published 2020 by John Wiley & Sons, Inc.
Companion website: www.wiley.com/go/monnet/gastrointestinal

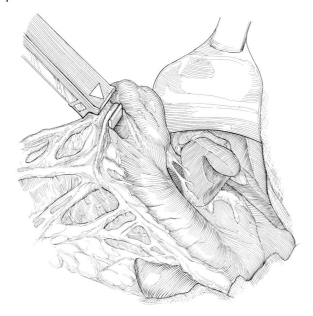

Figure 20.1

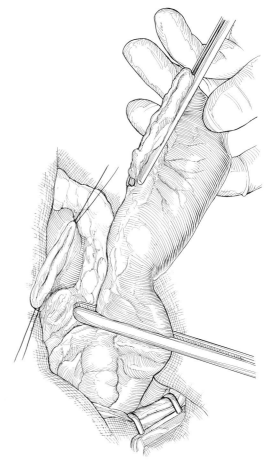

Figure 20.2

The body of the stomach is closed with a simple continuous apposition pattern. A 4-0 monofilament absorbable suture is used. An inverting pattern can be used as a second layer for the closure (Figure 20.4a). The stump of the duodenum is closed with a simple continuous apposition pattern with 4-0 absorbable monofilament suture (Figure 20.4b).

If stapling equipment is available a TA 4.8 mm stapler or a GIA stapler is used to close and incise the stomach and the duodenum (Figure 20.5a and b). If a TA stapler is used, crushing or Doyen clamps are necessary to close the distal part of the stomach to prevent contamination. With the GIA stapler the body of the stomach and the distal part of the stomach are closed while it is cut which reduces the risk of contamination. After establishing decent margins in the duodenum, TA stapler is used to close the duodenal stump (Figure 20.4b).

20.2.3 Gastrojejunostomy

A loop of the proximal jejunum is then mobilized toward the dorsal surface of the stomach (Figure 20.6a). It is anastomosed to the stomach with a side-to-side anastomosis. The stoma should be between 1.7 and 2.9 cm in diameter (Ahmadu-Suka et al. 1988). After placing two stay sutures to maintain the loop of jejunum against the wall of the stomach, a #11 blade is used to perform a jejunotomy on the antimesenteric side of the jejunum and a gastrotomy. The length of the jejunotomy and the gastrotomy should match. The anastomosis is performed with two simple continuous appositional sutures with

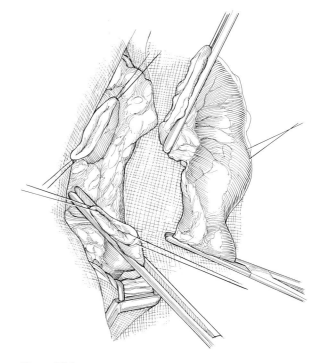

Figure 20.3

(a)

(b)

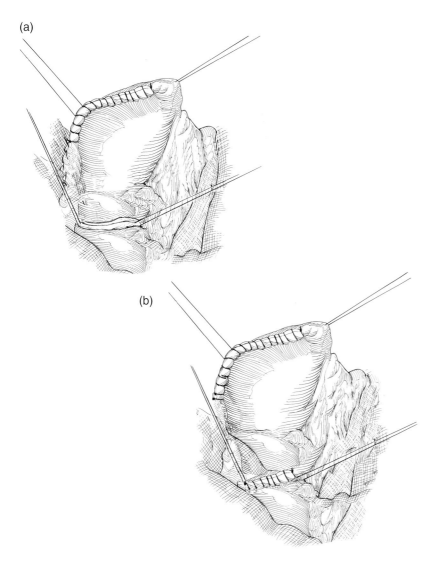

Figure 20.4

4-0 monofilament absorbable suture. The dorsal side of the anastomosis is completed first, followed by the ventral side (Figure 20.6b and c).

A GIA stapler can be used to perform the side-to-side anastomosis (Figure 20.7a) (Ahmadu-Suka et al. 1988). A hand suture is required to finish the anastomosis where the GIA was introduced (Figure 20.7b).

20.2.4 Cholecystoduodenostomy

A cholecystoduodenostomy is then performed as described in Chapter 36.

20.2.5 Feeding Tube

Gastrostomy and jejunostomy tubes are placed (see Chapter 4) at the end of the surgery to maintain the stomach decompressed and provide enteral feeding in the post-operative period. A J through G tube can be placed instead. The gastrostomy tube might be required for long-term support to supplement feeding because a lot of dogs are still anorexic for a long period of time after surgery.

The abdominal cavity is then lavaged with warm and sterile saline. The abdominal cavity is closed in a routine fashion.

20.3 Tips

Billroth II is rarely required in dogs and cats because the body of the stomach can be easily mobilized to allow a gastro-duodenal anastomosis. It has been recommended in human surgery that jejuno-gastric anastomosis be

(a)

(b)

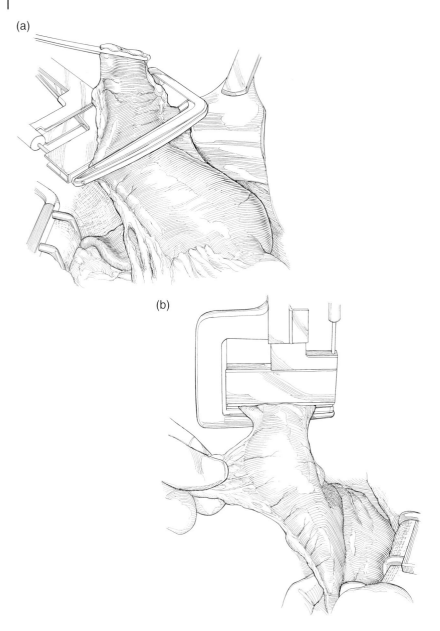

Figure 20.5

performed on the dorsal side of the stomach as this is more likely to help prevent dumping syndrome.

A vagotomy at the time of surgery will help to increase the gastric emptying time. Also, the vagotomy will reduce acid secretion in the stomach from the parietal cells.

It has also been recommended to completely remove the pyloric antrum, which is the major source of gastrin. Pyloric antrum distension stimulates gastrin secretion, which will increase acid secretion in the stomach (Dunlap et al. 1975; Turner and Mulholland 2007). The connection of the pyloric antrum and body of the stomach is identified at the connection of the left and right gastroepiploic arteries along the greater curvature.

It has been shown in a study on normal dogs that a stoma of 1.7–2.7 cm is recommended to prevent nausea and vomiting (Ahmadu-Suka et al. 1988).

Feeding tubes are very helpful in the post-operative period to support the patient and reduce the frequency of vomiting and the risk of aspiration pneumonia. Many dogs or cats are nauseated and anorexic after a Billroth II. The feeding tubes will help maintain caloric and protein intake. The jejunostomy tube is used to feed the patient while the gastrostomy tube is used to keep the stomach empty to minimize the dumping syndrome, reflux esophagitis and vomiting.

(a)

(b)

(c)

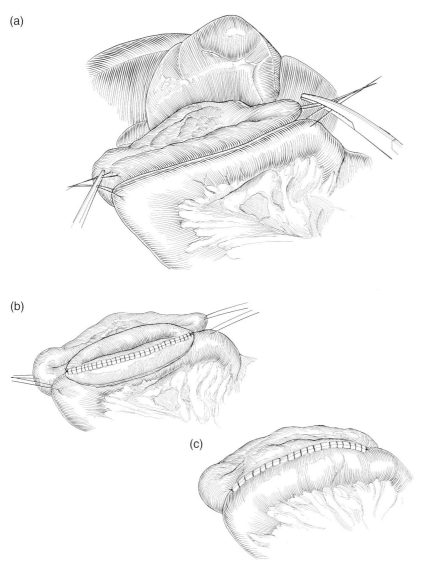

Figure 20.6

Medical treatment with ondansetron, omeprazole, and sucralfate is required after surgery to control the gastritis and the esophagitis.

20.4 Complications and Post-Operative Care

Post-operatively dogs and cats are monitored for signs of septic peritonitis due to leakage or dehiscence of the multiple anastomosis. Monitoring the patient with electrocardiogram and arterial pressure measurement is recommended. Venous blood gases with measurement of lactate should be evaluated regularly in the post-operative period. If the gastrostomy tube is suctioned to keep the stomach decompressed, electrolytes can be severely affected. Therefore electrolyte supplementation is required. Also, the amount of fluid withdrawn from the gastrostomy tube should be replaced to prevent dehydration.

Patients are maintained on ondansetron and pantoprazole intravenously, and sucralfate in the gastrostomy tube.

20.4.1 Dumping Syndrome

Dumping syndrome results from fast emptying of the stomach content in the jejunum. The stomach should accumulate food and mix it with acid and pepsin. It transforms the meal into an isosmotic gastric chyme that is slowly released in the duodenum. If the pyloric antrum has been removed and the jejunum has been

(a)

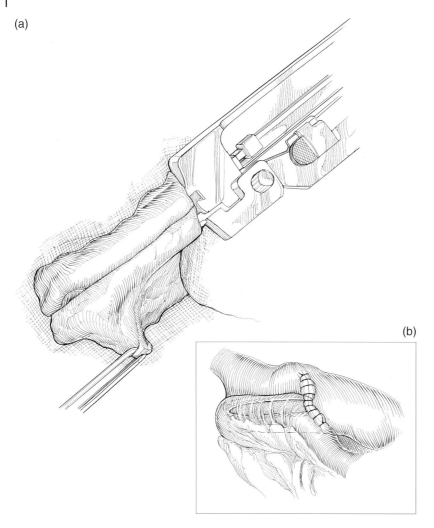

(b)

Figure 20.7

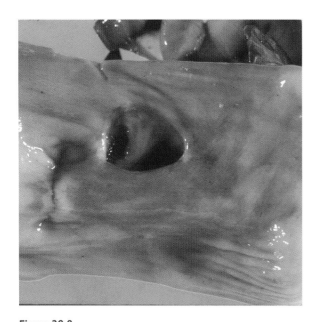

Figure 20.8

anastomosed to the stomach, the gastric emptying is severely affected. If the emptying is fast, hypertonic chyme is delivered to the small intestine (Dumon and Dempsey 2019).

The dumping syndrome can be biphasic: early dumping and late dumping. The early dumping occurs within 30 minutes of a meal. It is characterized by abdominal pain, nausea, bloating, and diarrhea. Tachycardia is commonly present. The early phase is mostly caused by the hyperosmolar chyme that attracts fluid in the small intestine. Early dumping syndrome is very common after a Billroth II in human patients (Miller and Savas 2007). The late dumping syndrome occurs usually two to three hours after a meal. It is also the result of rapid emptying of the hyperosmolar gastric content in the small intestine. The rapid delivery of carbohydrates triggers a massive release of insulin that results in hypoglycemia. The hypoglycemia triggers activation of the adrenal gland, with tachycardia, tachypnea, and nausea.

Medical treatment with small meals several times a day helps palliate the dumping syndrome. In human patients it has been shown that limiting absorption of liquid during a meal helps palliate the dumping syndrome. A diet with less carbohydrate is appropriate (Miller and Savas 2007).

Conversion of the Billroth II into a Billroth I might help palliate the clinical signs. An isoperistaltic or an anti-peristaltic loop of jejunum is interposed between the stomach and the jejunum to convert the Billroth II into a Billroth I (Vogel et al. 1988). The Roux-en-Y procedure seems to deliver the most durable options to palliate the dumping syndrome in humans (Vogel et al. 1988). It has been shown that the Roux-en-Y limb has electrical and mechanical activity to advance content toward the stomach instead of away (Cullen and Kelly 1993).

Also a selective vagotomy should help increase the gastric emptying time and slow the release of gastric chyme in the small intestine.

20.4.2 Afferent Loop Syndrome

Afferent loop syndrome results from the accumulation of bile and pancreatic fluid in the afferent loop of intestine going to the stomach after a Billroth II. Usually it results from a mechanical obstruction of the afferent loop. Either kinking of the loop or stenosis at the gastrojejunal junction create the syndrome. Severe abdominal pain occurs 30–60 minutes after a meal. The afferent loop syndrome results in copious vomiting of bile and resolution of the abdominal pain because the pressure in the afferent loop was released (Dumon and Dempsey 2019).

Mostly bile is vomited because the stomach is already empty 30 minutes after eating. It can result in perforation of the afferent loop if the distension is too severe. Bacterial overgrowth can also result in diarrhea. Acid secretion of the stomach is less buffered when it enters the jejunum and in the presence of bile the stoma of the afferent loop can get ulcerated (Figure 20.8).

The afferent loop syndrome requires a second surgery for the correction of the obstruction and/or creation of a Roux-en-Y.

20.4.3 Gastritis and Esophagitis

Bile reflux (alkaline reflux) in the stomach is frequent, resulting in severe gastritis and esophagitis if frequent vomiting is occurring. The creation of Roux-en-Y palliates the bile reflux in the stomach (Dumon and Dempsey 2019).

References

Ahmadu-Suka, F. et al. (1988). Billroth II gastrojejunostomy in dogs. Stapling technique and postoperative complications. *Vet. Surg.* 17 (4): 211–219.

Ali, A. et al. (2019). Surgery for peptic ulcer disease. In: Shackelford's Surgery of the Alimentary Tract (eds. C.J. Yeo et al.), 673–701. Philadelphia: Elsevier.

Cullen, J.J. and Kelly, K.A. (1993). Gastric motor physiology and pathophysiology. *Surg. Clin. North Am.* 73 (6): 1145–1160.

Dumon, K. and Dempsey, D.T. (2019). Postgastrectomy syndromes. In: Shackelford's Surgery of the Alimentary Tract (eds. C.J. Yeo et al.), 719–734. Philadelphia: Elsevier.

Dunlap, J.A. Jr. et al. (1975). The retained gastric antrum: a case report. *Radiology* 117 (2): 371–372.

Miller, T.A. and Savas, J.F. (2007). Postgastrectomy syndromes. In: Shackelford's Surgery of the Alimentary Tract (eds. C.J. Yeo et al.), 870–881. Philadelphia: Saunders Elsevier.

Turner, D.J. and Mulholland, M.W. (2007). Gastric resection and reconstruction. In: Shackelford's Surgery of the Alimentary Tract (eds. C.J. Yeo et al.), 831–861. Philadelphia: Saunders Elsevier.

Vogel, S.B. et al. (1988). Clinical and radionuclide evaluation of roux-y diversion for postgastrectomy dumping. *Am. J. Surg.* 155 (1): 57–62.

21

Pyloroplasty

Eric Monnet

Department of Clinical Sciences, College of Veterinary Medicine and Biomedical Sciences, Colorado State University, Fort Collins, CO, USA

21.1 Indications

Pyloroplasty and pyloromyotomy have been recommended to release a benign gastric outflow obstruction. Pyloric hypertrophy can be the result of muscular hypertrophy, mucosal hypertrophy, or both (Bellenger et al. 1990). Brachycephalic breeds seems to be more at risk than any other breeds for pyloric hypertrophy (Poncet et al. 2005). If neoplasia is suspected as the cause of the outflow obstruction, either a Billroth I or II, or a Roux-in Y are more appropriate (Chapters 19 and 20). Endoscopic evaluation of the pylorus is recommended before surgery with needle aspiration to further document the nature of the obstruction.

Several techniques of pyloroplasty have been described: Heineke–Mikulicz pyloroplasty, the Finney pyloroplasty and the Y-U pyloroplasty (Ali et al. 2019). The Y-U pyloroplasty is more likely the technique most commonly used in dogs (Bright et al. 1988). This technique has been shown to decrease gastric emptying time without increasing the risk of duodenogastric reflux in normal dogs (Bright et al. 1988). The Heineke–Mikulicz pyloroplasty has been used in the treatment of dogs with gastric dilatation volvulus (Greenfield et al. 1989). The pyloroplasty increased the complication rate and did not affect long-term outcome of dogs with gastric dilatation volvulus.

21.2 Technique

21.2.1 Y-U Pyloroplasty

After a midline incision and an abdominal exploration the stomach and the duodenum are isolated from the rest of the abdominal cavity with laparotomy sponges and towels to minimize contamination. The pyloric antrum is palpated to identify the extent of the hypertrophy.

Stay sutures are placed on the duodenum and the body of the stomach (Figure 21.1). A partial thickness incision over the serosa is made with a #15 blade to outline the Y incision. The black arrows and the four letters highlight the Y-shaped incision (Figure 21.2a). Then the full-thickness incision is made from the proximal duodenum over the pylorus into the stomach. This incision should be centered over the pylorus and extend 3–4 cm on each side (Figure 21.2b). Then two incisions are performed in the stomach from the end of the first incision, parallel to the lesser and greater curvature. This creates a U-shaped flap in the pyloric antrum (Figure 21.3a). The pyloric mucosa is biopsied. If mucosal hypertrophy is present, the mucosa and submucosa can be resected 360° at the level of the pylorus to increase the diameter of the pylorus (Figure 21.3a). Before starting the resection of the mucosa and submucosa it is recommended to place stay sutures in the mucosa on the side of the duodenum (Figure 21.3a and b). The resection is completed partial thickness (Figure 21.3c). The mucosa from the duodenum and the stomach are sutured with a 4-0 monofilament absorbable suture in a continuous pattern with the knots in the wall of the duodenum (Figure 21.3d).

Then the tip of the U flap created in the pyloric antrum is advanced and sutured to most distal point of the incision in the duodenum (Figure 21.2c). Simple interrupted full-thickness sutures are used to complete the closure of both arms of the U-shaped flap (Figure 21.2d). A monofilament absorbable suture size 4-0 is used for the closure.

Gastrointestinal Surgical Techniques in Small Animals, First Edition. Edited by Eric Monnet and Daniel D. Smeak.
© 2020 John Wiley & Sons, Inc. Published 2020 by John Wiley & Sons, Inc.
Companion website: www.wiley.com/go/monnet/gastrointestinal

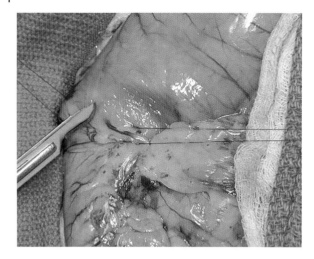

Figure 21.1

21.2.2 Other Pyloroplasty

For the Heineke–Mikulicz pyloroplasty a full-thickness incision centered over the pylorus is made in the proximal duodenum and the stomach. The total length of the incision is 4–5 cm. The incision is then closed in a perpendicular fashion with full-thickness simple interrupted sutures changing the longitudinal incision into a perpendicular suture line. A monofilament absorbable suture size 4-0 is used for the closure. This technique increases the diameter of the pylorus.

21.2.3 Pyloromyotomy

A Fredet–Ramstedt pyloromyotomy is indicated for a muscular hypertrophy of the pyloric region. A partial thickness incision center over the pylorus is made over 4 cm. The incision is through only the serosa and the muscularis region. When the incision is completed the submucosa and the mucosa are bulging through the incision. If the lumen of the stomach or the duodenum are entered during the procedure, the mucosa-submucosa are closed with simple interrupted suture with 4-0 monofilament absorbable suture. The omentum can be patched in the myotomy site. The serosa and the muscularis layers are left open.

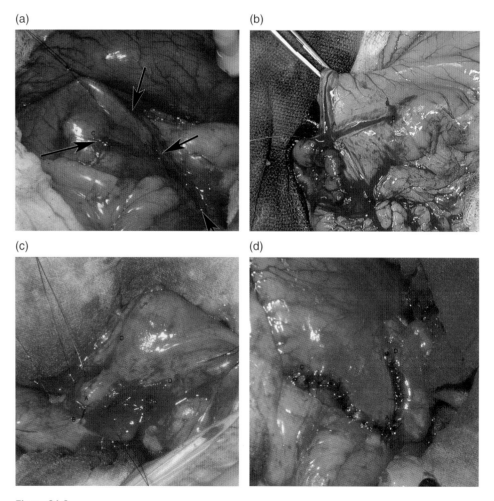

Figure 21.2

(a) (b)

(c) (d)

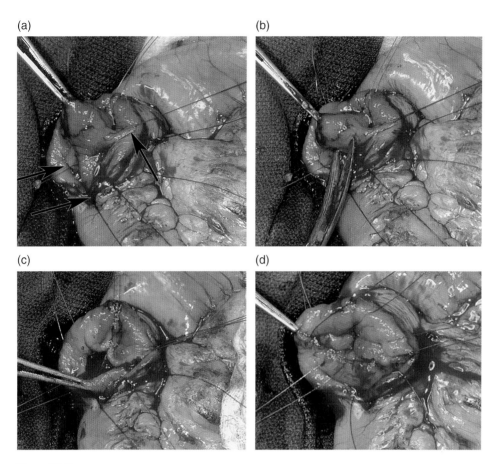

Figure 21.3

21.3 Tips

The Y-U pyloroplasty is most commonly performed in dogs with mucosal hypertrophy in the pyloric region because it has been shown to be associated with less biliary reflux in the stomach (Bright et al. 1988). If the hypertrophy is too severe, a Billroth I can be performed. If the disease process is infiltrative toward the duodenum a Billroth II or a Roux-en-Y should be attempted (Chapter 22).

The tip of the U flap from the pyloric antrum should be rounded to avoid necrosis of a narrow tip.

The closure of the U flap is better performed with simple interrupted sutures than with a continuous suture to avoid the formation of dog ears on each side. The author likes to divide each side of the U flap in half and keep adding sutures by dividing each segment by half.

Usually feeding tubes are not required for the post-operative support of those patients. However, a gastrostomy tube could be useful to keep the stomach decompressed after surgery and administer medications. A gastrostomy tube could be useful to keep the stomach decompressed in the post-operative period, especially if the stomach is very distended and flaccid at the time of surgery. A jejunostomy tube could be used to bypass the surgical site and feed a patient that is still vomiting in the post-operative period. A jejunostomy tube through a gastrostomy tube is appropriate for those cases.

21.4 Complications

In the immediate post-operative period dogs are monitored for signs of septic peritonitis. Dogs can eat orally immediately after surgery unless they are still vomiting because of gastritis. Ondansetron, omeprazole, and sucralfate are used after surgery to reduce the gastritis and the risk of vomiting.

Prognosis of dogs with benign pyloric hypertrophy is excellent. They may be nauseated because of duodeno-gastric reflux; however, the Y-U pyloroplasty has been shown to be associated with minimal reflux (Bright et al. 1988). It is not known if a very distended stomach because of chronic pyloric obstruction will regain normal size and function. Metoclopramide is recommended in the post-operative period to stimulate peristalsis in the stomach.

Dogs that had chronic vomiting gastritis and esophagitis should be treated in the post-operative period with sucralfate and omeprazole for at least 10 days.

References

Ali, A. et al. (2019). Surgery of peptic ulcer disease. In: Shackelford's Surgery of the Alimentary Tract (eds. C.J. Yeo et al.), 673–701. Philadelphia: Elsevier.

Bellenger, C.R. et al. (1990). Chronic hypertrophic pyloric gastropathy in 14 dogs. *Aust. Vet. J.* 67 (9): 317–320.

Bright, R.M. et al. (1988). Y-u antral flap advancement pyloroplasty in dogs. *Compend. Contin. Educ. Pract. Vet.* 10 (2): 139–144.

Greenfield, C.L. et al. (1989). Significance of the Heineke–Mikulicz pyloroplasty in the treatment of gastric dilatation-volvulus: a prospective clinical study. *Vet. Surg.* 18 (1): 22–26.

Poncet, C.M. et al. (2005). Prevalence of gastrointestinal tract lesions in 73 brachycephalic dogs with upper respiratory syndrome. *J. Small Anim. Pract.* 46 (6): 273–279.

22

Roux-en-Y

Eric Monnet

Department of Clinical Sciences, College of Veterinary Medicine and Biomedical Sciences, Colorado State University, Fort Collins, CO, USA

The concept of the Roux-en-Y procedure is the incorporation of a loop of jejunum into the upper gastrointestinal tract (Figure 22.1) to either reconstruct the upper gastrointestinal tract, reconstruct the biliary tract, or divert the gastrointestinal tract.

22.1 Indications

Roux-en-Y has been used mostly to replace the Billroth II in an effort to avoid the afferent loop syndrome and the reflux of bile in the stomach. It also helps prevent the ulceration of the afferent loop at the level of the stoma with the stomach (Morris et al. 1988; Namikawa et al. 2010; Zong and Chen 2011).

Biliary diversion can be performed with a Roux-en-Y procedure. Instead of creating a cholecystoduodenostomy, a cholecystojejunoduodenostomy, or cholecystojejunojejunostomy can be performed. A segment of jejunum is interposed between the gall bladder and the duodenum or the jejunum. This technique prevents duodenal content from refluxing in the gall bladder and thus the development of cholangiohepatitis.

Finally, diversion of the gastrointestinal tract with a Roux-en-Y technique can be used to palliate an obstruction of the upper gastrointestinal by a nonresectable pancreatic tumor.

22.2 Technique

22.2.1 Roux-en-Y for Upper GI Reconstruction

After performing the gastrectomy like for a Billroth II and the resection of the proximal duodenum, a 20 cm long segment of jejunum is isolated and transected after ligation of the arcadial vessels (Figure 22.2). The vascular supply to this segment of jejunum is maintained. Doyen clamps are used to prevent contamination of the peritoneal cavity. The distal part of the jejunum is then anastomosed to the dorsal part of the stomach with two simple continuous appositional suture patterns (Figure 22.3a and b). Monofilament absorbable suture size 4-0 is used. A #11 blade is used to perform a gastrotomy. The length of the gastrotomy should match the diameter of the jejunum (Figure 22.3a). Two stay sutures are placed to maintain the jejunum against the wall of the stomach at the level of the gastrotomy. The stay sutures are used to complete the anastomosis (Figure 22.3a). The anastomosis starts with the most dorsal side of the anastomosis followed by the ventral side (Figure 22.3b). Then the proximal end of the jejunum is anastomosed with end-to-side anastomosis to the distal jejunum (Figure 22.3c). Two simple continuous appositional suture patterns with 4-0 monofilament absorbable suture are used for this anastomosis. The anastomosis is performed 20 cm from the jejunogastric anastomosis. The efferent loop is then 20 cm long. If needed, a cholecystoduodenostomy is performed, like described for a Billroth II (Chapter 20).

As an alternative, stapling equipment can be used to complete the jejunogastric anastomosis. A gastrointestinal (GIA) stapler can be used for this anastomosis. One leg of the GIA stapler is introduced in the lumen of the stomach and the open end of the jejunum is advanced over the other leg of the GIA stapler (Figure 22.4a). The GIA is closed and after confirming the position of the stapler, the staples are applied. The GIA places six rows of staplers and a blade cut in the middle to create the anastomosis. The GIA is then removed and the entry site in the stomach and the jejunum are closed with a simple continuous suture (Figure 22.4b). An end-to-end anastomosis (EEA) stapler can also be used to perform the jejunogastric anastomosis (Figure 22.5). The EEA with its cartridge but without the anvil is introduced in the stomach through a gastrotomy on the ventral side of the stomach. Placement of a stay suture on each side of the gastrotomy helps the introduction of the EEA in the stomach (Figure 22.5a). The tip of the EEA is punctured through the dorsal side of the stomach. A purse-string is usually not needed in the wall of the stomach but can be placed. A purse-string suture is placed in the proximal jejunum. The anvil of EEA is attached to the distal tip of the EEA stapler and it is then advanced in the proximal jejunum. The purse-string of the jejunum is closed around the EEA and the EEA closed (Figure 22.5b). The staples are then applied. While the staples are applied a blade in the EEA cartridge cuts the wall of the stomach and the proximal jejunum, removing the purse-string suture. The EEA is then retrieved from the stomach and the gastrotomy can be closed with suture or a TA stapler.

22.2.2 Roux-en-Y for Biliary Diversion

With a cholecystoduodenostomy, ascending infection can occur, resulting in cholangiohepatitis. Chronic antibiotherapy is usually needed to control the clinical signs. To prevent this ascending infection in the biliary system, a Roux-en-Y diversion is possible. Two options are possible.

The first option is to create a cholecystojejunoduodenostomy (see Chapter 37) with the interposition of a loop of jejunum between the apex of the gallbladder and the duodenum. The second option is to perform a cholecystojejunojejunostomy (see Chapter 37). The proximal jejunum is transected distal to the duodenocolic ligament. The proximal end of the jejunum is anastomosed to the gallbladder. The distal part of the duodenum/proximal jejunum is anastomosed to the distal jejunum (Figure 22.6).

22.2.3 Roux-en-Y for Upper GI Diversion

The Roux-en-Y procedure can also be used to bypass a nonresectable obstructive lesion in the upper gastrointestinal

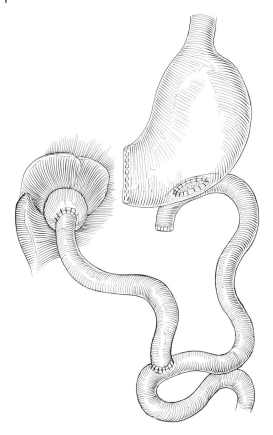

Figure 22.1

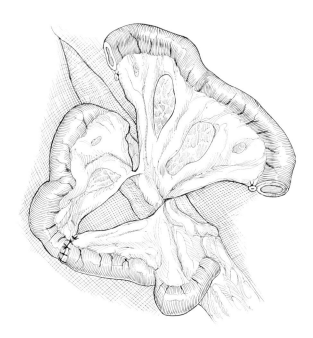

Figure 22.2

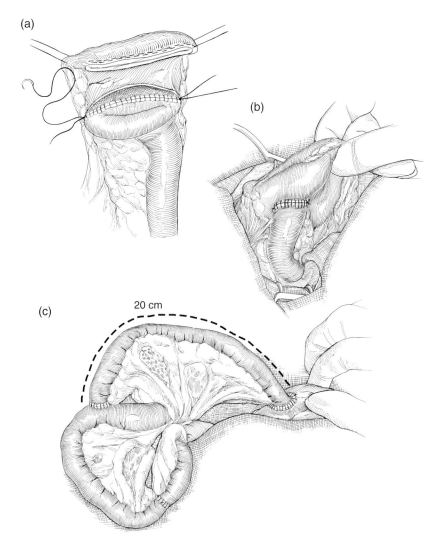

(a)

(b)

(c)

20 cm

Figure 22.3

tract. Pancreatic tumors obstructing the proximal duodenum, or a nonresectable gastric tumor obstructing most of the lumen of the stomach can be bypassed with a Roux-en-Y procedure. It is obviously a palliative procedure since the tumor is not resected.

As described above for upper gastrointestinal reconstruction, the proximal jejunum is transected. A gastrojejunostomy is then performed either at the level of the fundus of the stomach to bypass a gastric mass or on the dorsal side of the pyloric antrum to bypass a mass in the pancreas or in the proximal duodenum. Then an end-to-side anastomosis is performed to reconnect the proximal jejunum with the distal part of the jejunum.

22.3 Tips

Roux-en-Y procedure is rarely required to rebuild the upper gastrointestinal tract because the stomach and the duodenum are very mobile in dogs and cats. Several studies in human medicine have documented the benefit of the Roux-en-Y compared to the Billroth II. However, there is no data in the veterinary literature to

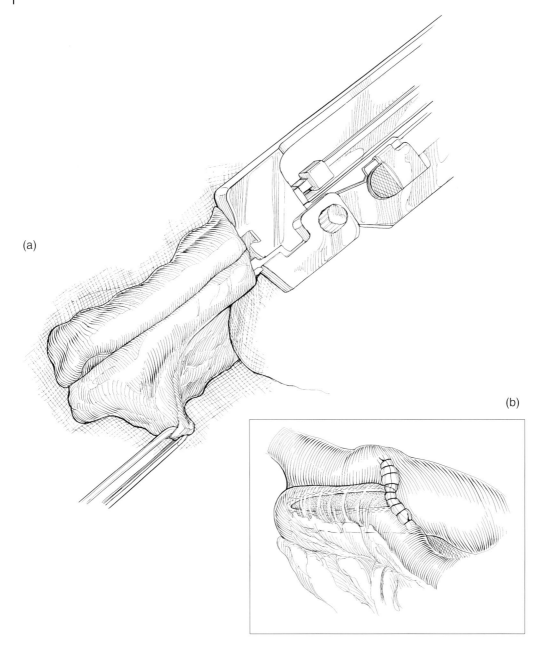

(a)

(b)

Figure 22.4

document long-term outcome associated with a Roux-en-Y procedure. In the author's experience this technique seems to be better tolerated than a Billroth II. It seems to reduce the afferent loop syndrome, with less biliary reflux in the stomach and less ulceration of the stomach and the jejunum at the level of the anastomosis.

The procedure is very useful for biliary diversion and reduces the risk of cholangiohepatitis.

Stapling equipment can be used to reduce the surgical time. However, the gastrointestinal stapler and the end-to-end anastomosis stapler are usually cumbersome and require closure of gastrotomy for their introduction.

(a)

(b)

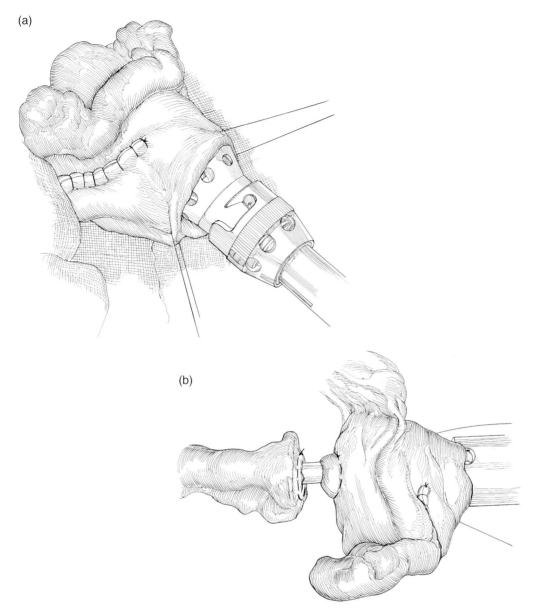

Figure 22.5

22.4 Complications

Post-operatively patients are monitored closely for signs of septic peritonitis.

Gastrostomy and jejunostomy tube should have been placed at the time of surgery and should be used in the post-operative period to keep the stomach decompressed and also feed the patient.

Since most of the patients requiring a Roux-en-Y procedure have severe gastritis, post-operative treatment requires sucralfate, omeprazole, ondansetron, and cisapride.

(a)

(b)

(c)

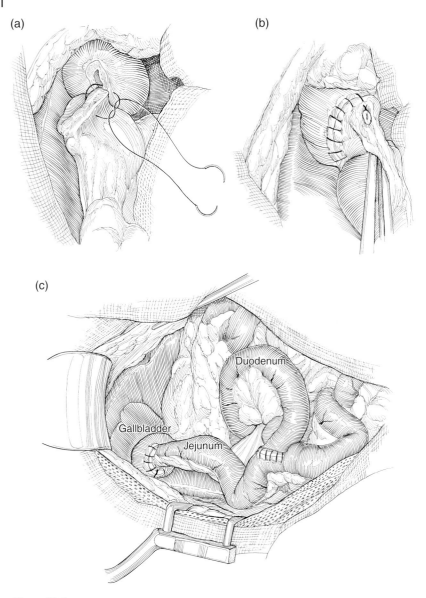

Duodenum

Gallbladder

Jejunum

Figure 22.6

References

Morris, D.L. et al. (1988). Gastric juice factors after roux-y reconstruction compared with Billroth II partial gastrectomy. *Am. J. Surg.* 156 (1): 21–25.

Namikawa, T. et al. (2010). Roux-en-Y reconstruction is superior to Billroth I reconstruction in reducing reflux esophagitis after distal gastrectomy: special relationship with the angle of His. *World J. Surg.* 34 (5): 1022–1027.

Zong, L. and Chen, P. (2011). Billroth I vs. Billroth II vs. Roux-en-Y following distal gastrectomy: a meta-analysis based on 15 studies. *Hepato-Gastroenterology* 58 (109): 1413–1424.

23

Gastropexy

Daniel D. Smeak

Department of Clinical Sciences, College of Veterinary Medicine and Biomedical Sciences, Colorado State University, Fort Collins, CO, USA

23.1 Indications

Gastropexy creates a permanent adhesion between the stomach and adjacent abdominal wall or adjoining viscera. Most gastropexies are performed as part of emergency treatment after stomach derotation in dogs with gastric dilatation volvulus (GDV), or to help prevent this condition (Cornell 2018). A left-sided gastropexy (gastric fundus to abdominal wall) is also occasionally performed as an adjunctive treatment in dogs with hiatal hernia. The adhesion helps prevent future stomach rotation in GDV or, in the case of hiatal hernia, it is thought to help keep the fundus of the stomach from migrating toward the hiatus during forced abdominal contraction and may help prevent gastroesophageal reflux (Pratschke et al. 2001).

Many gastropexy techniques have been described, including a variety of incisional gastropexies, the belt-loop and circumcostal gastropexy, gastrocolopexy, incorporating gastropexy (gastric wall is included in the linea alba closure), endoscopic-assisted gastropexy, and more recently, laparoscopic-assisted and intracorporeal gastropexy (Christie and Smith 1976; Fallah et al. 1982; MacCoy et al. 1982; Fox et al. 1985; Leib et al. 1985; Whitney et al. 1989; Meyer-Lindenberg et al. 1994; Rawlings et al. 2001; Steelman-Szymeczek et al. 2003; Eggertsdottir et al. 2008; Mayhew and Brown 2009; Runge et al. 2009; Dujowich et al. 2010; Spah et al. 2013; Imhoff et al. 2015; Coleman et al. 2016; Coleman and Monnet 2017).

A fundamental principle for most successful gastropexy techniques is joining exposed underlying raw muscle by scalpel incision or electrotomy through the antral serosa and adjacent abdominal wall. The stomach and abdominal wall are apposed and held together with suture until strong adhesions form. An important goal of successful gastropexy techniques for GDV is the creation of an anchor from the stomach and right abdominal wall in a functional stomach position.

Biomechanical testing of various gastropexy procedures that join the largest muscle surface area of the antrum to abdominal wall appear to result in the strongest adhesion formation (Fox et al. 1985; Hardie et al. 1996; Wilson et al. 1996; Waschak 1997; Rawlings et al. 2001). However, the amount of adhesion strength necessary to prevent the development of GDV has not been determined. Both the open and laparoscopic incisional gastropexies generally produce lower adhesion strength. However, retrospective studies have shown that incisional gastropexy, regardless of the approach, results in a consistent permanent adhesion with little ($<5\%$) to no incidence of GDV recurrence (Rivier et al. 2011; Benitez et al. 2013; Cornell 2018).

23.2 Surgical Procedures

23.2.1 Tube Gastropexy

The tube gastrostomy was one of the first procedures developed for gastropexy in dogs (Figure 23.1). This is considered an open gastropexy technique, and therefore, unlike the other closed procedures mentioned in this chapter, there is a risk of leakage from the tube site that extends into the stomach lumen. It is a relatively fast and technically easy technique, but the post-operative hospitalization can be lengthy, and the tube needs to be protected from premature dislodgement (the tube should remain in place for at least 7–10 days). A unique benefit of this technique is that it allows for continued gastric decompression in the early post-operative period

Gastrointestinal Surgical Techniques in Small Animals, First Edition. Edited by Eric Monnet and Daniel D. Smeak.
© 2020 John Wiley & Sons, Inc. Published 2020 by John Wiley & Sons, Inc.
Companion website: www.wiley.com/go/monnet/gastrointestinal

(a)

(b)

(c)

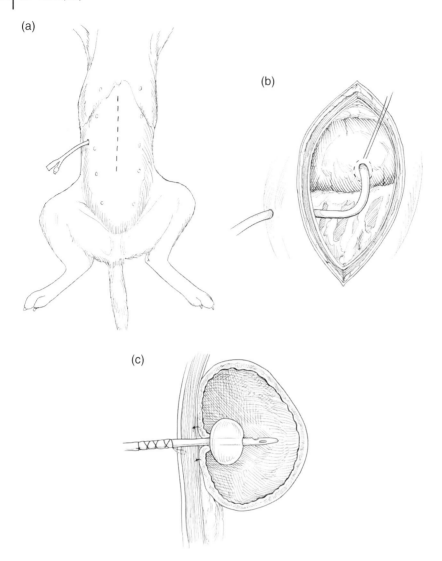

Figure 23.1

(if needed) and it provides access to the stomach for delivery of enteral nutrition and medications. A higher rate of recurrence and mortality rate when using this technique has been reported, so the procedure has largely been abandoned (Ellison 1993).

A 24 Fr Foley catheter is introduced through the right ventral abdominal wall 3–4 cm caudal to the last rib (Figure 23.1a). In the mid-antral area (similar location as the incisional gastropexy) a purse-string suture (about the 2.5 cm in diameter) is placed using 2-0 prolonged monofilament absorbable suture. A stab incision is created in the middle of the purse-string suture, the catheter is introduced into the stomach lumen, and the Foley bulb is inflated with an appropriate amount of saline (Figure 23.1b). The purse string is tied snugly around the tube. The stomach wall is sutured with four to five preplaced sutures to the abdominal wall such

that a seal is created around the tube. Some surgeons wrap omentum around the tube for extra insurance against possible leakage. Gentle traction is placed on the Foley catheter to draw the stomach wall firmly against the abdominal wall and a finger-trap suture is placed to fix the catheter to the skin (Figure 23.1c).

23.2.2 Incisional Gastropexy

23.2.2.1 Standard Incisional Gastropexy

During an incisional gastropexy two flaps in the pyloric antrum are sutured to the right transverse abdominalis muscle (MacCoy et al. 1982). A 3 cm incision is made in the pyloric antrum through the serosa and the mucularis midline between the greater and the lesser curvature of the stomach (Figure 23.2a). Flaps are elevated over 1 cm on each side of the incision. The submucosa and

(a)   (b)

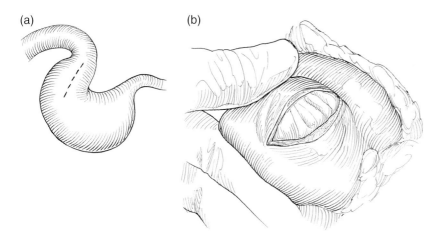

Figure 23.2

mucosa should bulge through the incision (Figure 23.2b). A 3 cm incision is then made in the right transverse abdominal muscle 2–3 cm caudal to the last rib along the direction of the muscle fibers. This incision is at the junction of the ventral third and middle third of the abdominal wall.

The pyloric antrum is then brought close to the abdominal wall. A 2-0 monofilament prolonged absorbable suture is then used to suture, with two separate simple continuous suture lines joining the two flap of the pyloric antrum with the two sides of the incision in the transverse abdominalis muscle.

23.2.2.2 Modified Incisional Gastropexy

This is a modification of the technique describe above and it is an efficient technique designed for the "solo" surgeon (Figure 23.3) (Touru and Smeak 2005). It holds advantages over other described incisional gastropexy techniques because it uses standard stomach and abdominal wall incision sites to reduce the likelihood of gastric malpositioning, or accidental diaphragm perforation during the abdominal wall incision.

The linea alba is incised on midline from the base of the xiphoid cartilage caudally to the umbilicus. Care is taken to prevent incising along the sides of the xiphoid cartilage (the linea is always incised *superficial* to the cartilage) to avoid accidentally perforating the diaphragm.

This cranial extension of the celiotomy incision helps the "solo" surgeon better expose the stomach, particularly in deep-chested dogs, and improves exposure of the incision site in the right abdominal wall.

The surgeon should stand on the *left* side of the patient to gain the best exposure to the right cranial aspect of the abdomen during the gastropexy procedure.

(a)

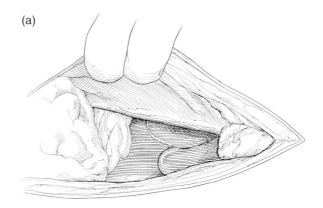

(b)

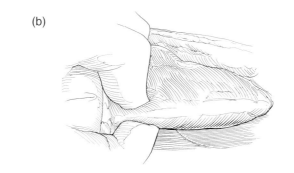

Figure 23.3

The abdominal wall incision site is exposed by grasping the right abdominal wall margin. The wall is everted and forcefully rolled to the right to allow exposure and palpation of the chondral aspect of the underlying rib just beneath the exposed transversus abdominis muscle (Figure 23.3a and b). The underlying 11th or 12th rib (depending on the breed conformation) is palpated approximately 5 cm caudal to the xiphoid cartilage at about the junction of the ventral and middle thirds of

(a)

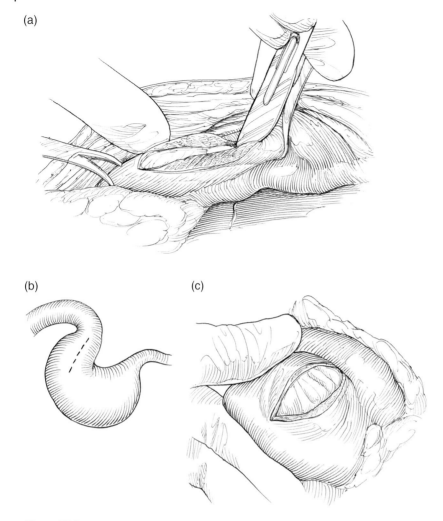

(b)   (c)

Figure 23.4

the abdominal wall. While isolating the rib with the index finger and thumb, two large towel clamps are placed through the transversus abdominis muscle just around the cartilage of the isolated rib. The first clamp is placed 5 cm caudal to the xiphoid and the second one 5 cm caudal to the first around the isolated chondral portion of the underlying rib. The clamps can be pulled up to the right by an assistant or rolled to the right and clamped to the drapes (for the solo surgeon) to keep the area well exposed for the wall incision and subsequent suturing.

An incision is made between the clamps directly onto the underlying cartilaginous portion of the isolated rib (Figure 23.4a). There should be no major arteries or nerves to contend with underneath the incision area. The clamps remain around the ribs for exposure throughout the later (suturing) part of the procedure.

Next, the pyloric antrum area is exposed in preparation for the gastric incision. A 5 cm antral incision is

created in the middle of the antrum, equidistant between the greater and lesser curvature, and *parallel* to the long axis of the antrum (Figure 23.4b). The "slip" maneuver helps eliminate the risk of accidentally perforating the mucosa when making the sero-muscular incision in the antrum. After drying the surgeon's gloves and antral area with dry sponges, the sero-muscularis layers are grabbed between two fingers and lifted. The submucosa and the mucosa can be felt slipping away ("slip" technique) from the sero-muscularis. With Metzenbaum scissors an incision is created fully through the isolated seromuscular layer such that the incision will run *parallel to the long axis of the antrum*. The incision is extended to create a 5 cm long mid-antral incision to match the length of the abdominal wall incision. Intact mucosa should freely bulge out of the incision (Figure 23.4c). Half centimeter bites (2-0 prolonged absorbable suture) are taken at the corner of the pyloric side of the antral incision and

(a)

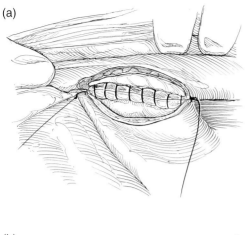

(b)

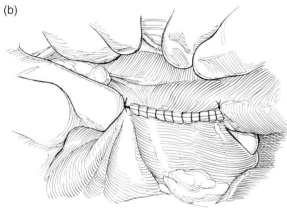

Figure 23.5

the cranial corner of the abdominal wall incision. Alternately, separate sutures are used to tack the cranial and caudal corners of the incisions for the two simple continuous lines (Figure 23.5a). This knotted stitch firmly fixes the stomach up and against the abdominal wall though out the suturing process. A simple continuous suture line is begun, incorporating 0.5 cm bites of the *dorsal* abdominal wall incision edge to the *greater curvature side* of the stomach incision edge. At the caudal corner of the incision, the line is knotted, and the loop is cut off. With the same needle connected to the knot, the ventral portion of the abdominal incision edge is apposed to the remaining free edge of the stomach incision (Figure 23.5b). Following knotting of the second continuous suture line, the position of the pylorus is inspected. It should extend from the gastropexy site in a *craniodorsal* direction.

23.2.3 Belt-Loop Gastropexy

In this technique, rather than creating a simple incision in the stomach, a seromuscular flap based on the greater

(a)

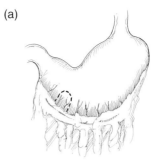

(b)

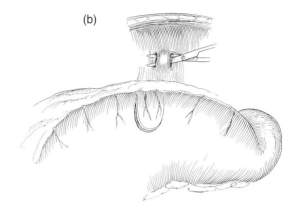

Figure 23.6

curvature of the stomach is created from the mid-pyloric antrum and passed through a tunnel created between two incisions in the right abdominal wall (Figure 23.6) (Whitney et al. 1989). If an assistant is available, two towel clamps can be placed on the incised right cranial abdominal wall (linea) edge to help pull up and retract the right abdominal wall and expose the proposed gastropexy site. At the midpoint of the gastric antrum on the greater curvature, two parallel seromuscular incisions 4 cm long and 3 cm apart are created. Another incision connects the cranial most aspect of the incisions creating a tongue-shaped seromuscular flap (Figure 23.6a and b). The flap base is located at the greater curvature incorporating a healthy blood supply from secondary branches of the gastroepiploic vessels. The "slip technique" (in the modified incisional gastropexy description) is utilized to safely incise through the seromuscular layer without invading the mucosa. The flap is carefully undermined from the bulging underlying mucosa. A region in the mid right abdominal wall adjacent to the normal position of the pylorus is chosen for the abdominal incisions. These incisions must be made caudal to the last rib and the diaphragm attachment to avoid accidental perforation and pneumothorax. Two parallel 3–5 cm long dorsal to ventral incisions are made through the transversus abdominis

(a)

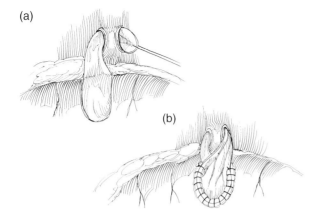

(b)

Figure 23.7

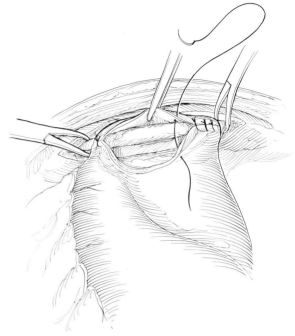

Figure 23.9

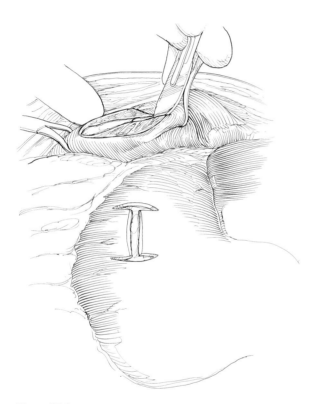

Figure 23.8

muscle about 3 cm apart (Figure 23.7a). The tissue under the incisions is bluntly undermined to create a tunnel through which the gastric flap will be passed.

It is helpful to place one or two stay sutures adjacent and on opposite sides of the flap base before advancing the flap through the abdominal wall tunnel. These sutures are first pulled through the tunnel to draw the flap base up against the abdominal wall and release tension in preparation for the next step (not shown in the figures). A stay suture placed at the distal aspect of the

flap can then be safely used to readily pull the flap through the tunnel in preparation for suturing (Figure 23.7b). The flap is advanced in a caudal to cranial direction.

The flap is sutured back to the defect from which it was created using simple interrupted 2-0 prolonged absorbable suture (Figure 23.7b).

23.2.4 Circumcostal Gastropexy

Seromuscular flaps at the mid-antral region are drawn *around* isolated portions of the chondral portion of the right caudal ribs (similar in position to the modified incisional gastropexy described previously) instead of through a tunnel in the transversus abdominis muscle (as described for the belt-loop gastropexy) (Figure 23.8) (Fallah et al. 1982).

The antrum is incised to make double-hinged mid-antral seromuscular flaps. A 5 cm incision is made directly over the chondral portion of the right eleventh or twelfth ribs and the exposed rib is bluntly undermined to create a tunnel (Figure 23.8). The seromuscular flaps are drawn around the isolated rib with the help of stay sutures. These seromuscular flaps are sutured back together with 2-0 prolonged absorbable suture (Figure 23.9). Since a tunnel is created completely around the rib in this technique, it is important to avoid perforating the diaphragm or fracturing the rib during blunt dissection.

23.2.5 Gastrocolopexy

With gastrocolopexy, a permanent adhesion is created between the greater curvature of the stomach and adjacent transverse colon (Christie and Smith 1976). Serosal surfaces of the apposing margins of the stomach and transverse colon are scarified with a #15 scalpel blade to remove the serosal layer. The greater omentum is tucked dorsolateral to the transverse colon so that the transverse colon can be sutured to the stomach just cranioventral to the attachment of the greater omentum. The scarified surfaces are apposed with sutures incorporating the seromuscular layers only. The reported recurrence rate with gastrocolopexy is higher (up to 20%) than with many other techniques described in this chapter (Eggertsdottir et al. 2001). This technique does not use incisions through the seromuscular layers of the stomach or colon, so the longevity and strength of the gastropexy has not been yet been verified (Cornell 2018).

23.2.6 Incorporating Gastropexy

The so-called "incorporating" gastropexy includes approximately 5 cm of the gastric wall near the pyloric antrum within the linea alba suture line during abdominal wall closure (Meyer-Lindenberg et al. 1994). The pyloric antrum site for incorporation is not incised or scarified. Sutures do not penetrate into the stomach lumen. Prolonged 0 to 2-0 prolonged absorbable sutures are used for the incorporating linea alba closure. The recurrence rate of GDV after this procedure is slightly higher than with other gastropexy techniques (6.6%). Although this is arguably one of the easiest and quickest gastropexy techniques available, the strength or permanency of this gastropexy has not been definitively documented. The stomach antrum is more ventrally located, and the stomach axis is somewhat malpositioned with this technique. This technique fails to "pexy" the pyloric antrum to the right side of the abdominal cavity. In addition, if abdominal exploration is necessary in the future, the stomach could be accidentally penetrated when entering the abdominal cavity.

23.2.7 Endoscopically Assisted Gastropexy

This technique requires a flexible endoscope to distend the stomach and push the pyloric antrum toward the right side of the abdominal cavity (Dujowich and Reimer 2008). With the dog in left oblique recumbency, a flexible endoscope is inserted into the stomach and the lumen is distended with insufflation. The pyloric antrum is viewed with the flexible endoscope while the surgeon palpates the right abdominal wall to locate the desired anatomic area for gastropexy. The stomach is stabilized with two stay sutures (#2 polypropylene with large half-circle cutting needle) passed percutaneously through the right abdominal wall immediately caudal to the right 13th rib into the gastric lumen and back out adjacent to the entrance site. The stay sutures should be placed lateral to the rectus abdominalis muscle. The edge of the muscle can be palpated. The stay sutures should incorporate at least 2 cm of gastric wall and are placed 5 cm apart in an orad to aborad direction. The endoscopist simultaneously views the needle passing within the gastric lumen to verify the correct location and size of gastric wall purchase. An incision is made between the two stay sutures directly through the abdominal wall to expose the underlying stomach wall. A 2 cm seromuscular incision is created in the underlying antrum. The incised edges of the stomach antrum incision are sutured to the edges of the abdominal wall approach with 2-0 prolonged absorbable sutures. Since the general technique is similar to other incisional gastropexies, permanent adhesion formation should be expected. All gastropexy sites were intact when re-examined with laparoscopy in one report (Dujowich et al. 2010). Since the gastropexy site is chosen via endoscopy only, there is the potential to create a gastropexy site in an inappropriate position particularly for the inexperienced surgeon and endoscopist. Placement of the stay suture needles is blind, so inadvertent damage or penetration of adjacent viscera, such as the spleen, could potentially occur.

23.2.8 Laparoscopic-Assisted Gastropexy

In contrast to the endoscopic-assisted gastropexy, a laparoscope is used to view proper positioning of the stomach, nearby structures, and the site on the pyloric antrum for gastropexy (Figure 23.10) (Rawlings et al. 2001; Rawlings et al. 2002). With the dog in dorsal recumbency, the entire ventral abdomen is prepared. The aseptic preparation is extended 7–10 cm further toward the right dorsolateral abdominal wall for aseptic surgery. The surgeon stands on the right side of the patient with the monitor placed cranially. A 5 mm trocar cannula is inserted on midline 2 cm caudal to the umbilicus for the camera port and a similar trocar is placed lateral to the right margin of the rectus abdominis muscle and 3 cm caudal to the last rib for the working port (Figure 23.10a).

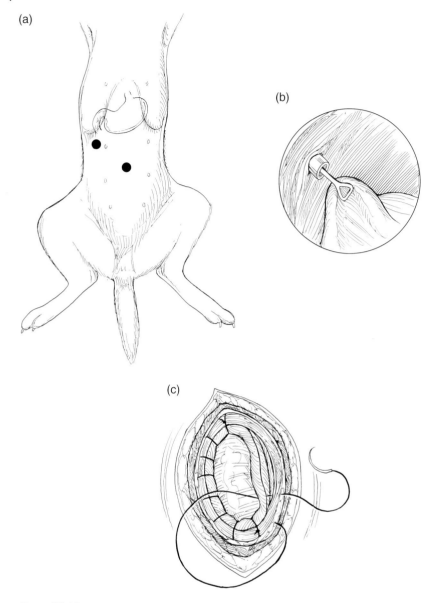

(a)

(b)

(c)

Figure 23.10

A modification of this technique uses a single-incision laparoscopic technique placing a single multiaccess port on the right side of the abdominal wall lateral to the right margin of the rectus abdominis muscle and 3 cm caudal to the last rib for the working port (Runge et al. 2013).

After insufflating the abdominal cavity with carbon dioxide, a 5 mm laparoscopic fine-toothed grasping forceps is passed through the working cannula. The middle of the pyloric antrum, equidistant between the lesser and greater curvatures is grasped and held securely (Figure 23.10b). The working cannula incision is extended through skin and underlying muscle parallel to the last right rib to create a 4 cm full-thickness abdominal wall incision. If a single-port multiaccess system is used, the port is removed once the antrum is grasped, and the pyloric antrum is exposed through the larger port incision.

When the pyloric antrum is exposed through the abdominal wall incision a stay suture is placed through wall of the pyloric antrum. The underlying incised abdominal muscle edges (from the port sites) are retracted with Gelpi retractors. Care is taken to be sure that the antrum is not twisted as it is exteriorized, and a 2.5–3 cm seromuscular incision is created in the mid-pyloric antrum region. Penetration of the gastric mucosa is avoided when creating the incision. The edges of the antral incision are sutured to the transversus abdominis muscle edges with continuous suture lines of 2-0 prolonged absorbable suture (Figure 23.10). The oblique muscle fascial layers are closed together with simple continuous 2-0 prolonged absorbable suture. The subcutaneous tissues are carefully closed to reduce any dead space and closure of the skin is routine. When separate cannulas are used, the abdominal wall fascia, subcutaneous layer, and skin are closed separately. This is a simple and quick gastropexy technique that is relatively easy to master. Few complications have been reported (Rawlings et al. 2001). Seroma is frequent in the post-operative period likely due to muscle dissection through the abdominal wall.

23.2.9 Laparoscopic Gastropexy

23.2.9.1 Stapled Technique

This technique requires a linear stapler to complete the gastropexy (Figure 23.11) (Hardie et al. 1996). With the dog in dorsal recumbency, three (10/12 mm) laparoscopic cannulas are placed in the caudal aspect of the abdomen to the right of midline. A 2 × 5 cm submucosal tunnel in the mid-antrum is made with Metzenbaum scissors and Kelly forceps using sharp and blunt dissection. A similar-sized tunnel is made in the adjacent right lateral abdominal wall between the transversus abdominis and internal abdominal oblique muscles caudal to the last rib and away from the diaphragm. A 35 mm laparoscopic linear stapler is inserted into the dissected tunnels and is used to staple the stomach to the right abdominal wall. Individual laparoscopic staples may be used to close the tunnel openings.

23.2.9.2 Intracorporeal Suturing Techniques

There are a variety of port sites described for intracorporeal gastropexy (Mayhew and Brown 2009; Corriveau et al. 2015; Coleman et al. 2016).

23.2.9.3 Three Port Technique

The first port is inserted 1 cm caudal to the umbilicus. The second port is placed 5–10 cm caudal to the rim of the xiphoid cartilage, the third is inserted midway between the other two port sites. For the author, the preferred port locations is 1 cm caudal to the umbilicus, 10 cm caudal to the xiphoid cartilage, and 3–5 cm caudal to the umbilical scar (Figure 23.12a). A 5 mm rigid endoscope is advanced through the middle port and the pyloric antrum is identified. The pyloric antrum is grasped with a 5 mm laparoscopic fine-toothed grasping forceps and the antrum is advanced to the right mid abdominal wall 2–3 cm caudal to the last rib. The line of insertion of the diaphragm is

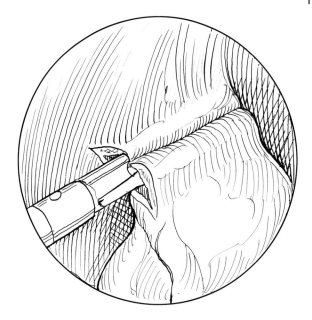

Figure 23.11

recognized. A percutaneous stay suture with a straight needle is advanced through the abdominal wall at this site at the level of the black arrow (Figure 23.12a). The straight stay suture needle is grasped intracorporeally with laparoscopic needle holders. A 5 mm fine-toothed grasping forceps are used to grab the mid-pyloric antrum and the straight needle is advanced through the pyloric antrum at that level. The needle is then returned through the abdominal wall adjacent to the original needle entrance site (Figure 23.12b). The pyloric antrum is lifted up to the abdominal wall with the stay suture to hold the regions together in preparation for incisional gastropexy. A 2.5–3 cm incision is made through the transversus abdominis muscle just caudal to the stay suture site with 5 mm laparoscopic Metzenbaum scissors. A seromuscular incision is created in the pyloric antrum along the long axis of the pyloric antrum equidistant between the lesser and greater curvature of the stomach. The seromuscular flaps are undermined about 5 mm on each side to facilitate placement of the suture without penetrating in the lumen of the stomach. In lieu of seromuscular incisions, some surgeons prefer to scarify the gastropexy sites with electrocoagulion (Takacs et al. 2017).

The flaps of the pyloric antrum and abdominal wall incisions (or scarified areas) are sutured together with a 2-0 barbed unidirectional suture using laparoscopic needle holders or an endoscopic suture assist device (Figure 23.12c) (Spah et al. 2013; Coleman et al. 2016; Coleman and Monnet 2017).

(a)

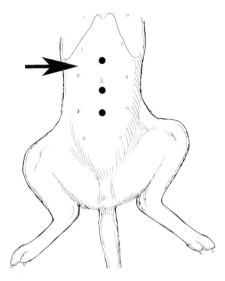

(b)

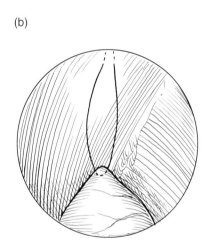

(c)

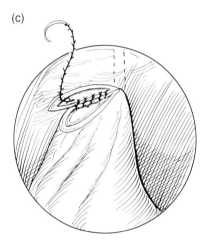

Figure 23.12

23.2.9.4 Single-Access Port Technique

Instead of using three separate ports on the abdominal midline, a single-access multiport can be placed on midline 2 cm caudal to the umbilicus. The single-access multiport allows placement of three cannulas (sizes 5 and 12 mm) through a single-port incision. Another cannula is very often required in the right lateral side of the abdominal cavity at the level of the single-access multiport (Coleman et al. 2016; Coleman and Monnet 2017).

With this technique the seromuscular flaps are made perpendicular to the long axis of the pyloric antrum. The flaps are 2–3 cm long. The incision in the rectus abdominalis muscle is also 2–3 cm and the incision is made in the direction of the muscle fibers. This incision is in the ventral third of the abdominal wall caudal to the last rib and the attachment of the diaphragm. A stay suture (black arrow) (Figure 23.13) is placed percutaneously with a straight needle as described above but in this case the pyloric antrum is fixed with a stay suture closer to the lesser curvature (Figure 23.14a).

Three-centimeters-long flaps in the pyloric antrum and the transverse abdominal muscle are created and undermined (Figure 23.14b and c). A 2-0 prolonged absorbable unidirectional barbed suture is used to complete the gastropexy. The strand of the suture should not be longer than 15 cm. Longer suture will be difficult to handle in the abdominal cavity. The lateral suture is completed first, followed by the medial suture (Figures 23.14d and 23.15). With this technique the needle holders or the laparoscopic suturing device are held in the same direction as the incision facilitating the procedure. A roticulated laparoscopic suturing

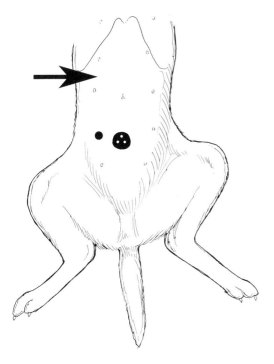

Figure 23.13

device can be used with the single-access port to facilitate the suturing (Figure 23.16) (Coleman et al. 2016; Coleman and Monnet 2017).

23.3 Tips

In the author's experience, several technical errors can complicate recovery of patients undergoing gastropexy. A gastropexy site can pull the stomach out of its normal anatomic position causing partial gastric outflow obstruction and recurrent gastric dilation, or the gastric gastropexy site is made to the body rather than the antrum of the stomach allowing excess antral rotation and GDV recurrence. It is easy for surgeons to secure open gastropexies too far ventral on the abdominal wall because it is the easiest area to expose for suturing (Cornell 2018).

It is paramount to permanently fix the pyloric antrum to the right side of the abdominal cavity to prevent a GDV or prevent a recurrence of an acute

(a)

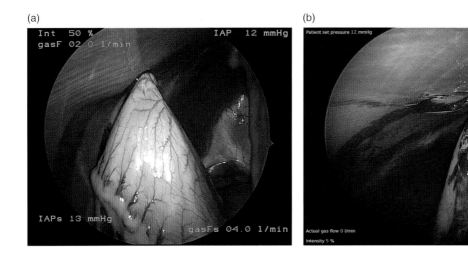

(b)

(c)

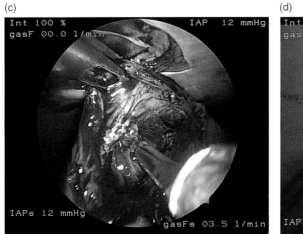

(d)

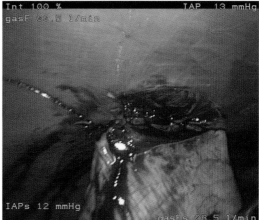

Figure 23.14

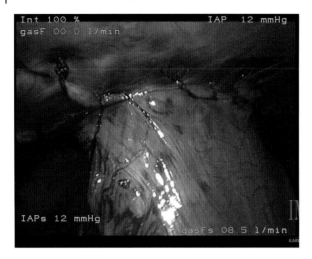

Figure 23.15

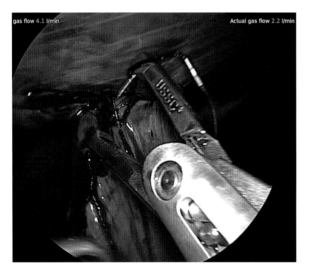

Figure 23.16

GDV. All the techniques describe above except the incorporating gastropexy have been shown to provide this security.

The adhesions resulting from the circumcostal gastropexy are stronger compared to most incisional gastropexies (Fox et al. 1985). However, it is not known how much strength is ultimately required to achieve a safe permanent gastropexy in the dog. The incisional gastropexy which is the weakest gastropexy provides excellent clinical results (Benitez et al. 2013; Przywara et al. 2014).

All the laparoscopic gastropexy technique requires experience and skill with laparoscopy instrumentation and techniques before it should be attempted in clinical cases. The unidirectional barbed suture greatly facilitates the procedure because no laparoscopic knot tying is required.

23.4 Post-Operative Care and Complications

Following prophylactic gastropexy, oral intake of food and water can be permitted once the dog has recovered from anesthesia and shows interest. Few complications have been reported overall for most gastropexy techniques, but gastric malpositioning causing partial outflow obstruction, pneumothorax from perforating the diaphragm during abdominal wall preparation for gastropexy, and minor self-limiting incisional problems such as seroma formation have been reported. Even with a properly performed gastropexy, gastric dilation can still occur. In these cases, it is important to confirm that the gastropexy is intact (with ultrasound), and the gastric position is normal (with a plain and contrast gastrogram, and endoscopic evaluation) (Sutton et al. 2015).

For dogs undergoing gastropexy for treatment of acute GDV, post-operative management involves maintaining fluid and electrolyte balance and blood pressure, administration of gastroprotective drugs, promotility agents, antiarrhymic drugs, and analgesics as required.

References

Benitez, M.E., Schmiedt, C.W., Radlinsky, M.G. et al. (2013). Efficacy of incisional gastropexy for prevention of GDV in dogs. *J. Am. Anim. Hosp. Assoc.* 49: 185–189.

Christie, T.R. and Smith, C.W. (1976). Gastrocolopexy for prevention of recurrent gastric volvulus. *J. Am. Anim. Hosp. Assoc.* 12: 173–1976.

Coleman, K.A., Adams, S., Smeak, D.D., and Monnet, E. (2016). Laparoscopic gastropexy using knotless unidirectional suture and an articulated endoscopic suturing device: seven cases. *Vet. Surg.* 45: O95–O101.

Coleman, K.A. and Monnet, A. (2017). Comparison of laparoscopic gastropexy performed via intracorporeal suturing with knotless unidirectional barbed suture using needle driver versus a reticulated endoscopic suturing device: 30 cases. *Vet. Surg.* 46: 1002–1007.

Cornell, K. (2018). Stomach. In: Veterinary Surgery Small Animal (eds. S.A. Johnston and K.M. Tobias), 1700–1730. St. Louis: Elsevier.

Corriveau, K.M., Runge, J.J., and Rawlings, C.A. (2015). Laparoscopic and laparoscopic-assisted gastropexy techniques. In: Small Animal Laparoscopy and Thoracoscopy (eds. A. Fransson and P.D. Mayhew), 125–133. Hoboken: Wiley Blackwell.

Dujowich, M., Keller, M.E., and Reimer, S.B. (2010). Evaluation of short- and long-term complications after endoscopically assisted gastropexy in dogs. *J. Am. Vet. Med. Assoc.* 236: 177–182.

Dujowich, M. and Reimer, S.B. (2008). Evaluation of an endoscopically assisted gastropexy technique in dogs. *Am. J. Vet. Res.* 69: 537–541.

Eggertsdottir, A., Stigen, O., Lonaas, L. et al. (2001). Comparison of the recurrence rate of gastric dilatation with or without volvulus in dogs after circumcostal gastropexy versus gastrocolopexy. *Vet. Surg.* 30: 546–551.

Eggertsdottir, A.V., Langeland, M., Fuglem, B. et al. (2008). Long-term outcome in dogs after circumcostal gastropexy or gastrocolopexy for gastric dilatation with or without volvulus. *Vet. Surg.* 37: 809–810.

Ellison, G.W. (1993). Gastric dilatation volvulus. Surgical prevention. *Vet. Clin. N. Am. Small Anim. Pract.* 23: 513–530.

Fallah, A., Lumb, W., Nelson, A. et al. (1982). Circumcostal gastropexy in the dog: a preliminary study. *Vet. Surg.* 11: 9–12.

Fox, S., Ellison, G., and Miller, G. (1985). Observations on the mechanical failure of three gastropexy techniques. *J. Am. Anim. Hosp. Assoc.* 21: 729–734.

Hardie, R.J., Flanders, J.A., Schmidt, P. et al. (1996). Biomechanical and histological evaluation of a laparoscopic stapled gastropexy technique in dogs. *Vet. Surg.* 25: 127–133.

Imhoff, D.J., Cohen, A., and Monnet, E. (2015). Biomechanical analysis of laparoscopic incisional gastropexy with intracorporeal suturing using knotless polyglyconate. *Vet. Surg.* 44 (Suppl 1): 39–43.

Leib, M., Konde, L., Wingfield, W. et al. (1985). Circumcostal gastropexy for preventing recurrence of gastric dilatation-volvulus in the dog: an evaluation of 30 cases. *J. Am. Vet. Med. Assoc.* 187: 245–248.

MacCoy, D.M., Sykes, G.P., Hoffer, R.E. et al. (1982). A gastropexy technique for permanent fixation of the pyloric antrum. *J. Am. Anim. Hosp. Assoc.* 18: 763–768.

Mayhew, P.D. and Brown, D.C. (2009). Prospective evaluation of two intracorporeally sutured prophylactic laparoscopic gastropexy techniques compared with laparoscopic-assisted gastropexy in dogs. *Vet. Surg.* 38: 738–746.

Meyer-Lindenberg, A., Harder, A., Fehr, M. et al. (1994). Treatment of gastric dilatation-volvulus and a rapid method for prevention of relapse in dogs: 134 cases (1988–1991). *J. Am. Vet. Med. Assoc.* 203: 1303–1307.

Pratschke, K.M., Bellenger, C.R., McAllister, H. et al. (2001). Barrier pressure at the gastroesophageal junction in anesthetized dogs. *Am. J. Vet. Res.* 62: 1068–1072.

Przywara, J.F., Abel, S.B., Peacock, J.T. et al. (2014). Occurrence and recurrence of gastric dilatation volvulus with or without volvulus after incisional gastropexy. *Can. Vet. J.* 55: 981–984.

Rawlings, C.A., Foutz, T.L., Mahaffey, M.B. et al. (2001). A rapid and strong laparoscopic-assisted gastropexy in dogs. *Am. J. Vet. Res.* 62: 871–875.

Rawlings, C.A., Mahaffey, M.B., Bement, S. et al. (2002). Prospective evaluation of laparoscopic-assisted gastropexy in dogs susceptible to gastric dilatation. *J. Am. Vet. Med. Assoc.* 221: 1576–1581.

Rivier, P., Furneaux, R., and Viguier, E. (2011). Combined laparoscopic ovariectomy and laparoscopic-assisted gastropexy in dogs susceptible to gastric dilatation-volvulus. *Can. Vet. J.* 52: 62–66.

Runge, J.J., Mayhew, P., and Rawlings, C.A. (2009). Laparoscopic-assisted and laparoscopic prophylactic gastropexy: indications and techniques. *Compend. Contin. Educ. Pract. Vet.* 31: 58–65.

Spah, C., Elkins, A., Wehrenberg, A. et al. (2013). Evaluation of two novel self-anchoring barbed sutures in a prophylactic laparoscopic gastropexy compared with intracorporeal tied knots. *Vet. Surg.* 42: 932–942.

Steelman-Szymeczek, S.M., Stebbins, M.E., and Hardie, E.M. (2003). Clinical evaluation of a right-sided prophylactic gastropexy via a grid approach. *J. Am. Anim. Hosp. Assoc.* 39: 397–402.

Sutton, J.S., Steffey, M.A., Bonadio, C.M. et al. (2015). Gastric malpositioning and chronic, intermittent vomiting following prophylactic gastropexy in a 20-month-old great Dane. *Can. Vet. J.* 56: 1053–1056.

Takacs, J.D., Singh, A., Case, J.B. et al. (2017). Total laparoscopic gastropexy using 1 simple continuous barbed suture line in 63 dogs. *Vet. Surg.* 46: 233–241.

Touru, S. and Smeak, D. (2005). A practical right-sided incisional gastropexy technique for treatment and prevention of gastric dilatation volvulus. *Suomen elainlaakaarilehti* 111: 63–68.

Waschak, M. (1997). Evaluation of percutaneous gastrostomy as a technique for permanent gastropexy. *Vet. Surg.* 26: 235–241.

Whitney, W., Scavelli, T., and Matthiesen, D. (1989). Belt-loop gastropexy: technique and surgical results in 20 dogs. *J. Am. Anim. Hosp. Assoc.* 25: 75–83.

Wilson, E., Henderson, R., Montgomery, R. et al. (1996). A comparison of laparoscopic and belt-loop gastropexy in dogs. *Vet. Surg.* 25: 221–227.

Section V

Intestine

24

Enterotomy
Daniel D. Smeak

Department of Clinical Sciences, College of Veterinary Medicine and Biomedical Sciences, Colorado State University, Fort Collins, CO, USA

24.1 Indications

Enterotomies are usually performed to remove foreign bodies, obtain full-thickness samples for biopsy, and to expose the bowel lumen for passing catheters up the common bile duct.

To rule out certain generalized benign inflammatory versus neoplastic intestinal conditions, a standard 3-site biopsy protocol is recommended. Separate biopsy samples are taken of the duodenum, jejunum, and ileum. For generalized disease processes, routine biopsies of the proximal duodenum are avoided, and instead it is preferred to take samples from the duodenum distal to the right limb of the pancreas. Repair of a biopsy site dehiscence in the proximal duodenum can be difficult and problematic due to shared blood supply of the duodenum and pancreas in that area, and adjacent pancreatic and common bile ducts must be preserved. The remaining biopsies are taken at areas of the jejunum and ileum the surgeon believes are most representative of the disease process. Obvious local processes, especially if there is evidence of neoplasia, obstruction, or impending perforation, are removed entirely with excisional biopsy (resection and anastomosis – see Chapter 25).

When considering removal of small intestinal foreign bodies and the affected bowel is considered viable, the decision where an enterotomy is made can influence intestinal healing and the risk of dehiscence. Intestinal foreign bodies can be subdivided into two types, lodged and movable. Lodged foreign bodies are those that cannot be moved by digital manipulation from the affected intestinal segment. When a foreign body can be "massaged" away from the most affected intestinal region, it is considered movable. If the foreign body can be gently moved either distally into the colon or proximally in an orad direction into the stomach without causing additional trauma to the intestine, this avoids creating an enterotomy altogether and is preferred. Otherwise, a movable foreign body can be moved orad to a healthier area for enterotomy and removal. Most foreign bodies that reach the colon can be expected to pass safely without colotomy. When a foreign body is pushed back into the stomach, a gastrotomy incision is preferred over enterotomy since stomach closures heal more consistently, and rarely leak. For lodged foreign bodies, if the bowel is not discolored, and the mesenteric blood supply appears healthy, an incision can be made directly over the foreign body. Enterotomies created aborad past the leading edge of a *lodged* foreign body should be avoided. Remember, lodged foreign bodies cannot be milked distally without extending the aborad incision directly over the most acutely damaged area of bowel, the leading edge. If there is any doubt about the bowel health over the foreign body, a resection and anastomosis is recommended.

Enterotomy can only be performed if the loop of intestine is viable. If the surgeon is not confident of the viability of the affected loop of intestine, an enterectomy should be chosen (Chapter 25).

A practical and consistent means of assessing intestinal viability to determine whether to remove a damaged area of bowel or not, continues to elude veterinary surgeons. Clinical factors surgeons currently use to assess viability such as presence of peristalsis, vascular pulsations at the mesenteric border, and intestinal color do not always correlate with histological evidence of intestinal damage (Brolin et al. 1989). Bruising, intramural hemorrhage and edema may cause surgeons to overestimate the degree of bowel damage and viability (Freeman et al. 1988). In most cases, overestimation of the length

Gastrointestinal Surgical Techniques in Small Animals, First Edition. Edited by Eric Monnet and Daniel D. Smeak.
© 2020 John Wiley & Sons, Inc. Published 2020 by John Wiley & Sons, Inc.
Companion website: www.wiley.com/go/monnet/gastrointestinal

of bowel for resection rarely causes a clinical problem. However, salvaging regions of intestines that have significant damage can greatly increase the risk of life-threatening leakage and intestinal dehiscence. Therefore, surgeons are inclined to remove questionable segments of bowel as a precaution (Lanzafame et al. 1983).

When removal of extensive regions of small bowel damage is being considered and short bowel syndrome is a concern, other more objective measurements of intestinal viability may be helpful, such as fluorescein dye infusion or surface oximetry. Intravenous fluorescein dye is nontoxic to dogs at a dose of 10–15 mg/kg. When injected at the time of celiotomy, the dye rapidly distributes in tissues within minutes, and is then excreted in urine. Using a Wood's lamp to illuminate the surface of intestines in a darkened surgery room, viable bowel appears as a uniform gold-green color, indicating ample vascular supply is present (Horgan and Gorey 1992). Non-viable bowel appears as patchy areas of nonfluorescence greater than 3 mm (Freeman et al. 1988). Fluorescence is considered more of an indicator of mucosal viability than full-thickness intestinal health, since some segments of viable intestine can fail to take up the fluorescein dye if smooth muscle in the region is not active (Mann et al. 1982; Lanzafame et al. 1983). Doppler ultrasound has been found to be an unreliable test to determine viability of ischemic intestine, especially if there is mesenteric venous occlusion (Mann et al. 1982). Surface oximetry may be useful for assessment of the health of bowel in a local region. Normal pulse oximetry reading compared to peripheral oxygen saturation reliably identified viable intestine in a canine model. The electrode of this instrument measures surface oxygen tension in a limited area, though it may not be reliable for assessing viability beyond 1 cm from the test site (DeNobile et al. 1990).

24.2 Surgical Techniques

24.2.1 Intestinal Biopsy

24.2.1.1 Punch Technique

Intestinal biopsy using a Baker's biopsy punch limits the defect size of the biopsy site, so fewer sutures are required for closure. No stay suture or forceps is required to take the sample, so it is considered an easy, minimally traumatic technique. A 4 mm Baker's punch is used to remove a full-thickness circular intestinal biopsy. After isolation of the region of intestine with laparotomy pads and Doyen forceps, an antimesenteric punch biopsy is performed. The punch biopsy can be obtained via two different techniques. With Doyens placed tangentially

across the middle of the chosen bowel segment, a punch can be taken directly downward toward the mesenteric side of the bowel (Figure 24.1). Since the Doyen forceps is situated just below the antimesenteric border, the punch sample will not drop away and get lost within the bowel lumen if it falls out of the punch barrel. This technique does not require an assistant since the forceps also helps hold the bowel while the sample is taken, and contamination is contained.

For the second punch technique, the isolated bowel segment is draped over a sterile wooden tongue depressor such that the sides of the bowel lay adjacent to one another. A Baker's punch is used to take a full-thickness biopsy perpendicular to the long axis of bowel at the antimesenteric border (Figure 24.2). The surgeon

(a)

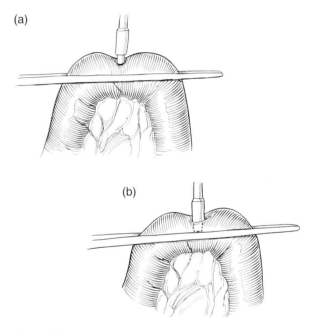

(b)

Figure 24.1

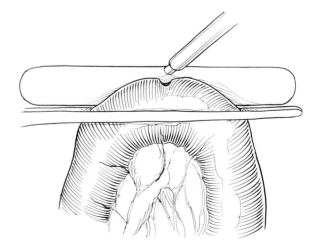

Figure 24.2

should be sure the punch barrel has included the deeper mucosal layer so that the sample taken is full-thickness. With either punch biopsy technique, the defect is closed perpendicular to the longitudinal axis of the bowel with simple interrupted sutures.

24.2.1.2 Incision Techniques

24.2.1.2.1 Longitudinal Incision Technique The chosen area for biopsy is isolated from the peritoneal cavity with multiple layers of laparotomy sponges. An atraumatic Doyen forceps isolate and block ingesta from soiling the surgery site. The Doyen forceps can be placed across the selected loop of bowel to help hold the bowel during biopsy and to contain contamination (Figure 24.3). Alternately, Doyen forceps are placed on either side of the proposed intestinal biopsy site. Using a #11

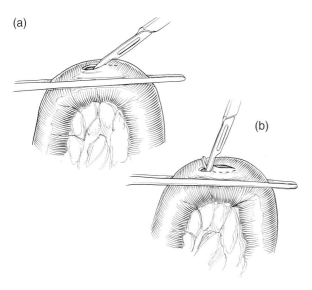

(a)

(b)

Figure 24.3

or #15 BP scalpel blade, a 0.75–1 cm longitudinal incision is made over the antimesenteric surface of the bowel. A full-thickness stay suture, oriented longitudinally, can be inserted just adjacent to the incision. While placing tension on the stay suture, a second incision is made to remove a small full-thickness elliptical sliver of intestine wall (2–3 mm wide) for biopsy. The defect is typically closed with a simple interrupted or simple continuous pattern using 4-0 monofilament absorbable suture. If there is concern that closure of the biopsy site could result in significant compromise of the lumen, the defect is closed transversely (Figure 24.4). Closure is begun with a simple interrupted suture joining adjacent corners of the linear defect. The remaining portion of the defect is closed with simple interrupted stitches to complete the transverse closure. This method can be expected to cause some buckling at the corners of the closure.

24.2.1.2.2 Transverse Incision Technique Some surgeons prefer to perform a transverse biopsy technique when bowel diameter is limited in size, for example for ferrets, small cats, and toy-breed dogs, since longitudinal biopsy/closure of even a thin biopsy defect could result in substantial lumen narrowing (Figure 24.5). A Doyen is positioned as described for the longitudinal technique. A stay suture is placed through the bowel wall perpendicular to the long axis of bowel at the antimesenteric border. Using a #15 scalpel blade, a full-thickness wedge of intestinal wall is removed by incising transversely on either side of the stay suture. This permits controlled removal of the biopsy sample without using damaging thumb forceps, and it prevents lumen narrowing during closure. The defect is closed with simple interrupted sutures.

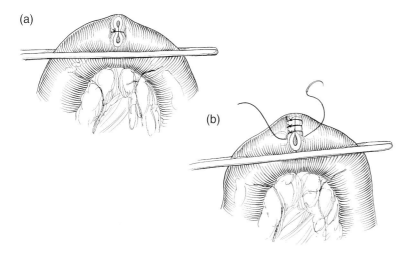

(a)

(b)

Figure 24.4

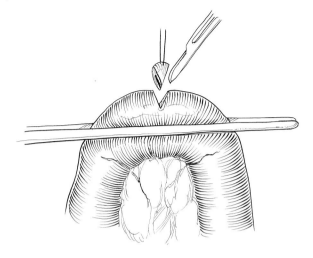

Figure 24.5

24.2.2 Enterotomy

An enterotomy is most commonly performed to remove intestinal foreign bodies. The opening is made in an area of bowel deemed healthy enough to support uncomplicated healing (see decision making for foreign body removal above) (Figure 24.6 a and b). Enterotomies can also be performed to gain access to an intraluminal mass for biopsy or excision, or for cannulation of the common bile duct.

The affected bowel is incised such that the foreign body can be removed easily without undue force, to avoid tearing the adjacent ends of the enterotomy incision. Torn intestinal margins may be difficult to close properly, and the added damage may increase the risk of dehiscence. The defect is closed with either simple interrupted or simple continuous appositional patterns using 4-0 monofilament absorbable suture with taper needles. Needle bites should include 3 mm of submucosa and are placed at intervals no greater than 3 mm. For simple continuous lines, start and end the pattern several mm outside the defect (Figure 24.6d).

Once the intestinal procedure is completed, before abdominal wall closure, surgeon's gloves are exchanged for sterile ones, and a new sterile pack is used to close the abdominal approach. Once the abdominal wall closure is completed, the subcutaneous tissues and exposed fascia are thoroughly lavaged. Subcutaneous tissue and skin are closed routinely (see Figure 24.6).

(a)

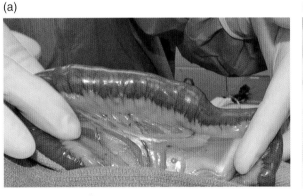

(b)

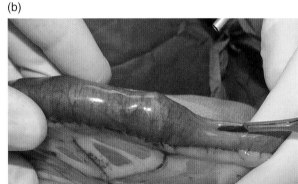

(c)

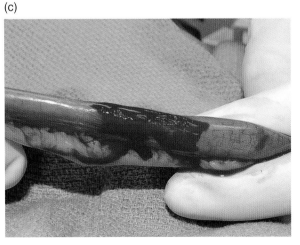

(d)

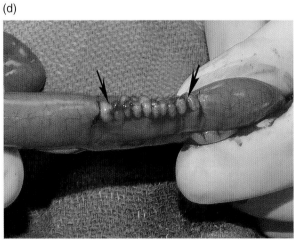

Figure 24.6

24.3 Tips

24.3.1 Leak Test

The so-called "leak test" has been recommended to assess intraoperative enteric suture and staple line security and to identify significant gaps in the closure (Pavletic and Berg 1996; Hedlund and Fossum 2007; Saile et al. 2010). Leak testing can be performed by injecting air or isotonic fluids intraluminally into an occluded intestinal segment while the suture line is observed for leaks (Saile et al. 2010). This is commonly performed after low colorectal anastomoses in humans since direct visual inspection of the entire suture or staple line within the pelvic canal is difficult. In these surgeries, the incidence of post-operative clinical and radiographic leaks has been reduced with intraoperative leak testing (Kwon et al. 2012). The canine small intestine is generally considered a low-pressure system with resting pressures falling below 4 mmHg. During peristalsis, pressures can rise to as high as 25 mmHg (34 cm H_2O) (Ellison 1993). A leak test procedure protocol has been developed to help identify significant gaps in closures of small intestinal biopsy sites without risking overexpansion. Fluid is injected within an isolated segment of bowel with an 18 gauge over-the-needle IV catheter attached to a water manometer. Either with Doyen forceps or digital occlusion isolating a 10 cm intestinal segment, it was determined that the volume of saline injected within the segment to achieve 34 cm H_2O pressure at the site of an intestinal repair was 16–19 ml with digital occlusion and 12–15 ml with the use of Doyen forceps. In cats, the volume necessary to achieve this maximal intraluminal pressure has not been determined. The author uses an arbitrary volume of 8–10 ml for leak testing in cats. If leaks are found after pressure testing and placement of additional sutures, serosal patching has been recommended (Saile et al. 2010). It can be argued that other factors besides gaps within an enteric closure are just as or even more significant in influencing dehiscence risk. Such factors as local blood supply, damage to the intestinal wall, tension, and the environment surrounding the healing intestinal repair (pre-existing contamination or peritonitis) have been shown to significantly affect intestinal healing and increase the risk of dehiscence. Furthermore, some surgeons argue that leak testing may produce a false sense of anastomotic integrity while others worry that the test may produce false positive results or even weaken the repair (Bruce et al. 2001).

Whether or not routine enteric leak testing will be shown to help reduce the risk of enteric dehiscence rates in small animal surgery remains to be determined. In the author's opinion, when inspection of the entire surgical repair site is challenging, or when gaping between sutures is a concern, leak testing may be considered.

24.3.2 Reinforcement of an Enterotomy

See Chapter 25 for the description of omentalization and serosal patching to reinforce an enterotomy.

24.4 Post-Operative Complications and Outcome

Complications following enterotomy closure include suture line dehiscence, peritonitis, adhesions, surgical site infections, and ileus (Pavletic and Berg 1996). Dehiscence after enterotomy closure is reported to occur in a range of 7–16% (Allen et al. 1992; Ralphs et al. 2003; Mouat et al. 2014). The reported incidence of dehiscence after intestinal biopsy is up to 11% (Harvey 1990; Shales et al. 2005; Smith et al. 2011). Cats appear to have a lower risk of dehiscence overall after intestinal anastomosis or biopsy compared to dogs (Ralphs et al. 2003; Smith et al. 2011). Many factors have been implicated in increasing risk of intestinal dehiscence including hypoalbuminemia, hypotension, use of blood products, longer length of bowel resected, and delayed enteral feeding post-operatively (Giuffrida and Brown 2018). The presence of pre-existing peritonitis is one of the most important risk factors in small animals (Allen et al. 1992; Ralphs et al. 2003; Giuffrida and Brown 2018); About 50% of dogs and cats die following intestinal dehiscence and septic peritonitis (Adams et al. 2010, 2014). Likely, this fatality rate is influenced by a high euthanasia rate because of the poor prognosis and expense related to post-operative treatment, and the high risk of complications.

Dogs and cats possess an active fibrinolytic system within their abdominal cavity that generally reduces the rate of significant adhesion formation after laparotomy. Adhesions form when there is a combination of the following factors: ischemia, hemorrhage, aggressive foreign body reaction, and severe inflammation and infection. Atraumatic tissue handling, keeping intra-abdominal tissues moist, strict asepsis, and hemostasis may minimize adhesion formation.

References

Adams, R.J., Doyle, R.S., Bray, J.P. et al. (2014). Closed suction drainage for treatment of septic peritonitis of confirmed gastrointestinal origin in 20 dogs. *Vet. Surg.* 43: 843–851.

Adams, W.M., Sisterman, L.A., Klauer, J.M. et al. (2010). Association of intestinal disorders in cats with findings of abdominal radiography. *J. Am. Vet. Med. Assoc.* 236: 880–886.

Allen, D.A., Smeak, D.D., and Schertel, E.R. (1992). Prevalence of small intestinal dehiscence and associated clinical factors: a retrospective study of 121 dogs. *J. Am. Anim. Hosp. Assoc.* 28: 70–76.

Brolin, R.E., Semmlow, J.L., Sehonanda, A. et al. (1989). Comparison of five methods of assessment of intestinal viability. *Surg Gynecol Obstet* 168: 6–12.

Bruce, J., Krukowski, Z., HAl-Khairy, G. et al. (2001). Systematic review of the definition and measurement of anastomotic leak after gastrointestinal surgery. *Br. J. Surg.* 88: 1157–1168.

DeNobile, J., Guzzetta, P., and Patterson, K. (1990). Pulse oximetry as a means of assessing bowel viability. *J. Surg. Res.* 48: 21–23.

Ellison, G.W. (1993). Intestinal obstruction. In: Disease Mechanisms in Small Animal Surgery, 2e (eds. M.J. Bojrab, D.D. Smeak and M.S. Bloomberg), 252–261. Philadelphia: Lea and Febiger.

Freeman, D.E., Gentile, D.G., Richardson, D.W. et al. (1988). Comparison of clinical judgment: Doppler ultrasound, and fluorescein fluorescence as methods for predicting intestinal viability in the pony. *Am. J. Vet. Res.* 49: 895–900.

Giuffrida, M.A. and Brown, D.C. (2018). Small intestine. In: Veterinary Surgery Small Animal (eds. S.A. Johnston and K.M. Tobias), 1730–1761. St. Louis: Elsevier.

Harvey, H.J. (1990). Complications of small intestinal biopsy in hypoalbuminemic dogs. *Vet. Surg.* 19: 289–292.

Hedlund, C.S. and Fossum, T.W. (2007). Surgery of the digestive system. In: Small Animal Surgery (ed. T.W. Fossum), 339–530. St. Louis: Mosby.

Horgan, P.G. and Gorey, T.F. (1992). Operative assessment of intestinal viability. *Surg. Clin. North Am.* 72: 143–155.

Kwon, S., Morris, A., Billingham, R. et al. (2012). Routine leak testing in colorectal surgery in the surgical care and outcomes assessment program. *Arch. Surg.* 147: 345–351.

Lanzafame, R.J., Naim, J.O., Tomkiewicz, Z.M. et al. (1983). The accuracy of predicting intestinal viability with fluorescein: experimental observations. *Curr. Surg.* 40: 292–294.

Mann, A., Fazio, V.W., and Lucas, F.V. (1982). A comparative study of the use of fluorescein and the Doppler device in the determination of intestinal viability. *Surg. Gynecol. Obstet.* 154: 53–55.

Mouat, E.E., Davis, G.J., Drobatz, K.J. et al. (2014). Evaluation of data from 35 dogs pertaining to dehiscence following intestinal resection and anastomosis. *J. Am. Anim. Hosp. Assoc.* 50: 254–263.

Pavletic, M.M. and Berg, J. (1996). Gastrointestinal surgery. In: Complications in Small Animal Surgery (eds. A.J. Lipowitz, D.D. Caywood, et al.), 365–398. Baltimore: Williams & Wilkins.

Ralphs, S.C., Jessen, C.R., and Lipowitz, A.J. (2003). Risk factors for leakage following intestinal anastomosis in dogs and cats: 115 cases (1991–2000). *J. Am. Vet. Med. Assoc.* 223: 73–77.

Saile, K.S., Boothe, H.W., and Boothe, D.M. (2010). Saline volume necessary to achieve predetermined intraluminal pressures during leak testing in small intestinal biopsy sites in the dog. *Vet. Surg.* 39: 900–903.

Shales, C.J., Warren, J., Anderson, D.M. et al. (2005). Complications following full-thickness small intestinal biopsy in 66 dogs: a retrospective study. *J. Small Anim. Pract.* 46: 317–321.

Smith, A.L., Wilson, A.P., Hardie, R.J. et al. (2011). Perioperative complications after full-thickness gastrointestinal surgery in cats with alimentary lymphoma. *Vet. Surg.* 40: 849–852.

25

Enterectomy

Daniel D. Smeak and Eric Monnet

Department of Clinical Sciences, College of Veterinary Medicine and Biomedical Sciences, Colorado State University, Fort Collins, CO, USA

25.1 Indications

The indications for intestinal resection and anastomosis include devitalization, irresolvable obstruction or dysfunction, and irreparable perforation. These conditions may be caused by foreign bodies, neoplasia, abscess, granuloma, trauma, intussusception, volvulus or torsion, herniation/strangulation, neurological disorders, ulceration/perforation caused by non-steroidal anti-inflammatory drug and corticosteroid administration, and rare congenital malformations (Weisman et al. 1999; Ralphs et al. 2003; Giuffrida and Brown 2018).

When considering removal of small intestinal foreign bodies and the affected bowel is considered non-viable, an enterectomy is recommended (see Chapter 24 for assessing intestinal viability).

25.2 Surgical Techniques

Following complete exploration of the abdomen, the diseased segment of bowel is identified and isolated from the abdominal cavity and adjoining viscera with moistened laparotomy sponges. If the diseased intestinal segment is freely mobile, it should be gently pulled out and exteriorized from the abdomen (Figure 25.1).

The disease segment is first isolated with crushing forceps such as Allen intestinal forceps or Carmalt forceps taking appropriate margins of healthy adjacent bowel. The crushing clamps are placed at an angle no more than 60° from the long axis of the segment, so the remaining bowel ends are longer on the mesenteric border than the opposite margin (Figure 25.2).

Blood vessels to the affected segment are ligated and divided, including connecting arcades in the mesenteric border of the intestine. The mesentery is incised, leaving as much of mesentery as possible alongside adjacent arcade vessels so that the thin sheets can be sutured closed after completing the anastomosis without damaging these vessels. Intestinal contents are milked well away proximally and distally from the proposed transection sites and contained with atraumatic intestinal forceps (Doyens) or an assistant's fingers (Figure 25.3).

If there is disparity between luminal diameters between intended bowel ends to be anastomosed, there are several methods to create similar bowel end diameters. For minimal luminal disparity, sutures on the larger diameter side of bowel are spaced slightly further apart than those on the smaller side. Spacing of sutures should not exceed 3 mm as a general rule. For greater luminal disparity, the smaller lumen end can be transected at a greater angle. Caution should be exercised when transecting the smaller segment at an acute angle because this makes closure of the mesenteric margin difficult. In this situation, the acutely sloped mesenteric margin of the smaller segment is "pointed" in shape and obtaining adequate needle purchase in this tip to appose with the opposite mesenteric margin of bowel is troublesome. Alternately, the author prefers to incise the antimesenteric border longitudinally to create a larger spatulated opening on the smaller side to match the opposing larger bowel margin (Figure 25.4). The resulting angled margins may be trimmed to create a smooth ovoid-shaped larger stoma. For marked luminal size differences, the larger segment diameter can be reduced by interrupted sutures placed from the antimesenteric side. Once the lumen sizes are approximately the same, anastomosis is performed routinely. The author generally avoids this technique since the region where the interrupted suture line meets the

Gastrointestinal Surgical Techniques in Small Animals, First Edition. Edited by Eric Monnet and Daniel D. Smeak.
Companion website: www.wiley.com/go/monnet/gastrointestinal

(a)

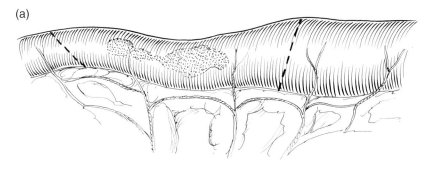

(b)

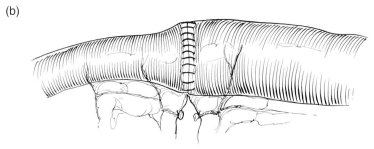

Figure 25.1

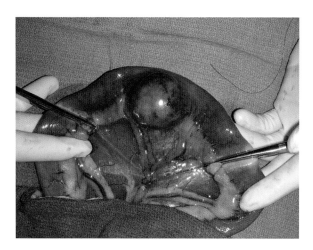

Figure 25.2

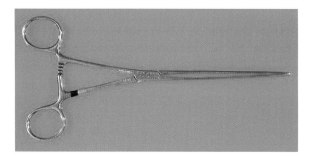

Figure 25.3

circular line can be difficult to create a leak-proof seal. An end-to-side anastomosis can also be performed. The larger segment is closed with a simple continuous suture, and the small segment is anastomosed on the

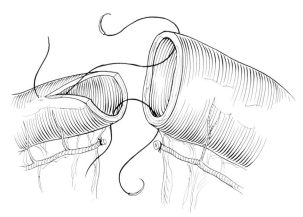

Figure 25.4

antimesenteric side of the larger segment. The anastomosis is performed 2–3 cm from the closed end of the larger segment (Figure 25.5).

25.2.1 Hand-Sewn Anastomosis

A hand-sewn, single-layer, simple interrupted apposition suture pattern is frequently used for end-to-end anastomosis in small animals because it produces minimal stenosis and leakage and heals rapidly (Jansen et al. 1981).

The surgeon must be confident that 3 mm of submucosa has been included in the needle purchases during intestinal closure. Alternatively, particularly when the mesentery adjacent to the bowel filled with thick fat, three preplaced interrupted sutures (with the ears left

(a)

(b)

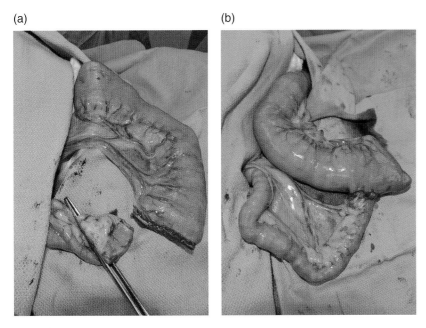

Figure 25.5

(a)

(b)

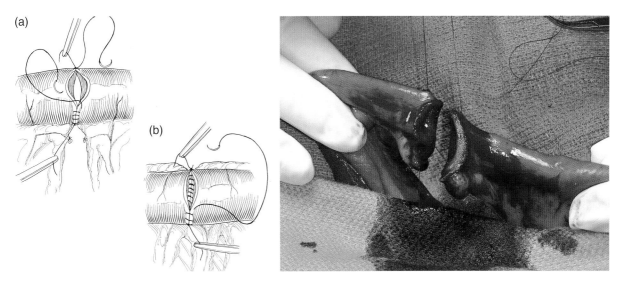

Figure 25.6

long to use as stay sutures) are inserted in the mesenteric side to reduce the risk of leaving gaps between the mesenteric sutures due to poor visualization. An opposing suture is placed on the antimesenteric side. Tension between the mesenteric and antimesenteric stay sutures helps with needle passage and consistent suture placement while avoiding excessive handling of the bowel with thumb forceps. Interrupted sutures, equally spaced approximately 3 mm apart, are used to close the remaining margins between the tensioned stay sutures.

Anastomoses have also been shown to be equally successful when performed with a continuous suture pattern (Weisman et al. 1999). Two separate monofilament absorbable sutures with taper needle are placed at the mesenteric and antimesenteric borders and are tied (Figure 25.6). One end of each knot ear is left at least 5–7 cm long to function as a stay suture. With firm tension maintained between the stay sutures held by an assistant, the opposing bowel walls are closed in a simple continuous suture pattern with full-thickness 3 mm bites spaced approximately 3 mm apart. Care is taken to keep firm constant tension on the suture line throughout the continuous pattern to avoid inadvertent gapping from unevenly tensioned areas. The continuous line can be either knotted to the stay suture at the opposite end of the pattern or the line completed with a separate penultimate loop-to-strand knot. The other side is completed in the opposite direction and knotted similarly (Figure 25.6 and 25.7).

Complications have been reported in several dogs when a circumferential continuous pattern was employed using *nonabsorbable* suture (polypropylene) for intestinal anastomosis. In these cases, the continuous suture line apparently broke over time within the lumen but remained anchored to the bowel, acting as a site for foreign body attachment, causing partial bowel obstruction (Milovancev et al. 2004). Therefore, when continuous patterns are used in bowel, an absorbable suture should be chosen.

Ideally minimal to no mucosa should be exposed after hand-sewn anastomosis. Excess mucosal eversion in an anastomosis increases the risk of both adhesion formation and leakage (Thompson et al. 2006). To reduce mucosal eversion during anastomosis, several methods have been described in the literature. When bowel ends have substantial eversion, the excess mucosa can simply be trimmed with sharp Metzenbaum scissors (Figure 25.8). Additionally, two suture insertion techniques have been described to help reduce mucosal eversion: the Gambee and modified Gambee stitch. Each technique can be utilized with both simple interrupted and simple continuous anastomosis patterns. The Gambee pattern has been shown to provide a more leak-proof closure than other suture patterns when performed by experienced surgeons (Kieves et al. 2014). With the Gambee technique, the needle is passed directly into the lumen 3 mm from the incised serosal, not mucosal, edge. The needle is slightly backed up and

passed up out from the lumen through the incised ipsilateral everted mucosal edge. The needle is re-established on the needle holders, and, on the opposing side, the needle is inserted beginning at the cut edge of the mucosa toward the lumen. Friction from the needle helps "push" the everted mucosa back into the lumen. Once this occurs, the needle is redirected to exit the intestinal wall with a full-thickness 3 mm bite (Figure 25.9a). Because the needle bites are full thickness with the Gambee technique, an adequate bite of submucosa is assured. For the modified Gambee technique (Figure 25.9b), the needle is inserted partial thickness through the intestine at least 3 mm from the edge of the incised serosal edge, through the muscularis and submucosa. It is highly important to feel the resistance to needle passage as it purchases the submucosa. The needle is passed parallel through the bowel wall to emerge between the submucosa and everted mucosa. Next, the needle is inserted into the opposing bowel wall at the mucosa–submucosa junction, catching the tougher submucosa, and then up through the muscularis and serosa to complete the 3 mm needle bite (Figure 25.9b). Since the modified Gambee stitch is partial thickness, care must be taken to assure enough submucosa has been incorporated in each bite. In an effort to avoid mucosal eversion, there is risk that novice surgeons may unintentionally miss achieving an adequate purchase of the submucosal layer. This renders the anastomosis at risk for premature tissue cut-out (Kieves et al. 2014). It should be the surgeon's highest priority during intestinal repair to include adequate purchase of submucosa for a reliably strong repair, instead of focusing more on avoiding mucosal eversion. In many cases it takes several Gambee or modified Gambee needle passes to eliminate mucosal eversion, after which

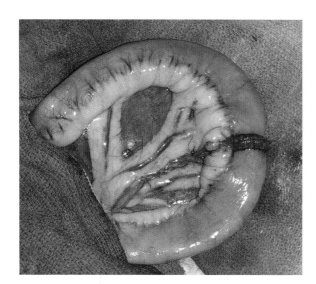

Figure 25.7

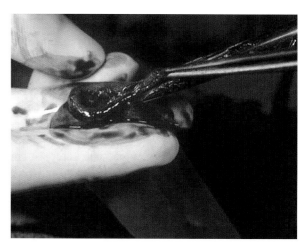

Figure 25.8

(a)

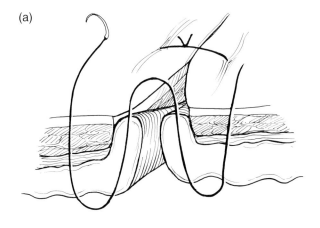

(b)

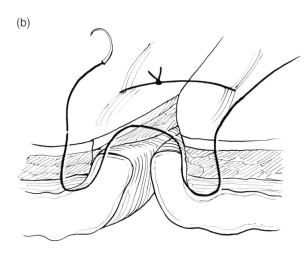

Figure 25.9

subsequent intestinal wall bites can be placed with a simple forehand, full-thickness, needle insertion technique. Suture bites should be firmly tensioned just enough to correct eversion. Once the stitch has been placed, the greater curvature of the needle can be used to "push down" on any mucosa that is still everted while the suture stitch is tensioned.

25.2.2 Anastomosis Using a Skin Stapler

Skin staplers have been used experimentally and clinically in dogs and humans to create technically simple and rapid end-to-end anastomoses. Up until the repair is begun, isolation and preparation of the bowel ends are similar to the description of the hand-sewn anastomosis. Starting at the mesenteric region, three full-thickness stay sutures are placed equidistant to one another around the circumference of the bowel ends (Figure 25.10).

An assistant gently places traction on the bowel between two stay sutures, and a regular-size skin stapler is used to place staples about 3 mm apart. Everted mucosa is gently pushed into the lumen with DeBakey thumb forceps during stapling. The procedure is repeated between the remaining adjacent stay sutures. The stapled anastomosis is complete when all quadrants of the intestinal edges are stapled closed. Skin stapled anastomoses are equivalent in bursting strength, lumen diameter, and quality of healing when compared to traditional hand-sewn repairs and can be completed significantly faster (Coolman et al. 2000). In a recent retrospective study, use of disposable skin staples in 63 dogs for intestinal anastomosis had an overall mortality rate similar to previous studies using hand-sewn techniques and a favorable dehiscence rate of 4.8% (Rosenbaum et al. 2016). In another prospective study, 2 of 14 dogs died of causes unrelated to the staple line; one dog developed a colonic stricture four weeks after surgery. There was no evidence of dehiscence in this series of dogs (Benlloch-Gonzalez et al. 2015).

25.2.3 Functional End-to-End Anastomosis (FEEA) with Stapling Equipment: Open Technique

Mechanical linear staplers offer a rapid and consistent means of intestinal anastomosis, so this method is often chosen in unstable patients or those with pre-existing peritonitis. The most commonly used linear stapling technique in small animal surgery is called FEEA (Ullman et al. 1991; Ullman 1994). The open technique described hereafter is generally preferred because it is easy and uncomplicated, requires only two staple cartridges, and does not cause any appreciable lumen compromise (Ullman et al. 1991). Linear stapling for anastomosis also minimizes the amount of bowel manipulation and potential for local contamination (White 2008). In addition, linear stapling permits anastomoses of two portions of bowel with considerable differences in diameter.

After routine resection of the damaged bowel, the two ends to be anastomosed are placed side-by-side. Monofilament 4-0 stay sutures are placed connecting the mesenteric and antimesenteric sides of the bowel ends (not shown in illustration). One limb of the GIA 60 stapler 3.8 mm is fully inserted into each intestinal lumen aided by traction on the stay sutures (Figure 25.11a). Staples can be fired between either the antimesenteric or lateral sides of the bowel walls. In any case, the mesenteric blood supply should not be included or damaged at the region of stapler cartridge compression. The stapler is compressed, locked, and fired. Four staggered rows of staples are released, and a

(a)

(b)

(c)

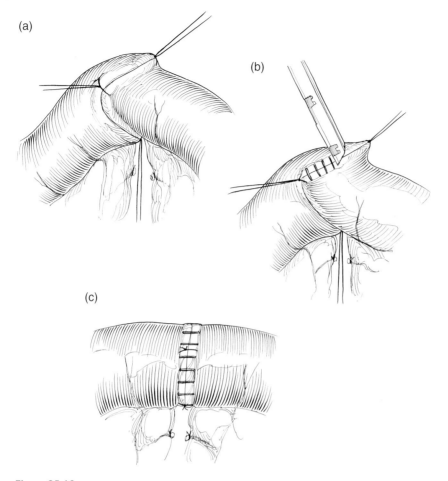

Figure 25.10

blade cuts between the two central rows of staples to create a stoma. The GIA stapler is released, and either a TA 3.5 mm or GIA instrument armed with 3.8 mm cartridges (60 mm length for smaller animals, 80 mm length for larger dogs) is placed transversely across the common intestinal opening. Before compression, the two initial GIA staple lines are offset such that the stoma is held open and only one staple line is included in the transverse staple line (Figure 25.11b and c). Stacking the initial GIA lines together when firing the transverse line is avoided, as this can increase the risk of leakage in those areas (Hansen and Smeak 2015). The transverse staple line is carefully inspected to be sure there is a uniform fringe of tissue extending several millimeters past the entire staple line. Excess tissue is removed with Mayo scissors for the TA staple line, or the GIA instrument will cut the line automatically. An anchoring suture (3-0 monofilament absorbable) is placed at the base or "crotch" of the GIA staple line to reinforce the terminal portion of initial GIA staple line (Figure 25.11c).

The anastomosis site should be inspected to ensure proper staple placement, which is dependent on passage of the staple fully through both layers of adjacent intestinal wall, and consistent closure of the B-shaped staple on the opposite tissue edge. The terminal end of the FEEA does not require oversewing with suture.

Dehiscence rates with linear staplers are similar to retrospective studies of hand-sewn anastomoses (Duell et al. 2016; Snowdon et al. 2016). Inflammatory bowel disease, anastomoses that connect small to large bowel, and intraoperative hypotension were risk factors for staple line dehiscence in one study (Snowdon et al. 2016). Increased thickening of bowel from inflammation and edema, or inflammatory bowel disease could have caused inconsistent engagement of staples or ischemic injury from over-compression of tissue within the anvil of the staple cartridge (Snowdon et al. 2016). Interestingly, stapling in the presence of septic peritonitis did not increase the risk of leakage in this case series. In another study, the researchers found no difference in the frequency of dehiscence between hand-sutured and stapled intestinal anastomosis, but stapling did reduce surgery duration (Chassin et al. 1978; Duell et al. 2016).

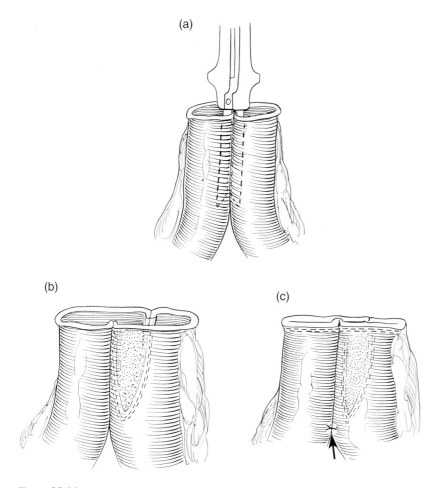

(a)

(b)

(c)

Figure 25.11

25.2.4 One-Stage FEEA

This technique requires less manipulation, and it is currently the preferred method of stapled anastomosis in human enteric surgery. It has been shown to be a fast and safe procedure even in the hands of non-expert but trained veterinarians (Jardel et al. 2011).

Mesenteric vessels supplying the segment to be resected are routinely ligated. The diseased intestinal loop is manipulated into a loop and crushing Carmalt forceps are placed across the base at the level of the planned resection (Figure 25.12). The two segments of intestine to be anastomosed are aligned side-by-side, apposing serosal surfaces without including vasculature in the mesenteric attachments. A Doyen atraumatic forceps is placed at least 8–10 cm away from the proposed resection site to reduce contamination during the stapling process. Stab incisions are made at the antimesenteric border of each intestinal segment beneath the isolated loop to allow full insertion of the two arms of the GIA (blue 3.8, 60 mm) cartridge (Figure 25.12a and b). The stapler is fired, and the staple line is inspected as

described previously. The surgeon should ensure that no mesentery is included in the staple line. The common lumen of the intestine is closed with a TA (blue 3.5 60- or 80-mm cartridge) stapling device placed transversely across the proposed excision line beneath the stab incisions (Figure 25.13a). Alternately, a GIA stapler (blue 3.8 cartridge) can be used to close the transverse line. A scalpel blade or scissors is used to resect the diseased loop using the device as a template (Figure 25.13b). There is no need to oversew the staple line (Jardel et al. 2011). A simple interrupted suture is again placed at the weak terminal aspect of the GIA line to bolster that area (Figure 25.13b).

With all anastomosis techniques, the mesenteric rent created during the anastomosis technique is closed with either simple interrupted or simple continuous suture pattern. Monofilament 4-0 suture material is used with taper needles (Figure 25.7). It is not important to create a water-tight seal, rather the mesentery is closed with no gapping, which could result in intestines migrating through the defect to become entrapped, obstructed, or

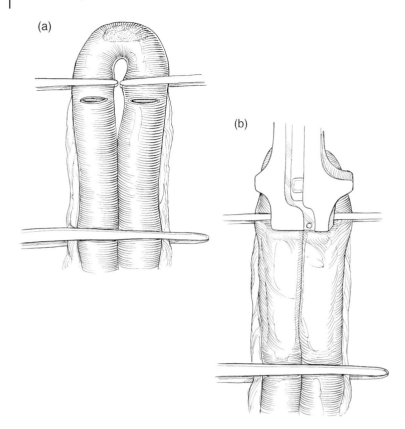

(a)

(b)

Figure 25.12

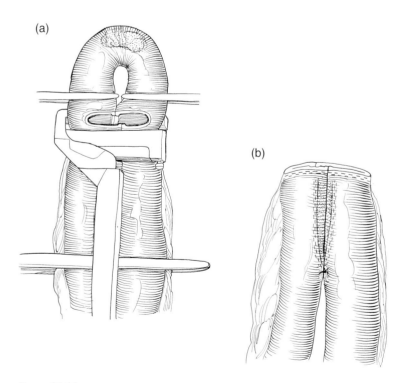

(a)

(b)

Figure 25.13

strangulated. Care is taken to avoid incorporating adjacent blood vessels within the mesenteric suture line.

Once the intestinal procedure is completed, before abdominal wall closure, surgeon's gloves are exchanged for sterile ones, and a new sterile pack is used to close the abdominal approach. Once the abdominal wall closure is completed, the subcutaneous tissues and exposed fascia are thoroughly lavaged. Subcutaneous tissue and skin are closed routinely.

25.3 Tips

25.3.1 Anatomical Considerations

25.3.1.1 Duodenum

The duodenum is relatively fixed in the abdominal cavity by a short mesentery and the duodenocolic ligament at the initial portion of the ascending duodenum. This ligament is important, since it is a common area of perforations from linear foreign bodies in dogs and cats and therefore must be examined carefully during abdominal exploration. Careful incision in the ventral-most firm band region of this ligament is safe and necessary when contemplating intestinal resection of a lesion in this region. Resection should continue along the antimesenteric attachment of the ligament directly adjacent to the ascending duodenum wall to avoid the interruption of vasculature to the colon or duodenum.

In the first 5 cm of the proximal duodenum, vital openings of the common bile duct and pancreatic ducts are found, and preservation of these structures are considered during surgical decision making for lesions in this region. Unless absolutely necessary, resection of the proximal duodenum is avoided, since aggressive and complicated "re-routing" procedures are required. Techniques to "patch" perforations (see serosal patch technique) or methods to bypass obstructive lesions in this region may be viable options in select cases.

25.3.1.2 Vasculature of the Intestine

Mesenteric artery and vein branches anastomose with each other in a series of arcades, and short vasa recta extend directly into the intestinal wall. Vasa recta bifurcate within the intestinal wall and extend on either side of the intestine to nourish the serosa and deeper layers of the wall. It is important to realize that there are relatively few longitudinal connections within the intestinal wall between these transversely oriented vasa recta vessels. Therefore, preservation of all vasa recti entering adjacent to the preserved ends of intestine after resection is important to ensure adequate perfusion of these ends during anastomosis.

25.3.2 Handling of Tissue

The author prefers using stay sutures to help manipulate and place tension on the bowel ends to facilitate accurate suture placement during anastomosis and help avoid using thumb forceps on the bowel edges. Intestinal ends are first apposed with two separate interrupted sutures connecting the antimesenteric and mesenteric borders. These first sutures are tied firmly, and the knot ears are left long to be used as stay sutures. Traction is placed between the stay sutures to pull the bowel ends together and help reduce excess mucosal eversion. In addition, the ends are held under some tension, which aids in needle passage and consistent suture spacing.

25.3.3 Utilization of Linear Stapler/ Staple Size

The author prefers to tack omentum over the everted transverse staple line after local lavage (Ullman 1994). When stapling grossly thickened or edematous intestinal walls use caution when choosing your linear staple size since this can increase the risk of poor staple purchase. In this instance, either choose a larger green cartridge (4.8 mm) for the transverse line, or the author prefers to hand-sew the open ends in a simple continuous pattern.

If the arms of the GIA device are too large to insert in the bowel lumen (common in toy-breed dogs and cats), an endoscopic linear cutting stapler (Endo GIA blue cartridge 3.5 mm) can be used in a manner similar to the standard GIA device description.

25.3.4 Suture Line Reinforcement

The omentum (omentalization) or an adjacent serosal-covered surface (serosal patch) can be used to reinforce an enterectomy or an enterotomy. The serosal patch technique can also be used to seal a defect in a hollow organ.

25.3.4.1 Omentalization

The omentum is a mesothelial membrane that has extensive vascular and lymphatic supply and exhibits angiogenic, immunogenic, and adhesive properties that can assist in restoring blood supply to ischemic tissue, controlling infection, and establishing lymphatic drainage (McLachlin and Denton 1973; Katsikas et al. 1977; Hosgood 1990). There is experimental evidence that the presence of viable omentum in contact with an enterotomy or anastomosis is important in reducing the risk of dehiscence. When intestinal anastomoses were wrapped in plastic sheeting to prevent the omentum from adhering to the repair, leakage and fatal septic peritonitis resulted. Vascularized omental wrapping provided significant protection against leakage when it was used to cover an avascular small bowel anastomosis (McLachlin and Denton 1973). In the same experiment, free (blood supply severed) omental wrapping was significantly less effective at preventing leakage. The free omentum did not adhere to the avascular intestine and became necrotic, offering no protection against leakage. In a rat model, omental wraps were shown to protect a compromised anastomosis by providing a biologically viable plug to prevent early leakage, and a source of granulation tissue and neovascularization for later wound repair (Adams et al. 1992). Since neovascularization from omentum provides significant bowel perfusion only after five days, leakage may occur before adequate neovascularization develops at areas of ischemic intestine (Enestvedt et al. 2006).

There is ample evidence in experimental studies to advocate routine use of omentum to prevent intestinal dehiscence, although its clinical efficacy remains unclear (Merad et al. 1998). In large human clinical studies, use of omentum to cover colorectal anastomoses after anterior resection for rectal cancer did not affect the incidence of anastomotic disruption, but it seemed to help contain the severity of the anastomotic leakage (Merad et al. 1998; Tocchi et al. 2000; Peeters et al. 2005). In another human study of 126 patients, anastomoses with omentoplasty had significantly less leakage, repeat operations, and mortality than those that did not have omentoplasty (Agnifili et al. 2004). Wrapping the anastomosis with omentum has been shown to reduce enterocutaneous fistula formation in humans, but it does not improve dehiscence rates (Galie and Whitlow 2006). Since it appears that covering the site of intestinal repair with healthy omentum does no harm and may have beneficial effects, and it does not appreciably prolong the surgical procedure, many surgeons choose to routinely perform omentoplasty after intestinal repair. Others argue that healthy omentum passively finds its way to areas of inflammation (Rothenberg and Rosenblatt 1942), so there is no need to surgically fix the omentum to an intestinal repair (Wilkie 1911).

A healthy vascularized segment of greater omentum is freed up, and the 2-ply sheet is draped over the anastomosis or enterotomy and tacked to the antimesenteric side of the intestines with a 4-0 monofilament absorbable suture, 3–5 cm orad and aborad to the site (Figure 25.14).

As an alternative, similar to the above draping procedure, following repair of an enterotomy or anastomosis,

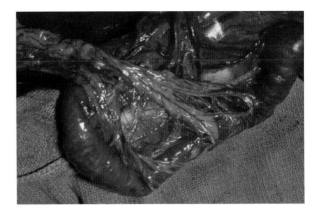

Figure 25.14

a 2-ply portion of the healthy greater omentum is freed up, and it is drawn through the mesenteric rent and loosely wrapped entirely (360°) around the circumference of the bowel. The terminal end of the omentum is tacked to the base of the omental flap and around the mesenteric margins being careful not to disturb blood supply to the repair site or omental flap (Weisman et al. 1999). Monofilament absorbable sutures (4-0) are placed approximately 1 cm apart, so there is no pathway for intestines to pass through the mesentery and become obstructed. At this time, there is no proof this technique reduces overall leak rates, but the author prefers this technique during intestinal anastomosis since it provides omental contact with the entire circumference of the repair, including the precarious mesenteric region.

25.3.4.2 Serosal Patch

Use of healthy adjacent serosal-covered tissue such as intestine or abdominal wall as a means of mechanical reinforcement of conventional suture or staple closure of a hollow organ, or as a primary means of patching open (unsutured) full-thickness defects has been termed "serosal patching." The serosal "patch" may help reduce the risk of dehiscence, since it helps provide a fibrin seal, increases resistance to leakage, and contributes additional blood supply to the damaged area (Hansen and Monnet 2013; Radlinsky 2013). The procedure was first described as a viable option for repairing large proximal duodenal perforations when primary closure would compromise the lumen (Kobald and Thal 1963). The antimesenteric border of the jejunum is most commonly used for serosal patching because of its long mesentery which allows its transposition literally anywhere in the peritoneal cavity. Other serosal-covered organs, such as the stomach or colon, can also be used provided the patch is directly adjacent to the defect so it can be sutured without tension

(Crowe 1984; Pozzi et al. 2006). The bladder has also been used clinically for serosal patching (Hosseini et al. 2009; Radlinsky 2013). When repair of hollow organ defects by conventional closure is challenging, serosal patching has been reported to be quite useful. It has been successfully used to repair intestinal perforations caused by bite wounds and gunshots, managing pyloroplasty dehiscence, and for buttressing repairs of the bowel, stomach, urinary bladder, colon, pancreas, uterus, and diaphragm (Jones et al. 1973; Crowe 1990; Pozzi et al. 2006). In an in vitro study, anastomoses supplemented with a serosal patch were able to sustain significantly higher leakage pressure than unsupplemented anastomoses (Hansen and Monnet 2013). However, in a clinical study, the efficacy of jejunal serosal patching to help reduce intestinal dehiscence in dogs with pre-existing septic peritonitis has been challenged (Grimes et al. 2011). In this retrospective study, there was no clear protective effect of serosal patching on either post-operative septic peritonitis or survival.

The use of omentum as a serosal sealing agent can be effective in many cases, but its use as a mechanical patch is limited because it is more likely to leak with increasing intraluminal pressure (Crowe 1984). In contrast to a serosal patch, using omentum for patching a defect will not reduce the risk of future defect contraction causing partial obstruction (Camp et al. 1968). In an experimental study comparing omentum versus jejunal serosal patches for repairing large open duodenal perforations, there was no evidence of leakage or obstruction with serosal patching, but one-third of the omental patches leaked, and half developed outflow obstruction (Isbell and Maher 1986). In another classic experimental study, the incidence of perforation or loosening of layered omental patches and the late development of strictures at the patch site made omentum unsatisfactory as a patching material in dogs. In contrast, results using jejunum to patch large duodenal defects were uniformly good (Camp et al. 1968). Therefore, when mechanical patching over a defect is important, serosal patches are recommended over using omentum.

Serosal patching is most useful when resection and anastomosis of a lesion would be difficult and complicated, and debridement and conventional hollow organ closure is likely to compromise the lumen, such as when large defects are encountered in the proximal duodenum. Serosal patches may also be used as an "insurance measure" in attempting repair of lesions involving the gastrointestinal tract with questionable viability or integrity, especially in the absence of healthy omentum. In addition, this technique may also be utilized under conditions when intestinal repair has greater risk of dehiscence, such as patients with pre-existing septic peritonitis, debilitated animals or those with significant hypoalbuminemia (Crowe 1990; Allen et al. 1992; Ralphs et al. 2003).

25.3.4.2.1 Serosal Patching Over Enterotomy Closure or Defect

Atraumatic intestinal clamps or an assistant's fingers are used during the procedure to prevent accidental contamination from ingesta leaking out of the defect. Devitalized edges of the perforation are carefully debrided. Use of adjacent jejunum to cover the unsutured defect will create a leak-proof patch and a surface, which will allow mucosa to cover the exposed serosa of the intestinal patch (Figure 25.15). Depending on the size of the defect, the defect will cover with healthy duodenal mucosa within three to eight weeks and will not contract substantially. A gently looped segment of healthy jejunum is laid longitudinally adjacent to the duodenal perforation.

A seromuscular stay suture is placed between the jejunum and duodenum orad and aborad about 5 mm from the defect (Figure 25.15b). This stay suture will keep the intestinal loops aligned during suture closure. The suture line is planned so the jejunal area for the patch will cover the defect without incorporating the mesenteric blood supply of either intestinal segment. The antimesenteric region of the jejunal patch should cover the center of the defect or closure line. Using a continuous or simple interrupted pattern, the lateral side of the jejunum is sutured to the deep side of the duodenum. In a similar fashion, the "near" side of the jejunal patch is closed over the opposite side of the defect (Figures 25.15c and 25.16).

25.3.4.2.2 Serosal Patching for Bowel Anastomosis

An intestinal anastomosis can be patched using the antimesenteric aspect of one or more adjacent healthy intestinal loops (Figures 25.17–25.19). The author prefers to use a single section of intestine laid perpendicular to the axis of the repaired intestinal segment for serosal patching (Figure 25.17). The jejunum is looped gently around the anastomosis line such that there is no kink that could cause an obstruction. Starting close to the mesenteric margin of the anastomosis parallel and 1 cm away from the anastomosis suture line, seromuscular bites are taken between the jejunum (patch) and the intestinal wall adjacent to the anastomosis. Seromuscular bites should be grasped 5 mm from the incision line, and care is taken to avoid catching the intestinal wall on the far side, which could cause an obstruction. Sutures

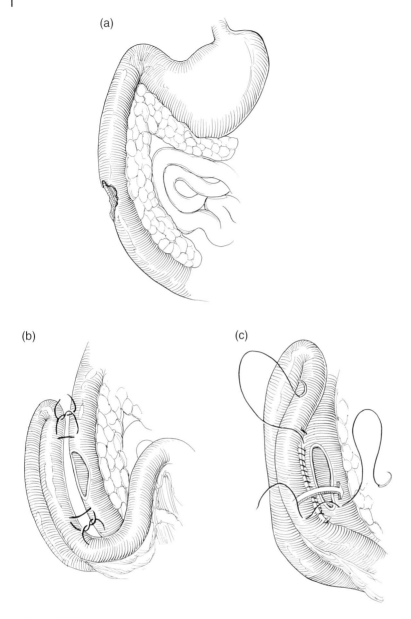

Figure 25.15

are placed in a simple continuous or interrupted pattern in sequence directed first toward the antimesenteric side and finally finishing across the mesentery from the initial knot. The antimesenteric aspect of the jejunum is rolled over the anastomotic site, and a second suture pattern is placed in a similar fashion 1 cm away from the anastomosis on the opposite side of the jejunal patch. Other methods of serosal patching using multiple loops of intestine to patch an intestinal anastomosis have been reported (Figure 25.18 and 25.19) (Radlinsky 2013).

25.4 Post-Operative Complications and Outcome

Complications following intestinal resection include suture line dehiscence, peritonitis, adhesions, short bowel syndrome, surgical site infections, and ileus (Pavletic and Berg 1996). Dehiscence after enterotomy closure or anastomosis is reported to occur in a range of 7–16% (Allen et al. 1992; Ralphs et al. 2003; Mouat et al. 2014). Cats appear to have a lower risk of dehiscence overall after intestinal anastomosis or biopsy compared

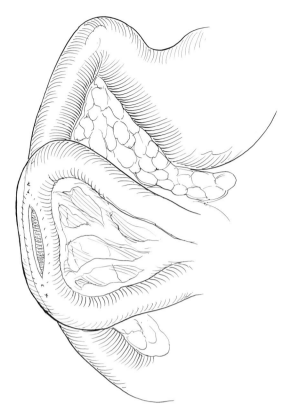

Figure 25.16

to dogs (Ralphs et al. 2003; Smith et al. 2011). Many factors have been implicated in increasing risk of intestinal dehiscence including hypoalbuminemia, hypotension, use of blood products, longer length of bowel resected, and delayed enteral feeding post-operatively (Giuffrida and Brown 2018). The presence of pre-existing peritonitis is one of the most important risk factors in small animals (Allen et al. 1992; Ralphs et al. 2003; Giuffrida and Brown 2018). About 50% of dogs and cats die following intestinal dehiscence and septic peritonitis (Adams et al. 2010, 2014). Likely, this fatality rate is influenced by a high euthanasia rate because of the poor prognosis and expense related to post-operative treatment and the high risk of complications.

Adhesions form when there is a combination of the following factors: ischemia, hemorrhage, aggressive foreign body reaction, severe inflammation, and infection. Atraumatic tissue handling, keeping intra-abdominal tissues moist, strict asepsis, and hemostasis may minimize adhesion formation.

A condition termed "short bowel syndrome" has been reported after extensive resection of small bowel (between 50 and 85% of the total small bowel length). Few intestinal disease disorders require extensive resection for treatment. Massive resections

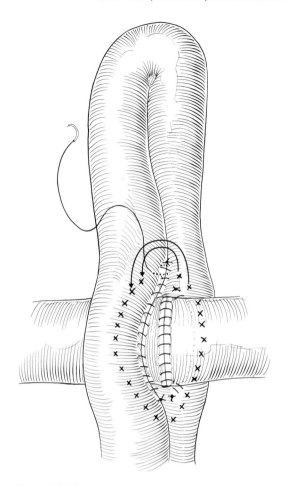

Figure 25.17

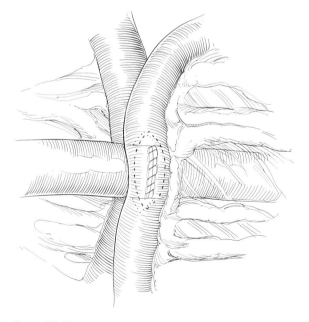

Figure 25.18

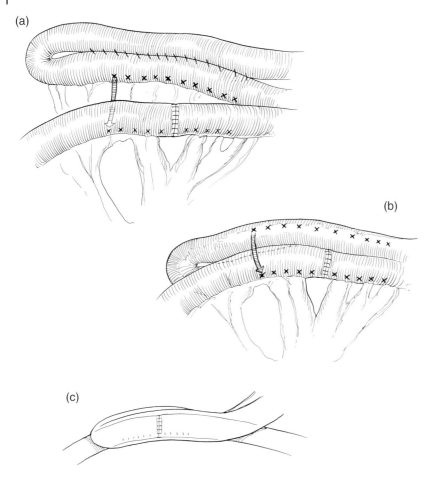

Figure 25.19

from global intestinal adhesions causing multiple areas of obstruction, chronic linear foreign bodies causing perforation of the majority of small bowel, and intestinal volvulus all have the potential to result in short bowel syndrome. With little bowel remaining, decreased transit time causes significant malabsorption and maldigestion resulting in severe fluid and electrolyte abnormalities, diarrhea, gastric ulceration, and weight loss. Intestinal adaptation may take weeks to months to occur before intractable diarrhea subsides, and the animal begins gaining weight. Enteral feeding appears to be important in promoting intestinal adaptation (Cuthbertson et al. 1970).

References

Adams, R.J., Doyle, R.S., Bray, J.P. et al. (2014). Closed suction drainage for treatment of septic peritonitis of confirmed gastrointestinal origin in 20 dogs. *Vet. Surg.* 43: 843–851.

Adams, W., Ctercteko, G., and Bilous, M. (1992). Effect of an omental wrap on the healing and vascularity of compromised intestinal anastomoses. *Dis. Colon Rectum* 35: 731–738.

Adams, W.M., Sisterman, L.A., Klauer, J.M. et al. (2010). Association of intestinal disorders in cats with findings of abdominal radiography. *J. Am. Vet. Med. Assoc.* 236: 880–886.

Agnifili, A., Schietroma, M., Carloni, A. et al. (2004). The value of omentoplasty in protecting colorectal anastomosis from leakage. A prospective randomized study in 126 patients. *Hepato-Gastroenterology* 51: 1694–1697.

Allen, D.A., Smeak, D.D., and Schertel, E.R. (1992). Prevalence of small intestinal dehiscence and associated clinical factors: a retrospective study of 121 dogs. *J. Am. Anim. Hosp. Assoc.* 28: 70–76.

Benlloch-Gonzalez, M., Gomes, E., Bouvy, B., and Poncet, C. (2015). Long-term prospective evaluation of intestinal anastomosis using stainless steel staples in 14 dogs. *Can. Vet. J.* 56: 715–722.

Camp, T.F., Skinner, D.B., and Connolly, J.M. (1968). Lateral duodenal defects. *Am. J. Surg.* 115: 291–294.

Chassin, J.L., Rifkind, K.M., and Sussman, B. (1978). The stapled gastrointestinal tract anastomosis: incidence of postoperative complications compared with the sutured anastomosis. *Ann. Surg.* 188: 689–696.

Coolman, B.R., Ehrhart, N., Pijanowski, G. et al. (2000). Comparison of skin staples with sutures for anastomosis of the small intestine in dogs. *Vet. Surg.* 29: 293–302.

Crowe, D.T. (1990). Serosal patching and jejunal onlay grafting. In: Current Techniques in Small Animal Surgery, 3e (ed. M.J. Bojrab), 252–255. Philadelphia: Lea and Febinger.

Crowe, D.T. (1984). The serosal patch clinical use in 12 animals. *Vet. Surg.* 13: 29–38.

Cuthbertson, E.M., Gilfillan, R.S., Burhenne, J.H. et al. (1970). Massive small bowel resection in the beagle, including laboratory data in severe undernutrition. *Surgery* 68: 698–705.

Duell, J.R., Thieman-Mankin, K.M., Rochat, M. et al. (2016). Frequency of dehiscence in hand-sutured and stapled intestinal anastomoses. *Vet. Surg.* 45: 100–103.

Enestvedt, C.K., Thompson, S.K. et al. (2006). Clinical review: healing in gastrointestinal anastomoses. Part II. *Microsurgery* 26: 137–143.

Galie, K.L. and Whitlow, C.B. (2006). Postoperative enterocutaneous fistula: when to reoperate and how to succeed. *Clin. Colon Rectal Surg.* 19: 237–246.

Giuffrida, M.A. and Brown, D.C. (2018). Small intestine. In: Veterinary Surgery Small Animal (eds. S.A. Johnston and K.M. Tobias), 1730–1761. St. Louis: Elsevier.

Grimes, J.A., Schmiedt, C.W., Cornell, K.K. et al. (2011). Identification of risk factors for septic peritonitis and failure to survive following gastrointestinal surgery in dogs. *J. Am. Vet. Med. Assoc.* 238: 486–494.

Hansen, L.A. and Monnet, E.L. (2013). Evaluation of serosal patch supplementation of surgical anastomoses in intestinal segments from canine cadavers. *Am. J. Vet. Res.* 74: 1138–1141.

Hansen, L.A. and Smeak, D.D. (2015). In vitro comparison of leakage pressure and leakage location for various staple line offset configurations in functional end-to-end stapled small intestinal anastomoses of canine tissues. *Am. J. Vet. Res.* 76: 644–648.

Hosgood, G. (1990). The omentum-the forgotten organ: physiology and potential surgical applications in dogs and cats. *Compend. Contin. Educ. Pract. Vet.* 12: 45–51.

Hosseini, S.V., Abbasi, H.R., Rezvani, H. et al. (2009). Comparison between gallbladder serosal and mucosal patch in duodenal injuries repair in dogs. *J. Investig. Surg.* 22: 148–153.

Isbell, S.A. and Maher, J.W. (1986). An experimental study to compare methods of closure of large duodenal defects. *Dig. Surg.* 3: 281–283.

Jansen, A., Becker, A.E., Brummelkamp, W.H. et al. (1981). The importance of the apposition of the submucosal intestinal layers for primary wound healing of intestinal anastomosis. *Surg. Gynecol. Obstet.* 152: 51–58.

Jardel, N.J., Hidalgo, A., Leperlier, D. et al. (2011). One stage functional end-to-end stapled intestinal anastomosis and resection performed by nonexpert surgeons for the treatment of small intestinal obstruction in 30 dogs. *Vet. Surg.* 40: 216–222.

Jones, S.A., Gazzaniga, A.B., and Keller, T.B. (1973). The serosal patch. A surgical parachute. *Am. J. Surg.* 126: 186–196.

Katsikas, D., Sechas, M., Antypas, G. et al. (1977). Beneficial effect of omental wrapping of unsafe intestinal anastomoses. An experimental study in dogs. *Int. Surg.* 62: 435–437.

Kieves, N., Thompson, D.A., and Krebs, A.I. (2014). Comparison of ex vivo leak pressures for single-layer enterotomy closure between novice and trained participants in a canine model. Scientific Presentation Abstracts: ACVS Surgery Summit October 16–18, San Diego, California.

Kobald, E.E. and Thal, A.P. (1963). A simple method for the management of experimental wounds of the duodenum. *Surg. Gynecol. Obstet.* 116: 340–344.

McLachlin, A. and Denton, D. (1973). Omental protection of intestinal anastomosis. *Am. J. Surg.* 125: 134–140.

Merad, F., Hay, J.M., Fingerhut, A. et al. (1998). Omentoplasty in the prevention of anastomotic leakage after colonic and rectal resection: a prospective randomized study in 712 patients. French associations for surgical research. *Ann. Surg.* 227: 179–186.

Milovancev, M., Weisman, D.L., and Palmisano, M.P. (2004). Foreign body attachment to polypropylene suture material extruded into the small intestinal lumen after enteric closure in three dogs. *J. Am. Vet. Med. Assoc.* 225: 1713–1715.

Mouat, E.E., Davis, G.J., Drobatz, K.J. et al. (2014). Evaluation of data from 35 dogs pertaining to dehiscence following intestinal resection and anastomosis. *J. Am. Anim. Hosp. Assoc.* 50: 254–263.

Pavletic, M.M. and Berg, J. (1996). Gastrointestinal surgery. In: Complications in Small Animal Surgery (eds. A.J. Lipowitz, D.D. Caywood, et al.), 365–398. Baltimore: Williams & Wilkins.

Peeters, K.C., Tollenaar, R.A. et al. (2005). Risk factors for anastomotic failure after total mesorectal excision of rectal cancer. *Br. J. Surg.* 92: 211–216.

Pozzi, A., Smeak, D.D., and Aper, R. (2006). Colonic seromuscular augmentation cystoplasty following subtotal cystectomy for treatment of bladder necrosis caused by bladder torsion in a dog. *J. Am. Vet. Med. Assoc.* 229: 235–239.

Radlinsky, M.A. (2013). Surgery of the Digestive System. Small Animal Surgery, 4e (ed. T.W. Fossum), 387–583. St Louis: Elsevier.

Ralphs, S.C., Jessen, C.R., and Lipowitz, A.J. (2003). Risk factors for leakage following intestinal anastomosis in dogs and cats: 115 cases (1991–2000). *J. Am. Vet. Med. Assoc.* 223: 73–77.

Rosenbaum, J.M., Coolman, B.R., Davidson, B.L. et al. (2016). The use of disposable skin staples for intestinal resection and anastomosis in 63 dogs: 2000 to 2014. *J. Small Anim. Pract.* 57: 631–636.

Rothenberg, R.E. and Rosenblatt, P. (1942). Motility and response of the great omentum. 1. Fluoroscopic observations on omental activity in dogs. *Arch. Surg.* 44: 764–771.

Smith, A.L., Wilson, A.P., Hardie, R.J. et al. (2011). Perioperative complications after full-thickness gastrointestinal surgery in cats with alimentary lymphoma. *Vet. Surg.* 40: 849–852.

Snowdon, K.A., Smeak, D.D., and Chiang, S. (2016). Risk factors for dehiscence of stapled functional end-to-end intestinal anastomoses in dogs: 53 cases (2001–2012). *Vet. Surg.* 45: 91–99.

Thompson, S.K., Chang, E.Y., and Jobe, B.A. (2006). Clinical review: healing in gastrointestinal anastomoses, part 1. *Microsurgery* 26: 131–136.

Tocchi, A., Mazzoni, G. et al. (2000). Prospective evaluation of omentoplasty in preventing leakage of colorectal anastomosis. *Dis. Colon Rectum* 43: 951–955.

Ullman, S.L. (1994). Surgical stapling of the small intestine. *Vet. Clin. North Am. Small Anim. Pract.* 24: 305–322.

Ullman, S.L., Pavletic, M.M., and Clark, G.N. (1991). Open intestinal anastomosis with surgical stapling equipment in 24 dogs and cats. *Vet. Surg.* 20: 385–391.

Weisman, D.L., Smeak, D.D., Birchard, S.J. et al. (1999). Comparison of a continuous suture pattern with a simple interrupted pattern for enteric closure in dogs and cats: 83 cases (1991–1997). *J. Am. Vet. Med. Assoc.* 214: 1507–1510.

White, R.N. (2008). Modified functional end-to-end stapled intestinal anastomosis: technique and clinical results in 15 dogs. *J. Small Anim. Pract.* 49: 274–281.

Wilkie, D.P.D. (1911). Some functions and surgical uses of the omentum. *Br. Med. J.* 2: 1103–1106.

26

Enteroplication/Enteropexy for Prevention of Intussusception

Daniel D. Smeak

Department of Clinical Sciences, College of Veterinary Medicine and Biomedical Sciences, Colorado State University, Fort Collins, CO, USA

26.1 Indications

Enteroplication (sometimes termed enteroenteropexy) is a procedure performed to help prevent recurrence of small bowel intussusception in dogs and cats (Olsen et al. 1977; Oakes et al. 1994). It is a modification of a procedure first described in humans by Noble to create planned adhesion sites to prevent obstructive adhesions after abdominal surgery (Noble 1937). The goal of enteroplication in small animals is to create staggered points of contact (or serosal to serosal adhesions) between adjacent bowel segments to prevent telescoping of bowel. An enteroplication can be complete (the entire jejunum and ileum are plicated) or partial (local plication of two loops of bowels together). Enteropexy is a procedure performed to create adhesions of bowel to adjacent viscera or the abdominal wall to prevent local recurrence of intussusception (Wolfe 1977). Complete enteroplication has been recommended if generalized enteritis is present or if the small intestines exhibit signs of hyperperistalsis. If enteroplication is considered, complete plication of the intestine, from the duodenocolic ligament to ileum, has been recommended since intussusception tends to recur at a site remote to the initial lesion or proximal to areas where limited enteroplication has been performed (Wilson and Burt 1974; Wolfe 1977; Levitt and Bauer 1992; Oakes et al. 1994). Since the descending duodenum has a short mesentery and is an area that is rarely found to undergo intussusception, plication is this segment of bowel is considered unnecessary (Wilson and Burt 1974; Levitt and Bauer 1992). Limited plication or enteropexy may be considered after reduction of an intussusception if during the procedure there is evidence of the original area of the intussusception re-telescoping in that local

area only. This occurs most often at the ileocolic junction in the author's experience.

Intussusception is the invagination of one portion of the gastrointestinal tract in the lumen of another adjoining segment. Affected animals are generally young and often less than one year of age. This condition has been associated with enteritis secondary to parasites, viruses, linear foreign bodies, intestinal masses, or previous enteral surgical sites (Rallis et al. 2008). In older animals this condition may be associated with enteral neoplasia. Post-operative intestinal intussusception is a frequent problem (up to 25%) associated with a variety of immunosuppressive protocols for experimental renal transplantation in dogs (Kyles et al. 2009). The recurrence rate of intestinal intussusception after surgical treatment in dogs ranges from 3 to 25% (Applewhite et al. 2002). When recurrence of intussusception is a concern, either local or global enteroplication may be considered. Experimental studies in dogs undergoing Noble plication have shown that intestinal motility and transit time are not altered (Ragins et al. 1966).

26.2 Surgical Procedures

26.2.1 Complete (Global) Enteroplication

The goal of this technique is to create gentle loops in the intestines to minimize the possibility of foreign material becoming lodged at the bends during transit (Figure 26.1) (Applewhite et al. 2002). Optimal loop length and suture interval for enteroplication have not been studied. Sutures chosen for plication can be either absorbable or nonabsorbable and should be placed at intervals that will help prevent entrapment and

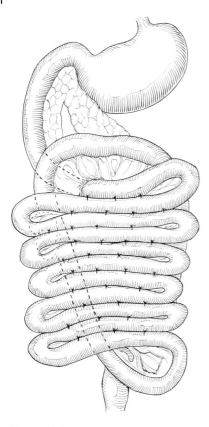

Figure 26.1

strangulation of other portions of bowel. Sutures should incorporate the submucosal layer for strength without penetrating the lumen. To prevent intussusception throughout the small bowel, the entire small intestine from the duodenocolic ligament to the ileocolic junction should be plicated (Oakes 1998). Cyanoacrylate glue has been studied as an alternative to suture in experimental enteroplication in cats. Use of glue was not supported in the report, the application was not as quick and simple as the authors had thought, and adhesion failure was a frequent complication (Nash and Bellenger 1998).

The small bowel is placed side-by-side to form a series of gentle back and forth 10–20 cm length loops from the duodenocolic ligament to the distal ileum. Adjacent loops of intestine are sutured to each other approximately 6 cm apart with 4-0 suture. Sutures are placed midway between the mesenteric and antimesenteric borders (or between antimesenteric borders) and are placed no less than 5–6 cm from each gentle bend, to avoid "kinking" at each loop turn.

26.2.2 Limited Enteroplication

For a more limited use of enteroplication, place the segment location where the intussusception was reduced

or resected at the bend of a 15–20 cm length loop of bowel. Place sutures between the adjacent loops of bowel as described for complete enteroplication.

26.2.3 Enteropexy

Following reduction or resection, a 10–15 cm orad segment of bowel (intussusceptum) just proximal to the leading edge of the intussusception is placed longitudinally along an adjacent area of healthy lateral abdominal wall. The antimesenteric border of the involved segment is sutured to the abdominal wall or adjacent bowel with an interrupted or simple continuous line using 3-0 to 4-0 absorbable monofilament suture. There is no need to incise or scarify the opposing serosal surfaces since temporary fixation rather permanent adhesion formation is necessary. This technique theoretically fixes the orad segment to the abdominal wall, so this portion of bowel will not allow propagation of an invagination leading to re-intussusception at the original site (Applewhite et al. 2001a). Whether enteropexy or limited enteroplication is effective at reducing the risk of local re-intussusception has not been studied (Wolfe 1977).

26.3 Tips

Enteroplication should be used with caution and is most indicated to prevent recurrence of intussusception when a predisposing cause is not apparent, or when the cause is not expected to be readily responsive to medical therapy (Brown 2012). Intussusception caused by a mural mass, for example, is remedied by removal of the mass with the intussusception, and most surgeons would choose not to preform enteroplication in this instance. A complete enteroplication may be indicated, on the other hand, in a dog or cat with several intussusceptions in the process of forming during surgical exploration. Until prospective studies identify risk factors for recurrence of intussusception and verify the efficacy of enteroplication in reducing this risk, the decision to perform enteroplication is at the discretion of the surgeon.

26.4 Post-Operative Considerations and Prognosis

Enteroplication has been implicated as a cause of several serious post-operative complications including abdominal abscess formation, partial intestinal obstruction, and even localized intestinal volvulus and strangulation (Kyles et al. 1998; Applewhite et al. 2001b; Jasani et al. 2005).

The clinical results of enteroplication techniques for prevention of intussusception have been varied. Two retrospective studies have reported no difference in recurrence rates with or without enteroplication for prevention of intussusception (Levitt and Bauer 1992; Applewhite et al. 2001a). However, in five other large retrospective studies, no dog that underwent enteroplication developed a recurrence of intussusception. Of the 63 dogs that did not receive enteroplication in those series of studies, 17% developed re-intussusception. In one prospective study to evaluate Noble plication as a means to prevent intussusception after immunosuppression and renal transplantation, those dogs that were plicated experienced no intussusception, compared to 3/14 dogs (21%) without plication. No complications related to the plication procedure were reported in that report (Kyles et al. 2009). Therefore, it appears that enteroplication is effective at reducing the risk of recurrence. However, as mentioned earlier, significant complications have been documented with this procedure, and these must be weighed against the possible benefits of plication (Wilson and Burt 1974; Weaver 1977; Levitt and Bauer 1992; Oakes et al. 1994; Applewhite et al. 2001b).

The prognosis for dogs and cats that have received appropriate preoperative stabilization and that have had reduction or resection of an intussusception is good (Oakes et al. 1994; Applewhite et al. 2002). Survival rates after surgical repair of intussusception are well over 80%. However, a more guarded prognosis is given for dogs with a perforated intussusception and septic peritonitis (Applewhite et al. 2002). Recurrence rates range from 6 to 27% after surgical intervention for intussusception (Weaver 1977; Lewis and Ellison 1987; Levitt and Bauer 1992; Applewhite et al. 2000, 2002). Recurrence was reported in 22% of 18 dogs having undergone manual reduction alone and in 17% of 88 dogs having undergone resection and anastomosis for intussusception (Applewhite et al. 2002). Without enteroplication, most intussusceptions recur within three days, but some have been reported up to three weeks after surgery. Most recurrences have been reported remote and orad to the original site of the intussusception. Complications related to enteroplication generally have been reported to occur within a few months from surgery (Applewhite et al. 2002).

Butorphanol tartrate has been reported to decrease the occurrence of intussusception formation in a canine model of renal transplantation (Klinger et al. 1990). The incidence of intussusception in this model was decreased from 17 to 3% when this opioid agent was administered during the perioperative period. A more recent retrospective study during which opioids were administered consistently perioperatively also showed a lower risk of recurrence of intussusceptions following initial correction of the lesion (Applewhite et al. 2001a). It is hypothesized that opioid administration increases tone of the small intestine and reduces local bowel inhomogeneity and segmental ileus, thereby decreasing the likelihood of intussusception.

Bibliography

Applewhite, A.A., Cornell, K.K., and Hawthorne, J.C. (2000). Benefit versus risk for prevention of intestinal intussusception. *Vet. Surg.* 29: 456.

Applewhite, A.A., Cornell, K.K., and Selcer, B.A. (2001a). Pylorogastric intussusception in the dog. A case report and literature review. *J. Am. Anim. Hosp. Assoc.* 37: 238–243.

Applewhite, A.A., Hawthorne, J.C., and Cornell, K.K. (2001b). Enteroplication for the prevention of intussusception recurrence in dogs. A retrospective study (1989–1999). *J. Am. Vet. Med. Assoc.* 219: 1415–1418.

Applewhite, A.A., Cornell, K.K., and Selcer, B.A. (2002). Diagnosis and treatment of intussusceptions in dogs. *Compend. Contin. Educ. Pract. Vet.* 24: 110–126.

Brown, D.C. (2012). Small intestine. In: Veterinary Surgery Small Animal, 2e (eds. K.M. Tobias and S.A. Johnston), 1513–1541. St Louis: Elsevier.

Jasani, S., House, A.K., and Brockman, D.J. (2005). Localized mid-jejunal volvulus following intussusception and enteroplication in a dog. *J. Small Anim. Pract.* 46: 398–401.

Klinger, M., Cooper, J., and McCabe, R. (1990). The use of butorphanol tartrate for the prevention of canine intussusception following renal transplantation. *J. Investig. Surg.* 3: 229–233.

Kyles, A., Schneider, T., and Clare, A. (1998). Foreign body intestinal perforation and intra-abdominal abscess formation as a complication of enteroplication in the dog. *Vet. Rec.* 143: 112–113.

Kyles, A.E., Gregory, C.R., Griffey, S.M. et al. (2003). Immunosuppression with a combination of the lefunomide analog, FK778, and microemulsified cyclosporine for renal transplantation in mongrel dogs. *Transplantation* 75: 1128–1133.

Kyles, A.E., Gregory, C.R., Griffey, S.M. et al. (2009). Modified Noble plication for the prevention of intestinal intussusception after renal transplantation in dogs. *J. Investig. Surg.* 16: 161–166.

Levitt, L. and Bauer, M.S. (1992). Intussusception in dogs and cats: a review of thirty-six cases. *Can. Vet. J.* 33: 660–664.

Lewis, D.D. and Ellison, G.W. (1987). Intussusception in dogs and cats. *Compend. Contin. Educ. Pract. Vet.* 9: 523–533.

Nash, J.M. and Bellenger, C.R. (1998). Enteroplication in cats, using suture or n-butyl cyanoacrylate adhesive. *Res. Vet. Sci.* 65: 253–258.

Noble, T. (1937). Plication of small intestines as prophylaxis against adhesions. *Am. J. Surg.* 35: 41–44.

Oakes, M.G. (1998). Enteroplication to prevent recurrent intestinal intussusception. In: Current Techniques in Small Animal Surgery, 4e (ed. M.J. Bojrab), 254. Baltimore: William and Wilkens.

Oakes, M.G., Lewis, D.D., Hosgood, G., and Beale, B.S. (1994). Enteroplication for the prevention of intussusception recurrence in dogs: 31 cases (1978–1992). *J. Am. Vet. Med. Assoc.* 205: 72–75.

Olsen, P.R., Boserup, F., Mikkelsen, A.M., and Rorbech, U. (1977). Intussusception following renal transplantation in dogs (author's transl). *Nord. Vet. Med.* 29: 36–40.

Ragins, H., Freeman, L., Coomaraswamy, R., and Liu, S. (1966). Clinical and experimental comparison of the Noble and the Childs–Phillips plications of the small bowel. *Am. J. Surg.* 111: 555–558.

Rallis, T.S., Papazoglou, L.G. et al. (2000). Acute enteritis or gastroenteritis in young dogs as a predisposing factor for intestinal intussusception: a retrospective study. *J. Vet. Med.* 47: 507–511.

Sridhar, R., Thanikachalam, M., Manonar, B.M., and Sundararaj, A. (1994). Multiple intussusceptions in a puppy. *Can. Vet. J.* 35: 729.

Weaver, A.D. (1977). Canine intestinal intussusception. *Vet. Rec.* 100: 524.

Wilson, G.P. and Burt, J.K. (1974). Intussusception in the dog and cat: a review of 45 cases. *J. Am. Vet. Med. Assoc.* 164: 515–518.

Wolfe, D.A. (1977). Recurrent intestinal intussusceptions in the dog. *J. Am. Vet. Med. Assoc.* 171: 553–556.

Section VI

Colon

27

Colectomy and Subtotal Colectomy

Daniel D. Smeak and Eric Monnet

Department of Clinical Sciences, College of Veterinary Medicine and Biomedical Sciences, Colorado State University, Fort Collins, CO, USA

27.1 Indications

Surgery on the large intestine may be indicated for lesions that cause obstruction, perforation, colonic inertia (megacolon), entrapment, torsion, or volvulus, and for severe or long-standing inflammatory conditions. The most common causes of colonic obstruction in small animals include neoplasia, intussusceptions, and inflammatory/granulomatous masses. In most cases, foreign bodies that eventually reach the large bowel are usually safely expelled in the feces, so surgery is generally not necessary. In rare cases, sharp foreign bodies such as fish hooks or desiccated fecaliths can become lodged and may require endoscopic or surgical retrieval. Colonic perforations are dangerous and are often rapidly fatal, so they must be diagnosed and surgically managed on an emergent basis. Congenital lesions that require surgical resection, such as colonic duplication, are rare (Shinozaki et al. 2000; Williams 2012).

Chapter 1 describes the healing properties of the large intestine.

Megacolon in cats is mostly idiopathic, but it may result from mechanical obstruction, most commonly from pelvic malunion after fracture (Bright 1991). In one limited case series study, it was found that sufficient colonic motility may return if the obstruction is corrected within six months after the pelvic trauma. After six months, permanent intramural changes secondary to chronic distension prevent return of motility even after the obstruction is relieved (Schrader 1992). Most megacolon conditions in the dog and cat are idiopathic with no evidence of a distal colorectal obstruction (Nemeth et al. 2008). Occasionally, perineal hernias in cats can be the result or the cause of megacolon (Welches 1992). In the authors' experience,

if perineal hernia is found in a cat with concurrent megacolon, subtotal colectomy can be successful at alleviating the clinical signs long-term, with or without herniorrhaphy. When intractable constipation occurs and when megacolon is no longer responsive to promotility agents, lactulose, and periodic enemas, subtotal colectomy is considered in both dogs and cats.

The importance of preserving the ileocolic junction during subtotal colectomy remains unclear. The ileocolic orifice is felt to act as a sphincter to prevent reflux of colonic contents. The concern is that retrograde movement of colonic organisms into the small bowel will result in bacterial overgrowth. Some studies have documented an increased incidence of diarrhea after removing the ileocecal area for subtotal colectomy, but there is no evidence of greater risk of recurrent obstipation in cats when the junction was not removed (Bright 1991; Sweet et al. 1994). Preserving the ileocecal area during subtotal colectomy is recommended. However, in some cases, resection of the tethering proximal colon and cecum is necessary to reduce tension on the repair (Greenfield 1991; Sweet et al. 1994; Nemeth et al. 2008).

Key functions of the colon include fecal storage and maintenance of fluid and electrolyte balance through the colonic mucosa. Most of the absorption of water, Na, Cl, and short-chain fatty acids, and secretion of K, HCO_3, and mucus occurs in the proximal colon. The distal colon serves mostly as the storage region but also has some function in modulating fecal water content (Williams 2012). Removal of significant portions of the colon can cause chronic diarrhea and electrolyte disturbances. Continence is maintained; however, due to the loss of storage function, defecation is often more frequent (Nemeth et al. 2008).

Gastrointestinal Surgical Techniques in Small Animals, First Edition. Edited by Eric Monnet and Daniel D. Smeak.
© 2020 John Wiley & Sons, Inc. Published 2020 by John Wiley & Sons, Inc.
Companion website: www.wiley.com/go/monnet/gastrointestinal

27.2 Surgical Techniques

27.2.1 Preoperative Considerations

The patient should be well hydrated, and any electrolyte deficits should be corrected before general anesthesia. It is generally accepted in small animals that there is little indication for mechanical cleansing of the bowel in preparation for colonic surgery. To date, the value of colonic preparation before surgery has not been clearly demonstrated in small animal surgery. Firm feces can generally be manipulated into the segment of colon to be resected and subsequently removed. Preoperative enemas can liquefy otherwise easy-to-contain firm fecal material, and this can increase the risk of leakage and gross contamination of the surgical site (Holt and Brockman 2003). If enemas are being considered, they should be performed well before surgery (two to three days). Animals are fed a low residue diet up until 12–24 hours before surgery.

The risk of infection after colonic surgery is considered to be higher than other clean-contaminated procedures. Antibiotics chosen for prophylaxis should be especially effective against gram (−) aerobes and especially anaerobes that dominate the colonic flora. Second-generation cephalosporin antibiotics are given intravenously at anesthetic induction and every 90 minutes throughout the procedure. Alternately, provided there are no contraindications otherwise, some surgeons prefer administering a broader spectrum regimen consisting of an intravenous aminoglycoside, or fluoroquinolone and metronidazole during the surgical procedure.

27.2.2 Surgical Procedures

Suturing continues to be the most common technique of colonic repair in small animals. Other repair methods used in small animals include linear stapling, circular stapling, and biofragmentable rings. In experimental colonic injuries, the use of skin staplers, even in the presence of peritonitis, has been shown to be successful in primary repair (Edwards et al. 1999). In one recent clinical retrospective study, skin staplers were consistently successful in colonic repair in a limited number of dogs (Rosenbaum et al. 2016). The authors of this study concluded that disposable skin staples can be used to perform end-to-end anastomosis for a variety of clinical indications. The overall dehiscence rate (5%) with skin staplers was consistent with those of other studies using suture for colonic repair. No comparative studies to date have identified the most successful anastomotic method, though most surgeons including the author prefer hand suturing or linear stapling techniques.

27.2.2.1 Colonic Anastomosis Closure Methods
27.2.2.1.1 Suture
The most widely utilized suture pattern for closure of the colon currently in small animals is a single-layer, simple interrupted, appositional pattern (Ryan et al. 2006). Appositional anastomoses without excessive mucosal eversion were found to produce less scar tissue and morbidity than inverting or everting patterns. Simple appositional closure also provides the least reduction of luminal diameter (Ellison et al. 1982). Just as in enteric closure, simple continuous appositional patterns provide more histologic alignment of layers and decreased surgical time and tissue trauma from excessive handling, and this is also an acceptable means of colon repair (Weisman et al. 1999; Williams 2012). The suture material and needle for colonic surgery should be chosen to minimize trauma and tissue reaction. Preferably, colon wounds are closed with 4-0 monofilament absorbable sutures using a swaged-on taper needle. Multifilament sutures are generally avoided since they cause trauma due to their relatively rough surface when passed through friable colonic tissue, and they may also wick and trap bacteria within the interstices of the fibers (Niles and Williams 1999). Nonabsorbable monofilament suture use in the colon in a continuous pattern should be avoided because the suture can break and unravel, leaving a trailing strand anchored within the lumen. Fecal material has been reported to accumulate on the exposed suture strand and act as a linear foreign body (Milovancev et al. 2004; Williams 2012).

27.2.2.1.2 Linear Stapler
Stapling devices have been used successfully for anastomosis and closure of bowel. The risk of intestinal dehiscence in stapled repair is similar to hand-sutured anastomoses, but they do reduce surgical time (Snowden et al. 2016). Functional end-to-end anastomosis with a linear GIA stapler and TA stapler is a recognized acceptable method of colonic and ileocolic anastomosis. The technique of functional end-to-end anastomosis for colonic anastomosis is similar to that of the small intestine. The technique of intestine anastomosis using linear staplers can be reviewed in the small intestinal anastomosis chapter (Chapter 25).

27.2.2.1.3 EEA Stapler
The tubular-shaped EEA device creates a true inverting anastomosis by placing a circular, double row of steel staples (Figure 27.1). This device can be placed transcecally or transanally for anastomosis after colectomy (Kudisch and Pavletic 1993). For the transcecal approach, the cecum and colon are isolated carefully with multiple layers of laparotomy sponges.

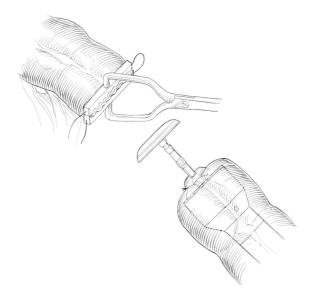

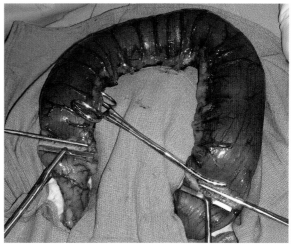

Figure 27.2

Figure 27.1

A Furniss purse-string instrument is used to place a purse-string at the proximal and distal limits of the colectomy (Figures 27.1 and 27.2). A straight taper point needle is used to feed 2-0 suture through the instrument at both sites. Use of this instrument is important since a short, uniform cuff of tissue allows even inclusion of the large intestine into the circular stapling device. The colon segment to be excised is isolated with crushing clamps and transected using the Furniss clamp as a cutting guide (Figure 27.3).

Following removal of the Furniss clamp, a 3 cm incision is made on the antimesenteric side of the cecum. An ovoid sizer is lubricated with sterile water-soluble gel, introduced through the cecal incision, and advanced normograde to the proximal colon margin. Sizers of different diameter exist to help determine the diameter of EEA to use for the patient. In Figure 27.4, the sizer was placed outside the lumen of the colon. Most cats and

dogs require either an EEA cartridge of 21 or 25 mm diameter with 4.8 mm staples. EEA cartridge with 3.5 mm staples might be appropriate for cats. The EEA stapler is advanced through the cecal access incision and advanced to the proximal colectomy site. The anvil is unseated. The purse-string is loosened, and the anvil is advanced through the proximal segment. After tightening the proximal purse-string suture around the unseated anvil shaft, the anvil is advanced and eased through the loosened purse-string suture in the distal segment. The purse-string sutures are firmly tied, and then the bowel segments are brought together using the EEA stapling device and the staples fired. As the staples are fired, the EEA stapler circular cutting blade removes inverted tissue inside the circular staple line. After firing, the stapler is opened slightly and rotated to ease it out from around the staple line, so it can be removed. The staple line is inspected for leakage or hemorrhage, and the excised doughnut of tissue within the stapler is inspected to be sure that it formed a complete ring

Figure 27.3

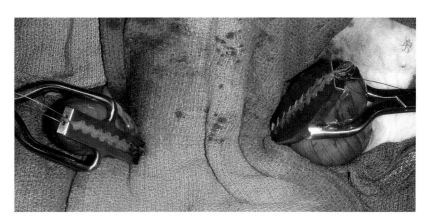

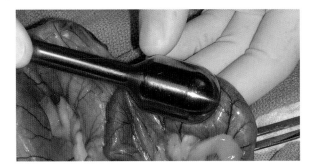

Figure 27.4

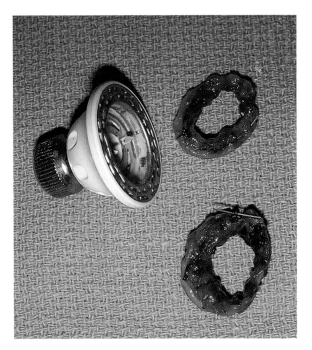

Figure 27.5

signaling adequate purchase of the inverted staple line (Figure 27.5). The cecal access incision is closed with either a TA linear 3.5 mm stapler, or it is sutured with an appositional suture pattern. A similar method of colocolic circular stapled anastomosis can be performed without an access incision. The EEA device is instead advanced in an opposite direction through the anus (Chapter 33).

27.2.2.1.4 Biofragmentable Ring
The biofragmentable anastomotic ring (Valtrac Medtronic, Minneapolis, MN) is a sutureless intestinal anastomosis technique that has been proven successful in human enterocolic surgery and for colocolic anastomosis in cats (Figure 27.6) (Hardy et al. 1985; Huss et al. 1994; Ryan et al. 2006). The technique is fast and easy to perform, and interoperative complications are generally

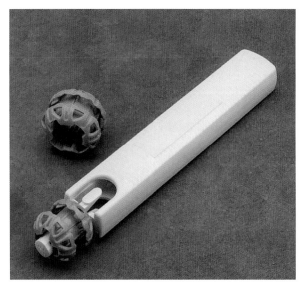

Figure 27.6

minor and mostly due to difficulty feeding the device into colonic segments. The rings consistently fragment and are passed in the feces within 10–12 days. Stricture formation has not been encountered in the limited number of case series published to date. For anastomosis with this biofragmentable ring device, colonic excision is performed using the same technique described for the EEA technique. Furniss purse-string sutures are placed at both blind ends after the affected colon segment is resected (Figure 27.2). The purse-string suture is loosened at the orad segment first and one ring is passed into the segment using a holding device (Figure 27.7a). The proximal purse-string is tied firmly and securely against the internal barrel of the biofragmentable anastomosis ring (Figure 27.7b and c). After removing the holding device, the exposed half of the biofragmentable ring is then placed in the aborad segment, and the distal purse-string is similarly tied (Figure 27.8a). Both halves of the biofragmentable anastomosis rings are snapped together and locked by placing digital pressure on each cap toward each other through the colonic wall (Figure 27.8b). Usually a biofragmentable anastomotic ring with a 1.5 mm gap between the two closed halves is used in cats (Ryan et al. 2006). This creates an inverting serosal to serosal anastomosis. The repair is inspected to be sure there is accurate apposition of the anastomosis and for any leakage or hemorrhage.

27.2.2.2 Surgical Techniques
27.2.2.2.1 Segmental Colectomy
The colon is isolated with multiple layers of laparotomy sponges, and colon contents are milked away from the proposed excision/biopsy segment (Figure 27.9a).

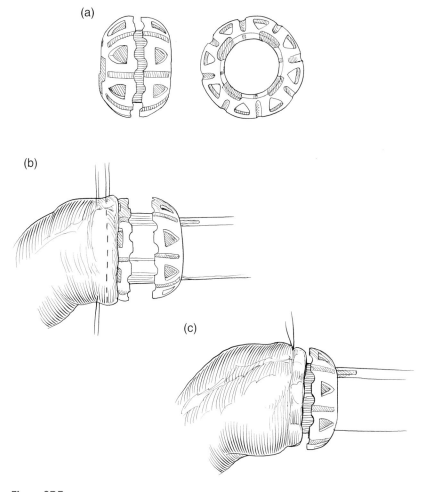

(a)

(b)

(c)

Figure 27.7

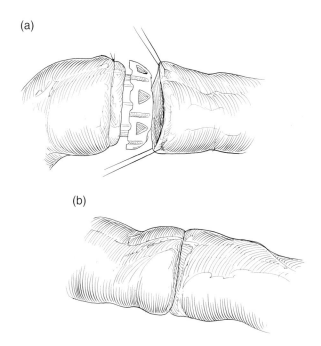

(a)

(b)

Figure 27.8

For segmental colectomy, the lesion to be resected is isolated with appropriate margins by straight Carmalt forceps. Feces are milked and held away from the area of resection with Doyen atraumatic forceps (black arrow) (Figure 27.9b). Individual vasa recti supplying blood to the area of resection are ligated (Figure 27.9b and c). Alternately, the left colic vessels are ligated proximally and distally to the isolated area in the descending colon region. A colocolostomy is performed with one of the aforementioned closure methods (Figure 27.9d).

27.2.2.2.2 Colectomy and Subtotal Colectomy for Megacolon

Surgery for megacolon is approached with a large ventral midline celiotomy. The entire abdomen should be explored first, and biopsy samples are collected, if indicated, before colectomy is initiated to reduce unnecessary fecal contamination. The colon is exteriorized, and the appropriate colic and caudal mesenteric vessels are ligated (Figure 27.10a and b). For the ileocolic anastomosis (A–C Figure 27.10a), appropriate branches from the caudal mesenteric pedicle are ligated, ensuring perfusion to the

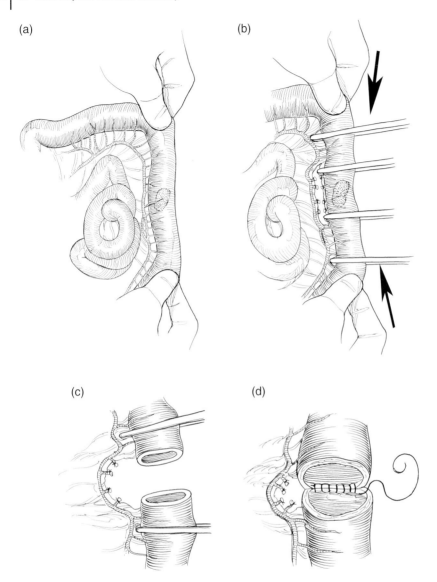

(a)

(b)

(c)

(d)

Figure 27.9

distal colic excision margin. The common trunk of the colic vessel is ligated, and the proximal blood supply to the terminal ileum, the ileal branch, is ligated at the proximal excision margin. For colocolic anastomosis (B–C in Figure 27.10a), the caudal mesenteric blood supply is preserved as described previously, but the left colic, middle, and the mid portion of the right colic vessels are ligated, leaving the proximal margin principally supplied by the right colic and ileocecocolic vasculature. The diseased bowel is isolated with laparotomy sponges or sterile towels. For a "trial fit" the proximal colon segment is carefully mobilized, and the ascending colon is pulled toward the terminal colon area. The author decides which level of resection is chosen (ileocolic anastomosis or colocolic anastomosis with sparing of the ileocolic valve) by determining whether excess tension is felt when pulling the proximal

colon to the proposed distal stump region. The longer and more mobile mesentery always allows free transfer of the ileocolic area to the distal segment if tension is a concern. Regardless of whether the ileocecocolic junction is removed or not as part of a megacolon resection, the distal colonic segment is resected in the same location, 3–5 cm from the pelvic brim (Sweet et al. 1994; Bertoy 1993). Enough distal colon is preserved to enable the surgeon to perform the anastomosis without difficulty or risk of retraction of the stump and potential contamination into the deeper pelvic cavity during repair. The author prefers to preserve the caudal mesenteric blood supply to the distal colonic segment if possible, rather than solely relying on the cranial rectal artery. Individual vasa recta vessels are ligated instead of sacrificing the main caudal mesenteric or cranial rectal vessels (Figure 27.10).

(a)

(b)

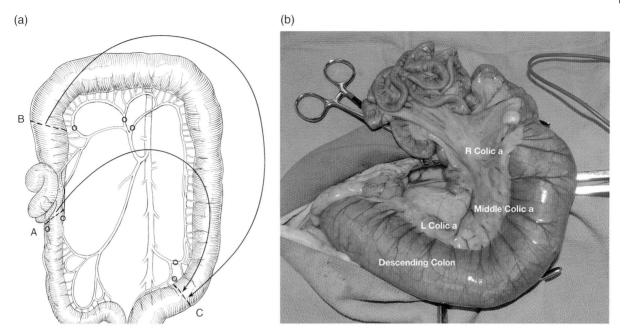

Figure 27.10

Subtotal Colectomy – Colocolic Anastomosis (Preservation of the Ileococcolic Junction) Most colocolic anastomoses do not have excessive luminal size disparity, so a simple end-to-end colocolic anastomosis is performed. When the surgeon wishes to preserve the ileocolic junction, the ascending colon is transected 2 cm distal to the cecum. The method chosen for the anastomosis is the surgeon's preference (see previously described anastomosis methods).

Subtotal Colectomy – Ileocolic Anastomosis Techniques used for successful ileocolic anastomosis after megacolon resection when there is large size discrepancy between the segments include end-to end (Figure 27.11a and b), end-to-side (Figure 27.11c), and side-to-side enterocolostomy with stapling equipment (Figure 27.12) (Bertoy et al. 1989; Matthiesen et al. 1991; Sweet et al. 1994; Bertoy 1993; Bright 1993; Williams et al. 1999). A GIA stapler is first used to perform the side-to-side anastomosis (Figure 27.12a and b), and then a TA stapler is used to complete the anastomosis (Figure 27.12c).

27.3 Tips

It is important to minimize contamination during colonic surgery. Introduction of the EEA stapler through the anus and the rectum results in some contamination of the peritoneal cavity. The biofragmentable device is placed in the surgical field without increasing the risk of contamination.

Placement of the biofragmentable device or the EEA is usually difficult because of the difference in diameter between the colon and the EEA device. Using warm saline to irrigate the surgical site and/or application of local anesthesia like lidocaine seem to help relax the wall of the colon.

Oversewing of the anastomosis is required after placement of the EEA or the biofragmentable device if tearing of the serosa is observed. Usually two simple continuous partial thickness sutures are placed.

27.4 Post-Operative Considerations and Prognosis

Hemorrhage and fecal contamination are the most common intraoperative complications after large intestinal surgery. Hemorrhage risk is reduced by proper ligation placement and careful inspection of the surgical site following repair. Fecal contamination is contained by isolating the surgical site with multiple layers of laparotomy sponges, milking fecal contents into the segment to be removed, use of atraumatic forceps to contain fecal matter orad and aborad to the resection, using new sterile gloves and instruments for closure of the abdominal approach, and copious local lavage. Post-operative complications include endotoxic shock, dehiscence, leakage, stricture, or death. Stricture risk can be minimized by avoiding excessively everting or inverting suture lines and eliminating any tension on the anastomosis. Fecal incontinence after colonic surgery should not be expected.

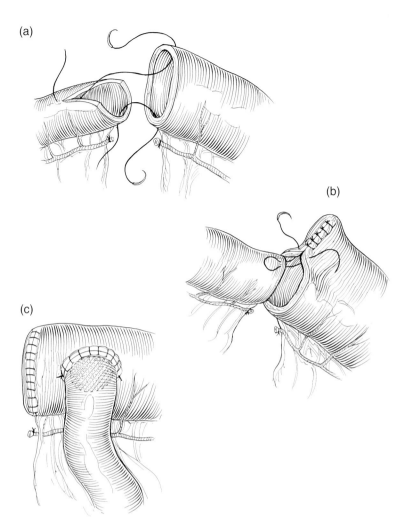

Figure 27.11

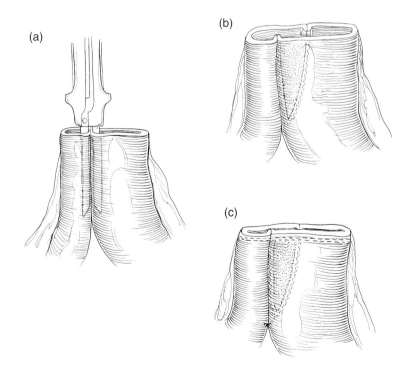

Figure 27.12

Patients are monitored carefully for anesthetic recovery and early signs of peritonitis or abscess formation. Depression, fever, excessive abdominal tenderness, vomiting, and ileus may indicate intraperitoneal infection. If these signs occur, serial blood cell counts should be performed, and abdominal ultrasound should be considered to scan the abdomen for free fluid and to guide fluid aspiration sampling. Rapid exploration is advised in animals with evidence of septic peritonitis after colectomy before signs of endotoxic shock occur. Patients are given appropriate post-operative analgesic drugs after surgery. NSAIDs are used with caution during and after colonic surgery, since these drugs may interfere with the early stages of colonic healing (Gorissen et al. 2012). A high-residue, low-fat diet is fed after colonic surgery to promote normal intestinal motility (Williams 2012).

After surgery for megacolon, loose stools can be expected initially due to reduced absorptive capacity and transit time (Jimba et al. 2002). Experimentally, normal colonic motility takes up to eight weeks to re-establish after subtotal colectomy in dogs. The remaining colon adapts over time by increasing villi height and enterocyte number and density in cats after total colectomy (Bertoy et al. 1989). In most cases, enteric function returns to near normal within two weeks after colocolostomy in experimental cats. Bowel movements are slightly more frequent but minimal changes in fecal volume or water content can be expected after several weeks (Gregory et al. 1990). It should be noted that permanent loose stools and incontinence following ileocolic anastomosis has been reported rarely after subtotal colectomy in cats (Webb 1985; Sweet et al. 1994; Ryan et al. 2006). Therefore, owners need to be warned that in rare instances cats may never fully recover and may have loose stools for years (Wells et al. 1995). In a study on 19 cats with idiopathic megacolon, two cats had persistence of loose stool at 254 and 1661 days after surgery (Ryan et al. 2006).

In one case series of eight dogs undergoing colocolic anastomosis for acquired megacolon, one dog died of septic peritonitis, seven dogs had resolution of signs, and normal defecation returned within seven weeks. No strictures or recurrence of signs developed in these dogs (Nemeth et al. 2008). Recurrence of megacolon was reported to be uncommon in several retrospective studies in cats, and in the authors' experience and that of others, most can be medically managed without surgery unless an obstruction is present (Rosin et al. 1988; Sweet et al. 1994; Ryan et al. 2006). In one case series of 22 cats undergoing colectomy with or without preservation of the ileocecal region there was recurrence of constipation in 45% of the cats, with some requiring repeat surgery (Sweet et al. 1994). Stricture after subtotal colectomy is rare, but when it develops, attributing signs occur usually within three weeks of surgery (Leighton and Grain 1978; Rosin et al. 1988). In a study on 19 cats with idiopathic megacolon, long-term survival of 90–100% was reported four years after surgery (Ryan et al. 2006).

The prognosis after colectomy for colonic neoplasia depends on the tumor type and whether clean surgical excision was obtained. In 18 cats undergoing subtotal colectomy for colonic adenocarcinoma treated with carboplatin, median disease-free interval was 251 days, and median survival time was 269 days (Arteaga et al. 2012). In dogs, the median survival time after resection of colorectal adenocarcinomas is 6–22 months. For stromal tumors, the survival time after resection can extend to greater than three years (Russell et al. 2007).

References

Arteaga, T., McKnight, J., and Bergman, P.J. (2012). A review of 18 cases of feline colonic adenocarcinoma treated with subtotal colectomies and adjuvant carboplatin. *J. Am. Anim. Hosp. Assoc.* 48: 399–404.

Bertoy, R.W. (1993). Megacolon. In: *Disease Mechanisms in Small Animal Surgery*, 2e (ed. M.J. Bojrab), 262–265. Philadelphia: Lea & Febiger.

Bertoy, R.W., MacCoy, D.M., Wheaton, L.G. et al. (1989). Total colectomy with ileorectal anastomosis in the cat. *Vet. Surg.* 18: 204–210.

Bright, R.M. (1991). Idiopathic megacolon in the cat: subtotal colectomy with preservation of the ileocolic valve. *Vet. Med. Rep.* 3: 183–187.

Bright, R.M. (1993). Treatment of feline colonic obstruction (Megacolon). In: *Current Techniques in Small Animal Surgery*, 3e (ed. M.J. Bojrab), 262–265. Philadelphia: Lea and Febiger.

Edwards, D.P., Warren, B.F., Galbraith, K.A. et al. (1999). Comparison of two closure techniques for the repair of experimental colonic perforations. *Br. J. Surg.* 86: 514–517.

Ellison, G.W., Jokinen, M.P., and Park, R.D. (1982). End-to-end approximating intestinal anastomosis in the dog: a comparative fluorescein dye, angiographic, and histopathologic evaluation. *J. Am. Anim. Hosp. Assoc.* 18: 729–736.

Gorissen, K.J., Benning, D., Berghmans, T. et al. (2012). Risk of anastomotic leakage with non-steroidal anti-inflammatory drugs in colorectal surgery. *Br. J. Surg.* 99: 721–727.

Greenfield, C.L. (1991). Idiopathic megacolon in the cat: subtotal colectomy with removal of the ileocolic valve. *Vet. Med. Rep.* 3: 182–185.

Gregory, C.R., Guilford, W.G., Berry, C.R. et al. (1989). Colonic function in cats after subtotal colectomy versus total colectomy for megacolon syndrome. *Vet. Surg.* 18: 69.

Gregory, C.R., Guilford, W.G., Berry, C.R. et al. (1990). Enteric function in cats after subtotal colectomy for treatment of megacolon. *Vet. Surg.* 19: 216–220.

Hardy, T.G., Pace, W.G., Maney, J.W. et al. (1985). A biofragmentable ring for sutureless bowel anastomosis. *Dis. Colon Rectum* 28: 484–490.

Holt, D.E. and Brockman, D. (2003). Large intestine. In: *Textbook of Small Animal Surgery*, 3e (ed. D. Slatter), 665. Philadelphia: Saunders.

Huss, B.T., Payne, J.T., Johnson, G.C. et al. (1994). Comparison of a biofragmentable intestinal anastomosis ring with appositional suturing for subtotal colectomy in normal cats. *Vet. Surg.* 23: 466–474.

Jimba, Y., Nagao, J., and Sumiyama, Y. (2002). Changes in gastrointestinal motility after subtotal colectomy in dogs. *Surg. Today* 32: 1048–1057.

Kudisch, M. and Pavletic, M.M. (1993). Subtotal colectomy with surgical stapling instruments via a trans-cecal approach for the treatment of acquired megacolon in cats. *Vet. Surg.* 22: 457–463.

Leighton, R.L. and Grain, E. (1978). Partial colectomy for the treatment of feline megacolon. *Feline Pract.* 3: 31–33.

Matthiesen, D.T., Scavelli, T.D., and Whitney, W.O. (1991). Subtotal colectomy for the treatment of obstipation secondary to pelvic fracture malunion in cats. *Vet. Surg.* 20: 113–117.

Milovancev, M., Weisman, D.L., and Palmisano, M.P. (2004). Foreign body attachment to polypropylene suture material extruded into the small intestinal lumen after enteric closure in three dogs. *J. Am. Vet. Med. Assoc.* 225: 1713–1715.

Nemeth, T., Solmymosi, N., and Balka, G. (2008). Long-term results of subtotal colectomy for acquired megacolon in eight dogs. *J. Small Anim. Pract.* 49: 618–624.

Niles, J.D. and Williams, J.M. (1999). Suture materials and patterns. *In Pract.* 21: 308–320.

Rosenbaum, J.M., Coolman, B.R., Davidson, B.L. et al. (2016). The use of disposable skin staples for intestinal resection and anastomosis in 63 dogs: 2000–2014. *J. Small Anim. Pract.* 57: 631–636.

Rosin, E., Walshaw, R., Mehlhaff, C. et al. (1988). Subtotal colectomy for treatment of chronic constipation associated with idiopathic megacolon in cats: 38 cases (1979–1985). *J. Am. Vet. Med. Assoc.* 193: 850–853.

Russell, K.N., Mehler, S.J., Skorupski, K.A. et al. (2007). Clinical and immunohistochemical differentiation of gastrointestinal stromal tumors from leiomyosarcomas in dogs: 42 cases (1990–2003). *J. Am. Vet. Med. Assoc.* 230: 1329–1333.

Ryan, S., Seim, H., MacPhail, C. et al. (2006). Comparison of biofragmentable anastomosis ring and sutured anastomoses for subtotal colectomy in cats with idiopathic megacolon. *Vet. Surg.* 35: 740–748.

Schrader, S.C. (1992). Pelvic osteotomy as a treatment for obstipation in cats with acquired stenosis of the pelvic canal: six cases (1978–1989). *J. Am. Vet. Med. Assoc.* 200: 208–213.

Shinozaki, J.K., Sellon, R.K., Tobias, K.M. et al. (2000). Tubular colonic duplication in a dog. *J. Am. Anim. Hosp. Assoc.* 36: 209–213.

Snowden, K.A., Smeak, D.D., and Chang, S. (2016). Risk factors for dehiscence of stapled functional end-to-end intestinal anastomoses in dogs: 53 cases (2001–2012). *Vet. Surg.* 45: 91–99.

Sweet, D.C., Hardie, E.M., and Stone, E.A. (1994). Preservation versus excision of the ileocolic junction during colectomy for megacolon: a study of 22 cats. *J. Small Anim. Pract.* 35: 358–363.

Webb, S.M. (1985). Surgical management of acquired mega-colon in the cat. *J. Small Anim. Pract.* 26: 399–405.

Weisman, D.L., Smeak, D.D., Birchard, S.J. et al. (1999). Comparison of a continuous suture pattern with a simple interrupted pattern for enteric closure. *J. Am. Vet. Med. Assoc.* 214: 1507–1510.

Welches, C.D. (1992). Perineal hernia in the cat: a retrospective study of 40 cases. *J. Am. Anim. Hosp. Assoc.* 28: 431–438.

Wells, K.L., Bright, R.M., and Wright, K.N. (1995). Cecal impaction in a dog. *J. Small Anim. Pract.* 36: 455–457.

Williams, J.M. (2012). Colon. In: *Veterinary Surgery Small Animal* (eds. K.M. Tobias and S.A. Johnston), 1542–1563. St Louis: Elsevier.

Williams, F.A., Bright, R.M., Daniel, G.B. et al. (1999). The use of colonic irrigation to control fecal incontinence in dogs with colostomies. *Vet. Surg.* 28: 348–354.

28

Colotomy

Daniel D. Smeak

Department of Clinical Sciences, College of Veterinary Medicine and Biomedical Sciences, Colorado State University, Fort Collins, CO, USA

28.1 Indications

Colotomy is rarely performed to collect full-thickness biopsies from the colon or to remove trapped foreign bodies that cannot be eliminated with the feces. In rare cases, sharp foreign bodies such as fish hooks or desiccated fecaliths can become lodged and may require endoscopic or surgical retrieval. Colonic perforations are dangerous and are often rapidly fatal, so they must be diagnosed and surgically managed on an emergent basis (Williams 2012).

Most biopsy attempts to determine the histological diagnosis of a colon lesion are performed by endoscopic means. This means of biopsy obtains samples that are only partial thickness; therefore, there is no risk of incisional dehiscence. However, this method of biopsy usually samples the only the mucosal layer, and therefore lesions that are deeper in the colonic wall or that are extraluminal in nature may be missed. The primary indication for colotomy is full-thickness biopsy when biopsy by other means, such as endoscopy or fine needle aspiration, is not possible or not definitive. In more rare circumstances, colotomy may be indicated *as a last resort*, if other methods are unsuccessful, for lodged foreign bodies or impacted fecoliths. As mentioned earlier, the unique and unforgiving nature of colonic healing explains why most surgeons will only consider open full-thickness biopsy of a colonic lesion or colotomy as a last resort.

28.2 Surgical Technique

28.2.1 Preoperative Considerations

See Chapter 27 for the similar pre-surgical considerations when planning a colotomy or colectomy.

28.2.2 Surgical Procedure

The colon is isolated with multiple layers of laparotomy sponges, and colon contents are milked away from the proposed excision/biopsy segment. Doyen forceps are used to hold fecal material well away from the resection site. Most biopsies for diffuse colonic disease are taken full-thickness by making an incision longitudinally on the antimesenteric border. When the lesion is focal, the biopsy is made directly over the lesion. If the lesion does not extend into the colonic lumen, a wedge biopsy is intentionally made without perforating the mucosa to reduce the risk of contamination and incisional dehiscence. To reduce any traumatic artifact on the full-thickness biopsy sample, a stay suture of 4-0 monofilament suture is placed full thickness through the proposed biopsy site, and elliptical incisions are made around the stay suture to remove the sample. Alternately, a 4 or 6 mm Baker's biopsy punch can be used to obtain a full-thickness colonic biopsy. The biopsy site is closed with 4-0 monofilament absorbable suture in a simple interrupted or continuous pattern (Figure 28.1). Mucosal eversion should be avoided during needle placement and at least 3 mm of colonic submucosa is caught with

Gastrointestinal Surgical Techniques in Small Animals, First Edition. Edited by Eric Monnet and Daniel D. Smeak.
© 2020 John Wiley & Sons, Inc. Published 2020 by John Wiley & Sons, Inc.
Companion website: www.wiley.com/go/monnet/gastrointestinal

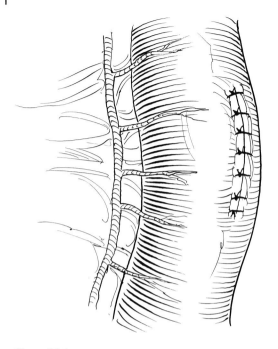

Figure 28.1

each bite. Sutures are placed consistently about 3 mm apart. To help avoid colotomy leakage, some surgeons prefer to complete the colotomy closure with a second inverting suture line provided it does not narrow the colonic lumen significantly. Omentum can be tacked over the site or a serosal patch can be performed if the surgeon desires (Hao et al. 2008). Surgeon's gloves are replaced, and the laparotomy is closed using a sterile closure pack.

28.3 Post-Operative Considerations and Prognosis

Fecal contamination is the most common intraoperative complication after colotomy. Fecal contamination is contained by isolating the surgical site with multiple layers of laparotomy sponges, milking fecal contents into the segment to be removed, use of atraumatic forceps to contain fecal matter orad and aborad to the colotomy, using new sterile gloves and instruments for closure of the abdominal approach, and copious local lavage. Post-operative complications include endotoxic shock, dehiscence, leakage, or death. Patients are monitored carefully during anesthetic recovery and for early signs of peritonitis or abscess formation. Depression, fever, excessive abdominal tenderness, vomiting, and ileus may indicate intraperitoneal infection. If these signs occur, serial blood cell counts should be performed and abdominal ultrasound considered to scan the abdomen for free fluid and to guide fluid aspiration sampling. Rapid surgical exploration is advised in animals with evidence of septic peritonitis after colotomy before deteriorating signs of endotoxic shock occur. Patients are given appropriate post-operative analgesic drugs after surgery. NSAIDs are used with caution during and after colonic surgery, since these drugs may interfere with the early stages of colonic healing (Gorissen et al. 2012). A high-residue, low-fat diet is fed after colonic surgery to promote normal intestinal motility (Williams 2012).

References

Gorissen, K.J., Benning, D., Berghmans, T. et al. (2012). Risk of anastomotic leakage with non-steroidal anti-inflammatory drugs in colorectal surgery. *Br. J. Surg.* 99: 721–727.

Hao, X.Y., Yang, K.H., Guo, T.K. et al. (2008). Omentoplasty in the prevention of anastomotic leakage after colorectal resection: a meta-analysis. *Int. J. Color. Dis.* 23: 1159–1165.

Williams, J.M. (2012). Colon. In: *Veterinary Surgery Small Animal* (eds. K.M. Tobias and S.A. Johnston), 1542–1563. St Louis: Elsevier.

29

Typhlectomy and Ileocecocolic Resection

Daniel D. Smeak

Department of Clinical Sciences, College of Veterinary Medicine and Biomedical Sciences, Colorado State University, Fort Collins, CO, USA

29.1 Indications

Diseases of the cecum that require resection are uncommon in the dog and cat. Surgical conditions of the cecum in small animals include neoplasia, cecal inversion, ileocolic intussusception with cecal inversion, cecal impaction, and cecal perforation (Clark and Pavletic 1992; Eastwood et al. 2005). The cecum can be removed at one of three levels: at its attachment to the proximal colon by simple typhlectomy, at its base through a proximal colotomy, or through entire ileocecocolic junction with an ileocolic anastomosis (Clark and Pavletic 1992; Williams 2012).

The level of excision is dictated by the disease process involving the cecum and regional bowel. Small peripheral cecal masses, cecal impaction, and reducible cecal inversions can be removed by simple typhlectomy. With cecal impaction excision, additional small bowel biopsies may be indicated depending on the suspected underlying cause of the cecal disease such as a generalized enteropathy (Wells et al. 1995; Eastwood et al. 2005; Russell et al. 2007). In most cases, cecal inversion cannot be reduced, so the cecum is removed via an adjacent colotomy and typhlectomy. The treatment of cecal neoplasia is excision. Provided an adequate margin of tissue can be obtained, for example with a more peripheral cecal mass, simple typhlectomy may be elected in this instance. More invasive masses or those involving the base of the cecum or proximal colon may require ileocecocolic resection and anastomosis. When cecal inversion is associated with ileocolic intussusception, the ileum, cecum, and proximal colon are excised if the bowel is devitalized or irreducible (Guffy et al. 1970; Bhandal et al. 2008).

29.2 Surgical Techniques

29.2.1 Simple Typhlectomy

Simple typhlectomy for a distal cecal perforation, cecal impaction, or tumor is begun by ligating several cecal branches of the ileocolic artery (if present) located at the base of the ileocecal fold. The ileocecal folds are dissected sharply toward the base of the cecum, freeing the cecum from the ileum and colon. A straight Carmalt clamp is placed across the base of the cecum. Intestinal contents are milked away from the proximal colon and ileum, and the contents are isolated away from the excision site with Doyen atraumatic forceps. The entire region is well "packed off" with several layers of laparotomy sponges. The cecum is transected where it joins the colon. The defect is closed with simple interrupted 4-0 monofilament absorbable sutures. Alternatively, an atraumatic clamp is placed across the cecal base, the cecum is resected distal to the clamp, and a Parker–Kerr oversewing technique is used to close the defect. The oversew technique produces a secure and sealed inverted closure of the defect, and it helps reduce intraoperative contamination during closure since the pattern is placed while the defect remains clamped. If linear staples are available, an appropriate length TA or GIA (blue cartridge) can be used to staple across the base of the cecum (Figures 29.1 and 29.2) (Clark and Wise 1994). The cecum is resected and submitted for biopsy, and the staple line is inspected to be sure the staples engage both bowel edges well (Figure 29.2). There is usually no need to oversew the staple line. The resection area is irrigated locally with warm saline.

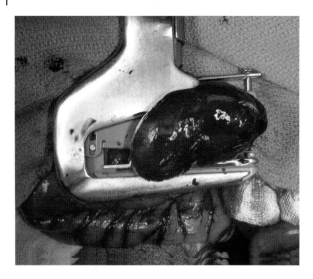

Figure 29.1

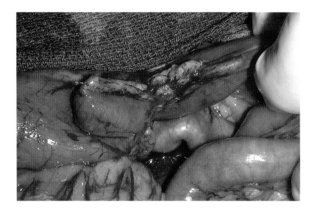

Figure 29.2

29.2.2 Colotomy and Typhlectomy Technique

If possible, an attempt is made first to gently manually reduce the cecum. If this is achievable, the cecum is removed as described for a simple typhlectomy. If the cecum is swollen, necrotic, or irreducible, and there is no evidence of a concurrent ileocecocolic intussusception, a separate colotomy and typhlectomy is indicated. Feces at the ileocecocolic region are milked away and isolated with atraumatic Doyen clamps as described for simple typhlectomy. The area is well "packed off" with laparotomy sponges. A 2–3 cm incision is made in the antimesenteric side of the colon just aborad to the "dimple" where the cecal inversion is located. The full-thickness incision is extended closely around the base to free the inverted cecum. After the cecum is excised, the defect is closed with a simple interrupted or continuous line of 4-0 monofilament absorbable suture. The resection area is irrigated locally with warm saline. Sterile

gloves are exchanged, and a separate sterile closure pack is used to close the abdominal approach.

29.2.3 Ileocolic Resection and Anastomosis

It is important to understand the terminal small bowel and large bowel vascular anatomy to preserve blood supply when considering bowel resection in this complex region. In obese animals the blood vessels within the mesocolon often cannot be isolated well at the time of surgery, so knowledge of the vascular anatomy is important. Blood supply to the ileocecocolic region begins with the cranial mesenteric artery. The common colic and jejunal arcade branch from this artery. The common colic artery branches into several colic vascular loops (colic, right colic, middle colic) as well as the left colic branch (from the caudal mesenteric artery), which supply the ascending and proximal transverse colon. The ileocecocolic branch forms a vascular loop running close to the mesenteric border of the ileum and cecocolic junction. It is supplied by the terminal jejunal artery (ileal artery-orad) and the terminal branch of the common colic (aborad).

To remove the terminal ileum, cecum, and proximal colon, the affected ileum and proximal colon borders are isolated with Carmalt forceps. As much of the healthy ileum is preserved as possible. The ileal artery is ligated just orad to the clamp on the ileum. Depending on the level of transverse colon to be removed, branches of the common colic artery are ligated as they run toward the mesenteric border of the affected colonic segment. Care is taken that the remaining stumps of the ileum and colon are healthy and that the supplying vasa recti have visible arterial pulsations. Intestinal contents are milked away, and atraumatic Doyen clamps are placed 5–10 cm orad and aborad to the Carmalt clamps on the isolated segment. The entire region is packed off with laparotomy sponges. The isolated portion of bowel is excised just outside the crushing clamps. The antimesenteric border of the ileum is incised to "fish mouth" the stump, so it is approximately the same diameter as the colon segment. There is usually plenty of bowel length remaining after excision of this region, so there is rarely tension encountered at the anastomosis site. An ileocolic anastomosis is performed with either a single-layer simple interrupted or simple continuous suture pattern using 4-0 monofilament absorbable suture. Some surgeons prefer a functional end-to-end anastomosis of the ileum and proximal colon using a linear cutting stapling device. The resection area is irrigated locally with warm saline. Gloves are exchanged, and a separate sterile closure pack is used to close the abdominal approach.

29.3 Tips

When a colotomy is performed it is helpful to use stay sutures just proximal and distal to the incision for retraction and to hold the colotomy under tension to ease closure.

The mesentery to the ileocecocolic region is often fat-laden. This obscures the rather substantial vascular supply coursing to this region. It is best to stay as close as possible to the mesenteric border when isolating the blood supply to the region. This will help avoid accidental damage to the proximal blood vessel branches that perfuse the portions of the bowel to be anastomosed.

When using linear and linear-cutting stapling devices, either a TA 3.5 or GIA 3.8 mm staple cartridge is chosen for most bowel resections in dogs and cats. If the bowel is highly edematous or thickened, a larger staple size (TA 4.8, GIA 4.8 mm) may be chosen or, in this instance, the author prefers to close the bowel using hand suturing.

29.4 Post-Operative Considerations and Prognosis

Hemorrhage and fecal contamination are some of the more common intraoperative complications encountered with typhlectomy. Surgeons must use extreme measures to reduce contamination during large bowel surgery to reduce the risk of peritonitis and wound infection. Clinically significant strictures of the anastomosis are uncommon. Anastomotic leakage is of utmost concern, since peritonitis results in peracute signs of septic shock and a high mortality risk. Careful monitoring of the patient's vital signs, blood pressure, blood glucose, and white blood cell parameters are important to alert the clinician of possible early dehiscence of the anastomosis. Sampling of free peritoneal fluid is considered when detected using "cage side" ultrasound scanning. The prognosis is excellent for most cecal impactions, neoplasms, and inversions provided there is no evidence of peritoneal contamination at the time of surgery (Russell et al. 2007; Williams 2012).

References

Bhandal, J., Kuzma, A., and Head, L. (2008). Cecal inversion followed by ileocolic intussusception. *Can. Vet. J.* 49: 483–484.

Clark, G.N. and Pavletic, M.M. (1992). Typhlectomy in dogs using a stapling instrument. *J. Am. Anim. Hosp. Assoc.* 28: 511–517.

Clark, G.N. and Wise, L.A. (1994). Stapled typhlectomy via colotomy for treatment of cecal inversion in a dog. *J. Am. Vet. Med. Assoc.* 204: 1641–1643.

Eastwood, J.M., McInnes, E.F., White, R.N. et al. (2005). Caecal impaction and chronic intestinal pseudo-obstruction in a dog. *J. Vet. Med.* 52: 43–44.

Guffy, M.M., Wallace, L., and Anderson, N.V. (1970). Inversion of the cecum into the colon of a dog. *J. Am. Vet. Med. Assoc.* 156: 183–186.

Russell, K.N., Mehler, S.J., Skorupski, K.A. et al. (2007). Clinical and immunohistochemical differentiation of gastrointestinal stromal tumors from leiomyosarcomas in dogs: 42 cases (1990–2003). *J. Am. Vet. Med. Assoc.* 230: 1329–1333.

Wells, K.L., Bright, R.M., and Wright, K.N. (1995). Cecal impaction in a dog. *J. Small Anim. Pract.* 35: 455–457.

Williams, J.M. (2012). Colon. In: Veterinary Surgery Small Animal, 2e (eds. K.M. Tobias and S.A. Johnston), 1542–1563. St. Louis: Elsevier.

30

Colostomy and Jejunostomy

Daniel D. Smeak

Department of Clinical Sciences, College of Veterinary Medicine and Biomedical Sciences, Colorado State University, Fort Collins, CO, USA

30.1 Indications

Colostomy and jejunostomy are techniques designed to either temporarily or permanently bypass the lower large intestine. Use of colostomy has been rarely reported for clinical treatment of dogs and cats because it requires highly dedicated owners to commit to important management requirements associated with fecal incontinence (Williams et al. 1999). Colostomy has been successfully used to permanently bypass obstructive nonresectable rectal neoplasia and invasive intrapelvic cancers (Hardie and Gilson 1997). These fecal diversion techniques have also been used to temporarily redirect feces from an area of rectal trauma, and to help with wound management and healing of rectal perforations and fistulation from anal atresia (Tobias 1994; Chandler et al. 2005; Tsioli et al. 2009).

30.2 Surgical Technique

Two colostomy technique types have been described in dogs and cats to bypass the distal intestinal tract: the end colostomy or laparoscopic-assisted end jejunostomy (Figure 30.1a), and the loop colostomy (Figure 30.1b). With end colostomy/jejunostomy the complete end of the proximal segment of colon or jejunum is brought full thickness through the body wall at a right angle and sutured to the skin in the flank region. The distal segment can either be preserved for reconnection at a later time (Chandler et al. 2005) or removed when the distal colorectal area is considered end-stage – for example, after excision of extensive neoplastic conditions (Lewis et al. 1992; Kumagai et al. 2003; Tsioli et al. 2009). With a flank loop colostomy, the colon is left intact, and a small segment is isolated and exteriorized through the left flank (Hardie and Gilson 1997).

The anesthetized patient is placed in dorsal or lateral recumbency depending on the technique chosen, and the region is prepared for aseptic surgery.

30.2.1 Flank Diverting Loop Rod-Supported Colostomy

30.2.1.1 Creation of the Loop Colostomy

The patient is placed in right lateral recumbency (Figure 30.2). Before surgery, the left flank is clipped, and a permanent marker is used to make a 4 cm circle in a flat region free of skin folds (usually at or above the level of the mid-abdominal wall). After standard aseptic preparation of the left flank region, the circle of skin and underlying subcutaneous tissue are excised to the level of the abdominal fascia. A muscle separating flank approach through the abdominal wall is made at the site just beneath the excised skin or, alternately, a linear incision can be made through the abdominal wall. The size of the abdominal incision should be generous enough to allow unimpeded blood flow to the exposed intestinal segment. The descending colon is grasped through the incision with Babcock forceps and exteriorized (Figure 30.2a).

Use of a supporting rod is recommended to help reduce tension during the early phases of colostomy healing. A straight plastic loop ostomy rod (90 mm loop ostomy rod, Convatec, Squibb Co. Princeton NJ) is placed at a right angle through the mesentery just below the segment of bowel to be used for colostomy. Subcutaneous tissue is dissected dorsal and ventral to the excised skin so the rod can be situated in these "pockets." The rod is sutured to the subcutaneous tissue

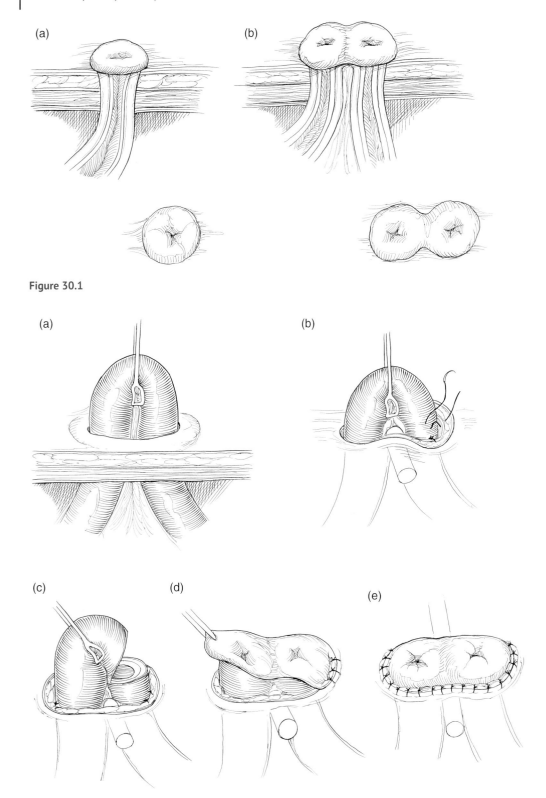

Figure 30.1

Figure 30.2

and underlying fascia using the loops at either end of the rod. Alternately, the transverse-oriented rod is fixed with suture on the skin surface under the colostomy and not implanted, and it is removed when the stoma matures, in approximately 10–14 days. The seromuscular/submucosal layer at the base of the exposed colon is sutured with 3-0 monofilament absorbable sutures to the abdominal wall fascia at the borders of the approach

(Figure 30.2b). A longitudinal or transverse incision (Figure 30.2c) is made in the colon, and the incised seromuscular edges are sutured with 4-0 monofilament nonabsorbable sutures to the skin, allowing the mucosa to evert over the skin edges (Figure 30.2d). This creates a nipple-like mucosal protrusion that extends through the flange of the colostomy appliance, minimizing fluid contamination at the flange-skin interface (Figure 30.2e). An appropriately-sized colostomy flange is attached to the skin surrounding the stoma, and a colostomy bag is attached to the flange. Alternately, the stoma is left uncovered, and skin protectants are used to help avoid dermatitis. Stoma irrigation may be used to help reduce fecal bulk and reduce stomal cleaning (see postoperative care).

30.2.1.2 Reversal of the Loop Colostomy

When the colostomy is not needed any longer, it is reversed. The patient is placed in lateral recumbency with the stoma side positioned upward. An elliptical incision is made about 1 cm around the exposed stoma site. The exteriorized colon segment is dissected free from surrounding tissue. Stay sutures are used to maintain exteriorization of the colon, and the rod is detached (if implanted) and removed. The edges of the colostomy are trimmed, and the colon is closed transversely with 4-0 monofilament absorbable sutures in a simple interrupted pattern (Hardie and Gilson 1997). The suture line is inspected for gaps, locally irrigated, and replaced into the abdominal cavity. Alternately, the colostomy site is excised, and the ends are anastomosed routinely (see Chapter 27). The region is lavaged, and the abdominal incision is closed routinely.

30.2.2 End-on Colostomy

The patient is placed in dorsal recumbency. Before surgery, a flat area in the left lateral flank region is marked with a permanent marker in an area that has no skin folds. After preparation of the patient for aseptic surgery, the descending colon is identified through a midline laparotomy. Intestinal contents are milked away from the proposed colon transection site, and the region is packed off with laparotomy sponges. Doyen forceps can be used to temporarily isolate fecal contents from the surgical site. The mid-descending colon is transected. The distal colon end is either stapled closed with a linear stapling device, or the end is oversewn with a Parker–Kerr pattern or double inverting pattern using 4-0 monofilament absorbable suture. The proximal end is temporarily closed with a simple continuous pattern using similar suture material or with a linear stapling device. A dorsoventrally oriented incision (usually about 4 cm in size to fit the diameter of the colon/ileum) is made through the skin and abdominal musculature at the marked "ostomy" site. The blind-ended proximal colon is brought through the abdominal incision with stay sutures. Care is taken to be sure the colon is not twisted during this maneuver. After donning new sterile gloves and using a sterile instrument pack, the laparotomy incision is closed routinely. The circumference of the seromuscular layer of the exteriorized colon is sutured to the flank abdominal fascial incision edges with 3-0 prolonged absorbable monofilament suture in a simple interrupted pattern. A stump of 2–3 cm is left extending from the abdominal wall suture line. A 0.5 cm margin of the terminal stump is excised including the temporary suture or staple line. The incised edge of the exteriorized colon is sutured in quadrants to the skin using 4-0 monofilament nonabsorbable suture (Figure 30.3a). These sutures are first placed at 90° from each other, and the remaining gaps are sutured closed. For suturing the bowel end to adjacent skin, a specific suture three-bite pattern is recommended to create a "nipple-like" end (Figure 30.3b). The first bite pierces the skin full-thickness, and a separate bite travels through a partial thickness 3 mm bite of bowel at the base of the exposed end. The final bite includes a 3 mm full-thickness

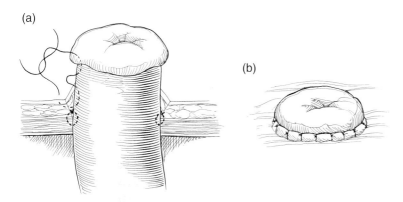

(a)

(b)

Figure 30.3

bite of the everted bowel edge (Figure 30.3a). An adhesive ostomy flange and bag (New Image Two-Piece Ostomy System, Hollister Inc. Libertyville Ill) are attached around the stoma (Figure 30.4).

Post-operatively, the stoma region is irrigated and cleaned, and the colostomy flange and bag are positioned (see 30.4). If the end-on colostomy needs to be reversed, the jejunostomy site is excised and the stoma is closed. The site is lavaged thoroughly and replaced in the abdominal cavity temporarily. The resultant abdominal wall defect is closed routinely. Through a separate midline abdominal approach, the blind-ended portions of the proximal and distal segments are excised, and an end-to-end anastomosis is performed.

30.2.3 Laparoscopic-Assisted End-on Jejunostomy

30.2.3.1 Creation of the Jejunostomy

A 5 mm trocar cannula is placed 2–3 cm caudal to the umbilicus, and the abdomen is insufflated. A rigid endoscope is introduced through this cannula. Another port (SILS multiple access port) is placed about 3 cm lateral to midline at the intended site for the jejunostomy. A blunt probe and a 5 mm laparoscopic fine-toothed grasping forceps are inserted in the paramedian port. The jejunoileal junction is identified using the cecum and antimesenteric ileal artery as landmarks, and the junction is grasped with fine-toothed grasping forceps. The section of intestine is exteriorized through the paramedian port incision while making sure no tension is present. Doyen forceps are placed orad and aborad to the jejunoileal junction, and the ileum (distal segment) is first closed with a thoraco-abdominal 3.5 linear autostapler and then oversewn (if desired) with an inverting continuous

pattern using 4-0 monofilament absorbable suture. The distal segment can be "tagged" to the proximal segment with nonabsorbable suture for easy retrieval later during stoma reversal (if indicated). The closed distal segment is irrigated and returned to the abdominal cavity. The multiple access port is removed, and the proximal end is pulled through the port site until 2–3 cm is exposed. The base of the exposed proximal segment is sutured in an interrupted pattern to the incised body wall edges, leaving 2–3 cm of the incised end exposed. The proximal bowel end is sutured to form a nipple-like stoma as shown and described for Figure 30.3. An adhesive ostomy flange and bag (New Image Two-Piece Ostomy System, Hollister Inc. Libertyville Ill) are attached around the jejunal stoma (Chandler et al. 2005) (Figure 30.4).

30.2.3.2 End-on Jejunostomy Reversal

The patient is placed in lateral recumbency with the stoma side positioned upward. A circular incision is made around the stoma site and extended 3 cm caudally. The jejunum is freed from surrounding tissue and exteriorized, and the stoma site is resected. The "tagged" blind-ended distal jejunal-ileum segment is identified and exteriorized from the abdomen. The previously staple-closed distal end is resected. A standard anastomosis is performed outside the abdominal cavity between the distal jejunum and ileum. The region is lavaged, the repaired intestine replaced into the abdomen, and the abdominal incision closed routinely using new sterile gloves and instrument pack.

30.3 Tips

The author prefers to create a nipple-like stoma to help reduce fecal soilage around the stoma, particularly when using a flanged colostomy bag. See Figure 30.3 for a description of the three-bite sequence when suturing the exposed intestinal edge to skin. An everted "button-like" ostomy site is more easily sealed against leakage by the closer fitting colostomy bag flange and bag.

The end-on jejunostomy is a simpler procedure and likely has less risk of dehiscence, since the loose jejunum segment can be exteriorized with minimal tension on the stoma site and the colon not involved in the procedure.

End-on colostomies may be a better technique than the loop colostomy because prolapse of the colon may occur more frequently with loop colostomy (Kumagai et al. 2003).

The flange that is applied to the skin around the stoma needs to well-adjusted and trimmed to the

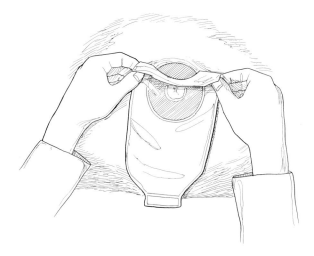

Figure 30.4

appropriate diameter to minimize exposure of skin to gastrointestinal contents. Stoma paste needs to be applied at each exchange of the stoma bag to protect the skin. A newer stoma bag comes with its own flange, so the flange is changed at each exchange which may help with stability of the flange over the skin surrounding the stoma.

30.4 Post-Operative Considerations and Prognosis

The patient is administered appropriate analgesics, crystalloid fluids, and electrolyte supplementation until it is comfortable, and eating and drinking on its own. The operative site is observed to be sure the color of the everted tissue is pink and healthy, and the site is monitored for infection and early dehiscence. The colostomy site may drain a bloody mucous discharge for the first 24–48 hours. Possible complications include peristomal dermatitis, intestinal prolapse, local wound infection, and peritonitis from dehiscence of the colostomy and leakage into the peritoneal cavity.

The ostomy site is cleaned, and the "ostomy" bag is changed every 12–24 hours (Figure 30.4). A major problem with colostomy collection systems available for human use is that the flange does not stay attached for more than several days at a time in small animals (Hardie and Gilson 1997). Soft, cloth-like backing on a flexible flange (Surfit Flexible, Convatec, Squibb Co.) stayed attached to the skin for longer periods of time than thicker flanges in one clinical study of dogs (Hardie and Gilson 1997). If fecal material leaks under the flange and stays in contact with the skin, severe irritation and infection can occur. This complication is treated by cleaning the skin and colostomy site thoroughly and replacement of the loose flange. Stoma paste is applied twice daily to areas of contact dermatitis surrounding the ostomy site, and the flange is not reapplied until the skin inflammation subsides. The owners are told to expect colostomy bag maintenance to take about 20 minutes per day. If the colostomy site is reversed, stricture of the repaired loop does not appear to be a common complication (Hardie and Gilson 1997).

All colostomies render the patient fecally incontinent since it bypasses the normal anal sphincter mechanism. Warm water enemas administered once daily may reduce the need for stomal care, since it may decrease fecal output over a 24-hour period (Williams et al. 1999). After the patient passes semi-solid feces from the stoma, peristomal irritation may be controllable even without the use of a colostomy apparatus (Tsioli et al. 2009).

References

Chandler, J.C., Kudnig, S.T., and Monnet, E. (2005). Use of laparoscopic-assisted jejunostomy for fecal diversion in the management of rectocutaneous fistula in a dog. *J. Am. Vet. Med. Assoc.* 226: 746–751.

Hardie, E.M. and Gilson, S.D. (1997). Use of colostomy to manage rectal disease in dogs. *Vet. Surg.* 26: 270–274.

Kumagai, D., Shimada, T., and Yamate, J. (2003). Use of an incontinent end-on colostomy in a dog with annular rectal adenocarcinoma. *J. Small Anim. Pract.* 44: 363–366.

Lewis, D.D., Beale, B.S., Pechman, R.D. et al. (1992). Rectal perforations associated with pelvic fractures and sacroiliac fracture-separations in four dogs. *J. Am. Anim. Hosp. Assoc.* 28: 175–181.

Tobias, K.M. (1994). Rectal perforation, rectocutaneous fistula formation, and enterocutaneous fistula formation after pelvic trauma in a dog. *J. Am. Vet. Med. Assoc.* 205: 1292–1296.

Tsioli, V., Papazoglou, G., Anagnostou, T. et al. (2009). Use of a temporary incontinent end-on colostomy in a cat for the management of rectocutaneous fistulas associated with atresia ani. *J. Feline Med. Surg.* 11: 1011–1014.

Williams, F.A., Bright, R.M., Daniel, G.B. et al. (1999). The use of colonic irrigation to control fecal incontinence in dogs with colostomies. *Vet. Surg.* 28: 348–354.

31

Colopexy
Daniel D. Smeak

Department of Clinical Sciences, College of Veterinary Medicine and Biomedical Sciences, Colorado State University, Fort Collins, CO, USA

31.1 Indications

Colopexy is mostly performed for treatment of chronic rectal prolapse and perineal hernia.

When prolapsed rectal tissue is considered viable and multiple treatment attempts with reduction and purse-string suture placement have been unsuccessful, a colopexy may be necessary. Colopexy is also indicated and is considered a first line treatment option when rectal prolapse is recurrent but no discreet predisposing factors can be identified, or if it is considered secondary to anal sphincter laxity.

Colopexy and/or cystopexy or vas deferens pexy have been performed as a successful adjunctive or sole treatment option for perineal hernia (Bilbrey et al. 1990; Dupre et al. 1993; Brissot et al. 2004; Grand et al. 2013). Colopexy combined with cystopexy have also been described as a two-step repair protocol for complicated and bilateral perineal hernias in dogs (Brissot et al. 2004; Grand et al. 2013). Laparotomy with colopexy ± cystopexy is performed first and definitive perineal hernia repair is usually delayed until the laparotomy wound is healed (approximately two weeks). Primary hernia repair was reported to be more easily performed because the hernia contained no obstructing viscera or periprostatic fat after the abdominal intervention.

31.2 Surgical Techniques

The goal of colopexy is to create a permanent adhesion between the descending colon and the left abdominal wall to prevent rectal prolapse or help reduce contents within a perineal hernia. An incorporating colopexy can be performed via a limited left paramedian abdominal approach when exploration of the abdomen is not necessary. Alternately, a laparoscopic or laparoscopic-assisted colopexy may be elected (Secchi et al. 2011; Zhang et al. 2013).

Sutures should incorporate at least 3 mm bites of submucosa when approximating the colonic wall to the abdominal incision. When a larger approach is important to achieve exposure or when a complete abdominal exploration is necessary, a standard ventral midline celiotomy is usually chosen.

31.2.1 Standard Ventral Midline Approach

The animal is placed in dorsal recumbency. A routine celiotomy is performed, and the peritoneal cavity and contents are systematically examined. The descending colon is identified and gently pulled cranially to help reduce the prolapse or reduce the contents within a perineal hernia. To help reduce an edematous rectal prolapse, an assistant outside the sterile field may be called upon to help manually push the prolapsed tissue forward while the surgeon gently pulls the colon forward through the celiotomy approach.

The descending colon is sutured to the left abdominal wall under moderate tension to form a permanent adhesion. Aggressive traction on the colon is avoided during the colopexy.

The goal is to form a permanent durable scar between the colon and abdominal wall, about 5–8 cm lateral to the linea alba without compromising the bowel wall. Two suture techniques have been described to form this colopexy (Popovitch et al. 1994) and both appear to be equally successful in avoiding rectal prolapse recurrence. In either technique, sutures are placed without penetrating the colonic lumen. The colopexy is made approximately 5–7 cm in length.

Gastrointestinal Surgical Techniques in Small Animals, First Edition. Edited by Eric Monnet and Daniel D. Smeak.
© 2020 John Wiley & Sons, Inc. Published 2020 by John Wiley & Sons, Inc.
Companion website: www.wiley.com/go/monnet/gastrointestinal

In the non-incision technique, 3-0 prolonged absorbable sutures are passed from the antimesenteric surface of the colon to the transversus abdominis muscle. The sutures are placed in two rows, with five to six simple interrupted or horizontal mattress sutures or simple continuous bites in each row.

The incision/scarification technique involves creating an incision through adjacent transversus abdominis muscle, and "scarifying" the proposed colonic "pexy" site. Scarification is created by taking a #15 scalpel blade and scraping off the thin serosa of the adjacent colon. Each edge of the scarified region is sutured separately to the corresponding edge of the transversus abdominis muscle incision.

31.2.2 Paramedian Incorporating

A left paramedian skin incision is made about 1 cm lateral to and parallel with the nipples from the level of the cranial aspect of the prepuce caudally, about 6–8 cm in length. The subcutaneous tissue is incised directly from the skin incision to the abdominal fascia. The first fascial incision is made parallel to the linea alba about 1 cm medial to the myofascial line of the external abdominal oblique muscle. Directly underneath, the internal abdominal oblique fascia is incised and the rectus abdominis muscle and peritoneum are bluntly separated to expose the abdominal cavity. The descending colon is identified, lifted out of the approach, and pulled cranially to help reduce the prolapse. At the proposed colopexy site, the serosal surface at the antimesenteric region of the exposed colon is scarified with a #15 BP blade. The "scarified" colonic wall is tacked firmly to the abdominal fascial layer closure using 3-0 monofilament, prolonged absorbable suture in a simple continuous pattern. Beginning at the caudal aspect of the approach, the two abdominal oblique fascial layers are closed while incorporating a 5 mm bite of the seromuscular layer of the "scarified" region of the colon with each needle pass. Subcutaneous and skin layers are closed routinely.

31.2.3 Laparoscopic Colopexy

A Veress needle is inserted on midline 1–2 cm cranial to the umbilicus. The abdomen is insufflated and a standard three-cannula laparoscopy technique is used. Alternately a single-incision laparotomy multiport access port can be inserted via a Hasson technique at the umbilical area, with an additional cannula added as needed. The first cannula is placed on ventral midline at the site of the Veress needle puncture. This site is used

for the camera. A brief abdominal exploration is performed to ensure that the Veress needle and subsequent cannula insertion did not cause visceral damage. The other cannulas are placed about 8–12 cm paramedian to the right about 5–8 cm caudal to the first cannula. These instrument cannulas are separated by 5–8 cm. The mid abdominal wall "pexy" site is incised parallel to the long axis of the body for 5 cm through the left transversus abdominis muscle adjacent to the respective colon "pexy" site. The antimesenteric border of the descending colon is grasped with laparoscopic forceps and pulled cranially. Once the rectal prolapse has been reduced, the adjacent colonic wall is sutured to the two muscle wall edges with two longitudinal continuous rows using 2-0 monofilament unidirectional barbed suture starting at the caudal aspect of the prepared colopexy site.

31.2.4 Laparoscopic-Assisted Colopexy

A two-port laparoscopic-assisted incisional colopexy technique has been described for successful treatment of rectal prolapse in a cat (Secchi et al. 2011). One port site is inserted on midline just cranial to the umbilicus (camera) and the other in the left inguinal region (instrument port). Through the inguinal cannula the descending colon is identified and grasped using atraumatic endoscopic forceps. The cannula is removed and the port site is enlarged with electrotomy for 2.5–5 cm. An incorporating colopexy is performed as described for the paramedian approach.

31.3 Tips

In the author's experience, suturing the colon under excessive tension can cause transient urinary incontinence, likely due to tension on the pelvic plexus within the peritoneal reflections.

31.4 Post-Operative Care, Complications

Appropriate analgesia is provided for patients undergoing colopexy. The prognosis after colopexy is good to excellent provided the primary cause of the condition is resolved, otherwise recurrence is a risk. Colopexy has not been reported to interfere with large intestinal function. In one retrospective study of 14 cats and dogs, there was no evidence of recurrence after colopexy;

however, several incisional complications were reported (Popovitch et al. 1994).

For staged colopexy and cystopexy with subsequent primary perineal hernia repair, a 10% hernia recurrence rate has been reported after surgery, which compares favorably with other studies (Brissot et al. 2004; Shaughnessy and Monnet 2015). However, mild but persistent post-operative urinary incontinence occurred in 17% of dogs, and tenesmus persisted in 10%. No fecal incontinence was reported. In a study on 41 cases with perineal hernia the addition of colopexy and cystopexy to an internal obturator transposition repair did not show any additional benefit, however (Grand et al. 2013).

References

Aronson, L.R. (2012). Rectum, anus, and perineum. In: *Veterinary Surgery Small Animal* (ed. K.M. Tobias), 1573–1575. St. Louis: Elsevier.

Bilbrey, S.A., Smeak, D.D., and DeHoff, W. (1990). Fixation of the deferent ducts for retrodisplacement of the urinary bladder and prostate in canine perineal hernia. *Vet. Surg.* 19: 24–27.

Brissot, H.N., Dupre, G.P., and Bouvy, B.N. (2004). Use of laparotomy in a staged approach for resolution of bilateral or complicated perineal hernia in 41 dogs. *Vet. Surg.* 33: 412–421.

Burrows, C.F. and Ellison, G.V. (1991). Recto-anal disease. In: *Textbook of Veterinary Internal Medicine*, 3e (ed. S.J. Ettinger), 1559–1575. Philadelphia: Saunders.

Corgozinho, K.B., Belchior, C., Moreira de Souze, J.H. et al. (2010). Silicone elastomer sling for rectal prolapse in cats. *Can. Vet. J.* 51: 506–510.

Dupre, G.P., Prat, N., and Bouvy, B.M. (1993). Perineal hernia in the dog: evaluation of associated lesions and results in 60 dogs. *Vet. Surg.* 22: 250.

Engen, M.H. (1990). Management of rectal prolapse. In: *Current Techniques in Small Animal Surgery*, 3e (eds. M.J. Bojrab, S.T. Birchard and J.L. Tomlinson), 259–263. Philadelphia: Lea & Febiger.

Gilley, R.S., Caywood, D.D., Lulich, J.P. et al. (2003). Treatment with a combined cystopexy-colopexy for dysuria and rectal prolapse after bilateral perineal herniorrhaphy in a dog. *J. Am. Vet. Med. Assoc.* 222: 1717–1721.

Grand, J.G. et al. (2013). Effects of urinary bladder retroflexion and surgical technique on postoperative complication rates and long-term outcome in dogs with perineal hernia: 41 cases (2002–2009). *J. Am. Vet. Med. Assoc.* 243 (10): 1442–1447.

Gunn-Moore, D., Bessant, C., and Malik, R. (2008). Breed-related disorders of cats. *J. Small Anim. Pract.* 49: 167–168.

Hosgood, G., Hedlund, C.S., Pechman, R.D. et al. (1995). Perineal herniorrhaphy: perioperative data from 100 dogs. *J. Am. Anim. Hosp. Assoc.* 31: 331–342.

Landon, B.P., Abraham, L.A., Charles, J.A. et al. (2007). Recurrent rectal prolapse caused by colonic duplication in a dog. *Aust. Vet. J.* 85: 381–384.

Matthiesen, D.T. (1989). Diagnosis and management of complications occurring after perineal herniorrhaphy in dogs. *Compend. Contin. Educ. Small Anim. Pract.* 11: 797–822.

Maute, A.M., Koch, D.A., and Montavon, P.M. (2001). Perineal hernia in dogs – colopexy, vaspexy, cystopexy, and castration as elective therapies in 32 dogs. *Schweizer Archiv fur Tierheilkunde.* 143: 360–367.

Niebauer, G. (1993). Rectoanal disease. In: *Disease Mechanisms in Small Animal Surgery* (ed. M.J. Bojrab), 271–284. Philadelphia: Lea & Febiger.

Popovitch, C.A., Holt, D., and Bright, R. (1994). Colopexy as a treatment for rectal prolapse in dogs and cats: a retrospective study of 14 cases. *Vet. Surg.* 23: 115–118.

Secchi, P., Castagnino, K.F., Feranti, J.P. et al. (2011). Laparoscopic-assisted incisional colopexy by two portals access in a domestic cat with recurrent rectal prolapse. *J. Feline Med. Surg.* 14: 169–170.

Shaughnessy, M. and Monnet, E. (2015). Internal obturator muscle transposition for treatment of perineal hernia in dogs: 34 cases (1998–2012). *J. Am. Vet. Med. Assoc.* 246 (3): 321–326.

Washabau, R.J. and Brockman, D.J. (1994). Recto-anal disease. In: *Textbook of Veterinary Internal Medicine*, 4e (eds. S.J. Ettinger and E.C. Feldman), 1398–1409. Philadelphia: Saunders.

Zhang, S.X., Wang, H.B., Zhang, J.T. et al. (2013). Laparoscopic colopexy in dogs. *J. Vet. Med. Sci.* 75: 1161–1166.

Section VII

Rectum and Anal Sac

32

Approaches to the Rectum and Pelvic Canal

Daniel D. Smeak

Department of Clinical Sciences, College of Veterinary Medicine and Biomedical Sciences, Colorado State University, Fort Collins, CO, USA

32.1 Indications

Rectal surgery is usually conducted to remove masses or non-viable bowel, and to repair prolapses, perforations, strictures, or rectal-cutaneous fistulas. It is imperative to achieve a definitive histologic diagnosis of a rectal mass and determine its local extent before contemplating surgery, as full-thickness rectal wall resection can have a high risk of complications including death (Nucci et al. 2014). Staging of neoplastic processes is also important to determine prognosis and whether ancillary therapy may be indicated after surgical resection. Thoracic radiographs and abdominal ultrasound, or CT imaging, is usually necessary before surgery to determine if there is evidence of metastasis and to help define the local extent of the neoplastic lesion. Following thorough cleansing of the terminal bowel, proctoscopy may be performed to biopsy and further assess the extent of the mass before surgery. Contrast enemas may be indicated to define rectal perforations, rectal fistulas, or other rectal wall abnormalities. In humans, transrectal ultrasound has been shown to be superior to computed tomography in preoperative assessment of depth of rectal wall invasion and adjacent organ involvement (Kim et al. 1999).

Perirectal (extramural) intrapelvic masses can also cause obstruction of the rectum within the restricted pelvic canal. These masses are best imaged with contrast CT or MRI. Fine needle aspirates and punch biopsies taken through the perineum outside the lumen of the rectum via digital or ultrasound guidance can often help definitively diagnose an intrapelvic mass. Cultures and cytology samples are submitted from aspirates of fluid collections within the pelvic canal.

Surgical access to a rectal lesion or the perirectal region can be challenging because most of the rectum is encased within the bony pelvic canal. Furthermore, important vessels and nerves are closely associated with the rectum and urogenital tracts, and inadvertent damage to these structures will not only increase the risk of rectal repair dehiscence, but also affect both fecal and urinary continence. Therefore, choosing the best approach to expose a rectal condition is paramount to successful surgical repair. Surgical access to lesions of the rectum may be achieved via a number of approaches, and determining the best approach depends upon location and extent/size of the lesion, and whether the disease process is benign or infiltrative. For the purposes of planning the surgical approach and procedure, rectal lesion location has been previously defined as colorectal junction, cranial rectum, mid rectum, and caudal rectum. The rectum can be approached or exposed via a ventral, dorsal, lateral, or caudal (transcutaneous or transanal) approach, or a combination of the listed approaches with celiotomy (Figure 32.1) (Baines and Aronson 2018).

In dogs, and less so in cats, the short mesocolon can limit caudal mobilization of the proximal colon segment, and extensive resections of the rectum may cause excess tension on the anastomosis, increasing the risk of dehiscence or stricture formation (Pavletic and Berg 1996).

The dorsal approach may be chosen for benign conditions that are intrapelvic but are not invading the rectal wall (extramural lesions), such as for abscesses, expansile lipomas, and for extraluminal benign mural masses

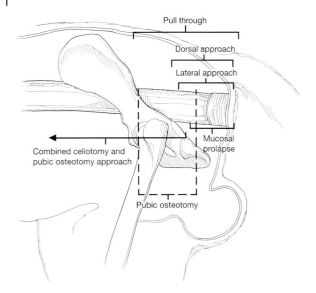

Figure 32.1

such as rectal leiomyomas or low-grade leiomyosarcomas. When the lesion is focal and at the dorsal mid to caudal third of the rectum, a partial rectal wall excision via a dorsal approach may be successful. When a benign lesion is narrow and circumferential, the mid to terminal rectal tube can also be resected and anastomosed via this approach. For more infiltrative rectal conditions necessitating larger surgical margins within the pelvic canal, a combined transanal ± ventral celiotomy approach may be a better choice.

The lateral approach offers limited exposure to one side of the caudal third of the rectum for repair of unilateral perforations or resections of limited benign mural lesions affecting the lateral wall of the rectum, such as for a diverticulum or rectocutaneous fistula removal.

A caudal ventral celiotomy approach extending from the umbilicus to pubis provides access to the descending colon and colorectal junction. The ventral approach via pubic osteotomy is useful for accessing most intrapelvic regions of the rectum. The surgeon should be prepared to extend a caudal celiotomy approach if more exposure is necessary for removal of colorectal or perirectal lesions that extend into the pelvic canal. This approach offers a rather restricted exposure to the intrapelvic rectum since urogenital structures must be carefully isolated and retracted to view the rectum through the limited boney window.

In some cases, these previously mentioned approaches to the rectum do not provide enough exposure particularly extensive full-thickness lesions that involve the mid to caudal rectal region. More novel transanal

and rectal eversion techniques allow for removal of lesions in this troublesome area (Chapter 33).

32.2 Surgical Approaches to the Rectum

32.2.1 Dorsal Approach

The dorsal approach to the rectum is relatively easy and it provides good exposure to the dorsal and dorsolateral aspects of the mid to caudal rectum (Figure 32.2) (McKeown et al. 1984; Anderson et al. 1987; Holt et al. 1991). However, it does not provide exposure to the anal canal. The dorsal approach is chosen for abscesses or expansile perirectal lipomas, and also for extraluminal, intramural noninfiltrative rectal masses such as rectal leiomyomas or low-grade leiomyosarcomas that do not require extensive full-thickness excision. When the lesion is focal and at the mid to caudal third of the rectum, a partial rectal wall excision via a dorsal approach may be attempted. A narrow circumferential rectal lesion (such as a benign stricture) in the mid to terminal portion of the rectum can be successfully resected and anastomosed via this approach.

The patient is positioned in ventral recumbency with the tail firmly fixed over the lumbar spine. The cranial aspects of the upper hind limbs are padded to prevent pressure damage to the femoral nerves on the firm edge of the surgery table. A purse-string suture is placed around the anus in most cases to prevent fecal soilage of the aseptic field during the procedure. After aseptic preparation of the patient, just medial to each ischiatic tuberosity, an inverted U-shape curvilinear skin incision is made which extends 1–2 cm dorsal to the cutaneous margin of the anus (Figure 32.2a). The subcutaneous tissue and thin perineal fascia are sharply dissected. The paired midline rectococcygeus muscles are transected between their origin on the dorsal rectal wall and ventral surface of the coccygeal vertebrae to improve exposure of the deeper, dorsal pelvic canal. The external anal sphincter and caudal edge of the levator ani muscles can be bluntly separated, if necessary, to improve exposure (Figure 32.2b). The caudal rectal nerves on the lateroventral aspects at the junction of the anal sphincter and levator ani are carefully identified and preserved if the procedure requires more ventral pelvic floor exposure. Damage to the peritoneal reflections on the lateral surfaces of the mid rectal region should be avoided. For more exposure at the mid-rectal region, incising completely through the levator ani muscles may be considered. Malleable or Gelpi retractors are used to improve

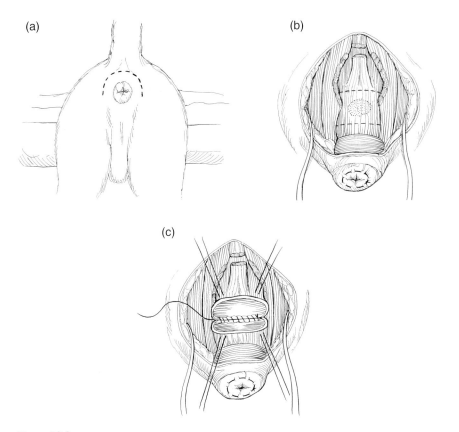

(a)

(b)

(c)

Figure 32.2

visualization when needed. The intrapelvic rectal segment is mobilized for the planned procedure. For circumferential excision of the rectum through this approach, stay sutures are placed cranial and caudal to the proposed resection site. Resection and anastomosis can be performed with either interrupted or continuous suture patterns (Figure 32.2c) or circular stapler (see Chapter 33) (Fucci et al. 1992; Banz et al. 2008). For closure, the levator ani muscles are reapposed with cruciate sutures (3-0 monofilament absorbable), if they were incised to gain exposure. The incised stumps of the rectococcygeus muscle are reapposed with cruciate sutures. The surgery bed is thoroughly lavaged before closure. In most cases, placement of a drain to manage dead space is not necessary. If significant contamination occurred during the rectal procedure, the wound bed is sampled for bacterial culture after thorough saline lavage, and a Jackson–Pratt active suction drain is placed within the wound dead space. Remember to avoid placing the drain tube directly against the rectal repair, since its presence may impair rectal healing. The subcutaneous and skin layers are separately closed in routine fashion, and the purse-string suture is removed.

32.2.2 Lateral Approach

The lateral approach is similar to the approach used for perineal hernia repair (Figure 32.3). It offers only limited exposure to one side of the caudal third of the rectum for repair of lateral perforations or resection of focal benign mural lesions of the rectum such as a diverticulum or rectocutaneous fistula (Fossum 1997). This approach should not be chosen for resection and anastomosis since the rectal wall opposite the approach cannot be adequately exposed.

The patient is placed in ventral recumbency with the tail fixed firmly over the lumbar spine. The lateral perineal region is draped, excluding the anus, after placement of an anal purse-string and aseptic preparation of the region. A vertical curvilinear incision is made 2–3 cm lateral to the anus, beginning just above the ventral tail base to just ventral to the middle of the ischial table (Figure 32.3a). Underlying subcutaneous tissues and the thin perineal fascia are sharply incised to expose the muscular perineal diaphragm. The ventrally located pudendal vessels and nerve (and caudal rectal nerve branch) are isolated and protected with an encircling

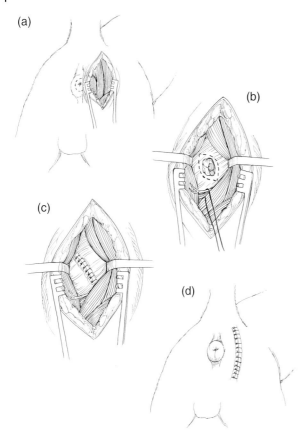

Figure 32.3

silk suture (Figure 32.3b). Depending on the location of the lateral rectal lesion, an incision is made between the levator ani and the anal sphincter (caudolateral lesions), or between the pubocaudalis and ishiocaudalis portions of the levator ani muscle (mid to caudolateral rectal lesions) (Figure 32.3b and c). The caudal rectal nerve branch located in the lower third of the anal sphincter attachment to levator ani muscle junction is avoided during muscle division. For closure, the divided muscle segments are reapposed with interrupted prolonged absorbable monofilament sutures to avoid creating a defect in the perineal diaphragm. Finally, the wound bed is lavaged and the subcutaneous tissues and skin are routinely closed (Figure 32.3d). Depending on the amount of wound contamination during the procedure, a Jackson–Pratt active suction drain can be inserted.

32.2.3 Ventral Approach with Pubic Osteotomy

The ventral approach via pubic osteotomy is useful for accessing most of the mid to cranial third regions of the intrapelvic rectum (Figure 32.4) (Davies and Read 1990; Yoon and Mann 2008). It is always wise to prepare for

this approach whenever dealing with rectal lesions that are close to the pelvic inlet since it may be necessary to help expose the terminal side of a colorectal mass that extends into the cranial portion of the pelvic canal from a caudal celiotomy approach. This approach is certainly helpful in obtaining exposure of the ventrolateral rectal wall, but the exposure is still limited due to overlying urogenital structures. These structures (urethra, prostate, vagina) must also be carefully isolated and retracted to view the rectum through this confined boney window. An alternative approach, pelvic symphysiotomy, involves complete separation of the pubis and ischium along their ventral midlines. Lateral retraction of the pubic and ischial bones is constrained by the flexibility of the bone and size of dog, so rectal exposure is even more limited because the pubic bone halves can be separated no more than 1.7 cm without causing subluxation of the sacroiliac joints (Schlicksup et al. 2013).

A large-bore urethral catheter should be placed at the time of surgery preparation for patients undergoing a ventral pubic osteotomy approach to help isolate and protect the urethra during the procedure. The patient is placed in dorsal recumbency and the entire abdomen and pubic area just cranial to the vulva or scrotum are prepared for aseptic surgery. One advantage of the ventral approach to the rectum is that it can be combined with a midline celiotomy, so a complete abdominal exploration can be performed before an extensive intrapelvic procedure. For neoplastic lesions, once exploration is complete, the terminal colon and cranial rectum are palpated carefully, and median iliac lymph nodes are examined to determine extent of involvement. The skin incision is carried back to end just cranial to the caudal ischial margin to begin the pubic osteotomy procedure. After sharp dissection is carried through the subcutaneous tissues, the entire length of the adductor/ gracilis muscle aponeurosis is incised on midline to the floor of the pubic bone. The adductor/gracilis muscles are bilaterally elevated from the pubic bone to the lateral limits of the obturator foramina (Figure 32.4a). The obturator nerves and vessels that lie at the craniolateral edge of each obturator foramina must be protected during the muscle elevation and osteotomies. Osteotomies (dashed lines) are created 2–3 mm medial to the lateral limit of the obturator foramina on each side of the pubis. Thin malleable retractors are preplaced under the osteotomy sites to help avoid damage to the obturator nerves (Figure 32.4b). After first protecting underlying soft tissues, a final transverse cut is planned caudally at the junction of the pubis and ischium. If exposure of the more caudal aspect of the pelvic area is additionally required, the adductor muscles are elevated off the

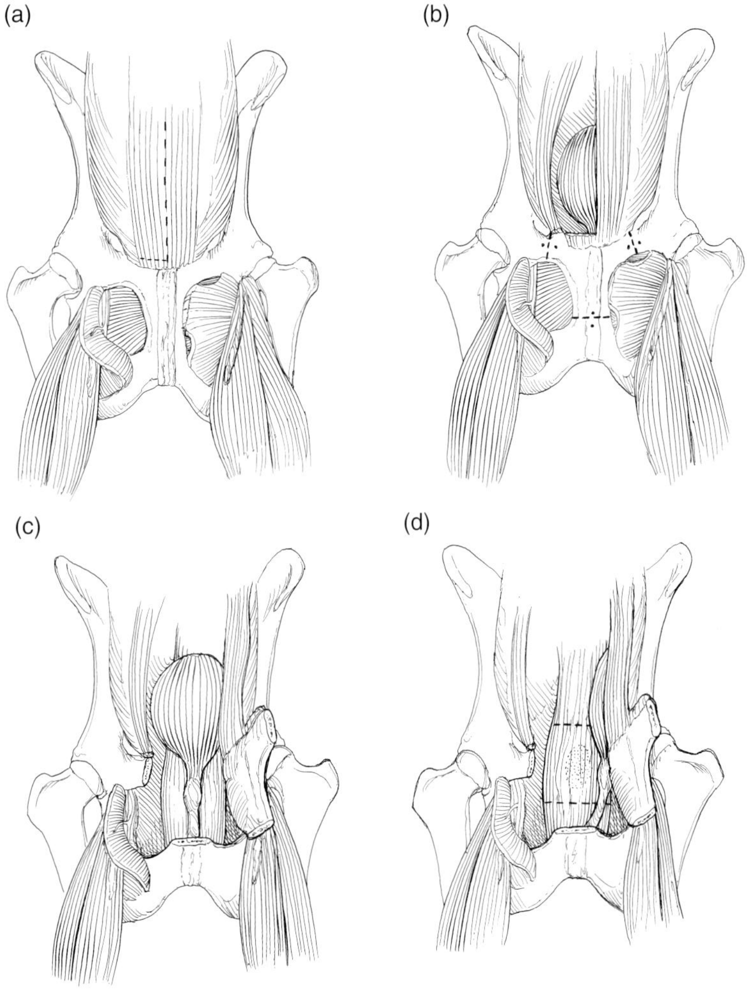

Figure 32.4   (a)   (b)

(c)   (d)

caudal ischial segment. Bilateral osteotomies are created at the level of the caudolateral aspect of each obturator foramina.

Before osteotomies are performed, it is best to predrill holes at least 5 mm away from the proposed osteotomy sites in preparation for wire fixation at the end of the procedure (Figure 32.4b). Drilling over a fixed bone surface is easier than attempting to drill on the free bone segment after the osteotomies are performed.

The author prefers to create a "hinged" pubic/ischial osteotomy approach rather than freeing up all soft tissues attached to the proposed pubic bone (Figure 32.4c). This leaves soft tissues attached to the pubis opposite the surgeon's view (in this case the view is from the dog's right side) and this helps facilitate caudal abdominal wall closure.

Using an oscillating saw, the pubic bone (and ischium if necessary) is fully cut through on both sides. One half of the prepubic tendon attachment of the rectus abdominis muscle is incised on the near side, but the tendon is left attached on the "hinged" side (Figure 32.4a). The bone segment is then easily hinged laterally (away from the surgeon's view) without the ipsilateral rectus abdominis muscle attachment draping over the approach, further limiting exposure. A 3–4 mm fringe of tendon is left on the pubis to allow suturing of the severed half of the rectus abdominis tendon back to the bone at the end of the procedure (Figure 32.4a). The pubic/ischial bone segment is pried up toward the side opposite the surgeon, leaving much of the soft tissue attachments on the opposite hinge side intact (Figure 32.4c). This maneuver helps leave a portion of the blood supply intact to the bone segment by preserving these remaining soft tissue attachments. Complete removal of the pubic bone from soft tissues may increase the susceptibility of the avascular bone to infection and subsequent sequestration (Orsher 1989). After the bone segment is hinged laterally to the side opposite the surgeon's view, soft tissues attached to the bone on the deep side of the segment are reflected off if necessary, to expose the urogenital tract overlying the rectum. The indwelling catheter is palpated to identify the location of the urethra and careful intrapelvic dissection is begun. Urogenital structures are freed up from their attachments on the *near side only* as needed to gain enough exposure for the rectal procedure. For rectal resection and anastomosis through this approach, the peritoneal reflection and pelvic nerves, located on the lateral walls of the mid pelvic rectum, are carefully separated close off the rectal wall by means of delicate blunt dissection (Figure 32.4d). The colon and rectum are isolated from the surrounding viscera with moistened laparotomy sponges. For detailed description of end-to-end anastomosis techniques of the rectum, refer to Chapter 33.

For closure, a segment of appropriately-sized orthopedic wire is fed between the opposing drill holes and once all wires are fed through the respective holes, the wires are uniformly twisted to firmly fix the bone in place. In toy-breed dogs and cats, large prolonged absorbable monofilament suture can be used instead of wire. If the rectum was entered during the procedure, the region is thoroughly lavaged, instruments are exchanged for sterile ones, and surgeons don sterile gloves before closure.

The severed prepubic tendon segments are sutured together with large monofilament prolonged absorbable suture in a cruciate pattern. The linea alba incision is closed on midline routinely. Incised adductor and gracilis muscle fascial edges are reapposed on midline with prolonged absorbable monofilament suture. Subcutaneous and skin closure is routine. If gross contamination is witnessed during the procedure, active wound drainage is advocated. Soft tissue should be interposed between the drain and rectal repair to help avoid impaired rectal healing from contact with the drain (Holt and Durdey 1999).

32.3 Post-Operative Care and Complications

The purse-string suture, if utilized, is removed upon anesthetic recovery. Post-operative care is tailored to the patient, surgical approach, and type of rectal procedure. Rectal thermometer use and digital rectal palpation is avoided for several weeks after rectoanal surgery. Antibiotics are not continued after surgery unless gross contamination occurred during the procedure or a source of infection is encountered. Appropriate analgesic agents are administered for five to seven days after surgery.

For patients undergoing pubic osteotomies that are showing signs of adductor weakness and "splaying out" of the hind limbs on slippery surfaces, hobbling the rear limbs for the first 10–14 days may be considered. Lameness and neurologic dysfunction from obturator nerve retraction may be seen for several days to weeks after pubic osteotomy.

References

Anderson, G.I., McKeown, D.B., Partlow, G.D. et al. (1987). Rectal resection in the dog. A new surgical approach and the evaluation of its effect on fecal continence. *Vet. Surg.* 16: 119–125.

Baines, S.J. and Aronson, L.R. (2018). Rectum, anus, and perineum. In: *Veterinary Surgery Small Animal* (eds. S.A. Johnston and K.M. Tobias), 1783–1827. St. Louis: Elsevier.

Banz, W.J., Jackson, J., Richter, K. et al. (2008). Transrectal stapling for colonic resection and anastomosis (10 cases). *J. Am. Anim. Hosp. Assoc.* 44: 198–204.

Davies, J.V. and Read, H.M. (1990). Sagittal pubic osteotomy in the investigation and treatment of intrapelvic neoplasia in the dog. *J. Small Anim. Pract.* 31: 123–130.

Fossum, T.W. (1997). Surgery of the perineum, rectum, and anus. In: *Small Animal Surgery* (ed. T.W. Fossum), 335–347. St. Louis: Mosby.

Fucci, V., Newton, J.C., Hedlund, C.S. et al. (1992). Rectal surgery in the cat: comparison of suture versus staple technique through a dorsal approach. *J. Am. Anim. Hosp. Assoc.* 28: 519–525.

Holt, P.E. and Durdey, P. (1999). Transanal endoscopic treatment of benign canine rectal tumours: preliminary results in six cases (1992–1996). *J. Small Anim. Pract.* 40: 423–427.

Holt, D., Johnston, D.E., Orsher, R. et al. (1991). Clinical use of a dorsal surgical approach to the rectum. *Compend. Contin. Educ. Small Anim. Pract.* 13: 1519–1528.

Kim, N.K., Kim, M.J. et al. (1999). Comparative study of transrectal ultrasonography, pelvic computerized tomography, and magnetic resonance imaging in preoperative staging of rectal cancer. *Dis. Colon Rectum* 42: 770–775.

McKeown, D.B., Cockshutt, J.R., Partlow, G.D. et al. (1984). Dorsal approach to the caudal pelvic canal and rectum: effect on normal dogs. *Vet. Surg.* 13: 181–184.

Nucci, D.J., Liptak, J.M. et al. (2014). Complications and outcomes following rectal pull-through surgery in dogs with rectal masses: 74 cases (2000–2013). *J. Am. Vet. Med. Assoc.* 245: 684–695.

Orsher, R.J. (1989). Problems and complications associated with colorectal surgery. In: *Problems in Veterinary Medicine* (ed. D.T. Matthiesen), 243–253. Philadelphia: JB Lippincott.

Pavletic, M.M. and Berg, J. (1996). Gastrointestinal surgery. In: *Complications in Small Animal Surgery* (eds. A.J. Lipowitz, D.D. Caywood, C.D. Newton, et al.), 390–398. Baltimore: Williams & Wilkins.

Schlicksup, M.D., Holt, D.E. et al. (2013). The effect of abaxial retraction on pelvic geometry after pubic symphysiotomy. *Vet. Surg.* 42: 958–962.

Yoon, H.Y. and Mann, F.A. (2008). Bilateral pubic and ischial osteotomy for surgical management of caudal colonic and rectal masses in six dogs and a cat. *J. Am. Vet. Med. Assoc.* 232: 1016–1020.

33

Surgery of the Rectum

Daniel D. Smeak

Department of Clinical Sciences, College of Veterinary Medicine and Biomedical Sciences, Colorado State University, Fort Collins, CO, USA

33.1 Indications

In dogs and cats, diseases of the rectum are relatively uncommon and include rectal neoplasms, strictures, diverticula, perforations, fistulae, prolapse, and trauma (Baines and Aronson 2018). Focal diseases, depending if they involve just the rectal mucosa or exhibit deeper wall invasion, may require local mucosal or full-thickness resection. For more circumferential or infiltrative masses, complete resection and anastomosis of the rectum may be required. A variety of external approaches have been previously described to help expose rectal lesions for resection (Chapter 32).

Extensive resection is particularly challenging when infiltrative lesions extend into the mid to distal region of the rectum. Due to the limited means to access this region, and the possibility of damage to important regional anatomic structures, the risk of post-operative complications is high (Nucci et al. 2014). In addition, lesions that involve the terminal rectum and anal canal cannot be accessed through the standard external approaches mentioned in Chapter 32, and require special transanal techniques. As mentioned previously, confirmation of the disease process with biopsy, combined with staging, radiographic imaging, and, when appropriate, endoscopic assessment of the extent of the rectal lesion are highly important for choosing the most appropriate surgical approach and excision technique.

Procedures that can be considered for removal of focal masses involving the terminal 2–3 cm of rectum include transanal endoscopic resection or rectal prolapse (eversion) and excision (Palminteri 1966; Holt and Durdey 1999). Transanal endoscopic resection is mainly indicated for small pedunculated masses. For more sessile

masses, transanal endoscopic resection can result in a somewhat "piecemeal" removal of the mass using a cauterizing endoscopic loop, which makes complete excision of the mass difficult to achieve. In addition, endoscopic loop resection may risk rectal perforation because the depth of the excision cannot always be determined intraoperatively. A more refined technique for removal of focal, partial thickness masses is transanal rigid endoscopic resection using a single-port access system.

Small, noninvasive (noncircumferential), focal, pedunculated or more sessile, terminal, rectal masses (1–3 cm from the anus), such as rectal polyps or adenomas and some focal carcinomas in situ, that are *readily exteriorized through the anus* can be resected successfully with a transanal prolapse and excision technique (Palminteri 1966). The benefit of this approach for mass removal is that the risk of wound contamination and damage to extra-rectal structures is limited. For known benign mucosal lesions, simple mucosal prolapse and excision is often successful. Focal masses (noncircumferential) that require full-thickness rectal wall excision can also be removed with the transanal prolapse and excision technique, but due to the limited access with this approach, surgical margins cannot be extensive. Besides mass recurrence, few surgical complications are encountered with this prolapse and excision technique. Excision via rectal prolapse can be successfully performed with electrosurgery (Palminteri 1966), a stapling device (Swiderski and Withrow 2009), laser (Shelley 2002), or cryosurgery (Valerius et al. 1997).

For an acquired rectal prolapse that cannot be reduced or when the wall of the prolapsed rectum is not viable or is associated with a mass, a resection is required. This is accomplished with a surgical

Gastrointestinal Surgical Techniques in Small Animals, First Edition. Edited by Eric Monnet and Daniel D. Smeak.
© 2020 John Wiley & Sons, Inc. Published 2020 by John Wiley & Sons, Inc.
Companion website: www.wiley.com/go/monnet/gastrointestinal

technique that is somewhat similar to the prolapse and mass excision technique.

More extensive circumferential and malignant masses within the terminal pelvic canal, or lesions that *cannot be readily exteriorized* and that have evidence of deeper rectal wall infiltration require wide, full-thickness excision. In these cases, to achieve appropriate surgical margins, transanal rectal pull-through techniques may be considered (Gerlach et al. 1992; Morello et al. 2008). These pull-through procedures are generally indicated for lesions involving the mid to terminal rectum but may be extended to include the cranial third of the rectum depending on mobility of the intrapelvic segment (Baines and Aronson 2018). Circumferential, benign, terminal, rectal strictures or sessile masses can also be readily excised with a pull-through technique. The difference between the rectal prolapse (eversion) and excision and pull-through techniques is that rectal prolapse and excision is performed completely within the lumen of the rectoanal canal and it does not involve circumferential dissection through perirectal attachments. Therefore, the prolapse and excision technique rarely results in significant surgical complications. Dissection just outside the involved full-thickness segment of rectal tube with the pull-through technique can result in contamination of the pelvic cavity, tension on the repair, and damage to perirectal tissue (such as the anal sphincter, or neurovascular tissue) which dramatically increases the risk of significant post-operative complications (Nucci et al. 2014). For these reasons, pull-through surgery should be performed only after an informed discussion with the owner, including risk of complications (both acute and long-standing), the impact these complications have on quality of life, and cancer-related outcomes.

33.2 Surgical Techniques

33.2.1 Transanal Techniques

The transanal approaches include prolapse and eversion, transanal endoscopic, pull-through, and combined transabdominal and transanal pull-through techniques.

33.2.1.1 Transanal Endoscopic Mass Excision

During colonoscopy with a flexible endoscope, a small pedunculated mass can be removed with a cauterizing loop wire or with grasping forceps and electrotomy.

33.2.1.2 Transanal Approach with a Rigid Endoscope and a Single-Port Access System

A single-port access system utilized for laparoscopy can be used to perform a transanal approach to the rectal lumen for partial thickness resection of a benign lesion or for biopsy (Figure 33.1a and b). This technique allows for insufflation of gas to distend the rectum affording more accurate exposure of a rectal mass for mucosal dissection and resection (van den Boezem et al. 2011; Aly 2014).

(a)

(b)

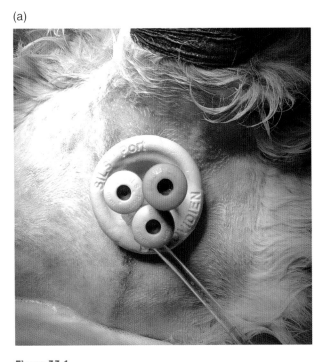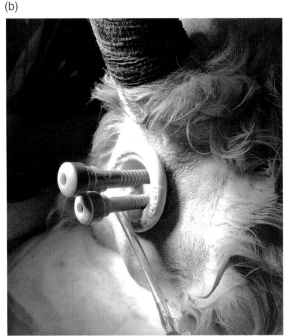

Figure 33.1

33.2.1.3 Transanal Prolapse and Mass Excision; Intraluminal Closure of a Distal Rectal Perforation

Before considering this technique, the focal lesion involving the caudal rectum or anal canal should be *readily exteriorized with digital eversion*. Perforations of the terminal rectum can also be exposed and closed with this technique provided the perforation was caught early, and no evidence of perirectal inflammation was present on physical examination. With this technique, the author generally does not attempt bowel preparation or enemas before surgery because the liquefied feces can obscure visualization during surgical excision. At the time of surgery, the terminal rectum and anal sacs are digitally evacuated, and several gauze sponges are inserted cranially up the rectum to help temporarily block stool from the surgery field.

With the patient in ventral recumbency (with the tail bandaged and secured dorsally and cranially, and pelvic limbs hanging freely over the end of a padded surgical table), the anal opening is dilated with four stay sutures (2-0 or 3-0 nylon) placed at the mucocutaneous junction (Figure 33.2a). Continual traction on these stay sutures will help keep the anus open for the remaining part of the procedure. The involved rectal wall is everted with stay sutures placed at least 1 cm *cranial* to the rectal lesion. Additional stay sutures are placed through the mass or adjacent to the mass if necessary, to help manipulate and expose the lesion (Figure 33.2b). These stay sutures are important since after mass resection the incised rectal mucosal edges can invert and often can be difficult to isolate for closure. Electrosurgery or a scalpel is used to remove the mass. The excision is made either full-thickness through the rectal wall (for locally invasive masses), or partial thickness through the mucosa only (benign polyps and adenomas). For benign masses, the lesion should be excised with at least 0.5 cm margins of healthy tissue (Morello et al. 2008). Mucosal defects are closed with 4-0 monofilament, absorbable sutures in a simple interrupted or simple continuous pattern (Figure 33.2c). Full-thickness defects are closed similarly being careful to purchase 3 mm of submucosa with

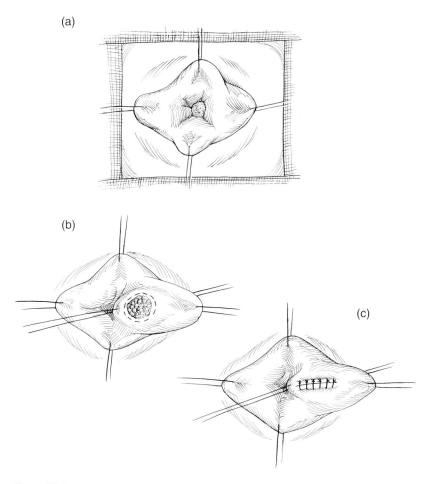

Figure 33.2

each full-thickness needle bite. For peracute uncomplicated rectal perforations, the focal tear is exposed with stay sutures, devitalized edges are debrided adjacent to the defect, and the defect is closed with full-thickness simple interrupted sutures (3-0 or 4-0 monofilament, absorbable sutures). The stay sutures and gauze sponges are removed, and the surgical site is allowed to retract back into the pelvic canal. Afterward, the rectal canal is digitally palpated gently to check for unintentional rectal canal narrowing from misplaced sutures.

33.2.1.4 Excision of a Rectal Prolapse

When a rectal prolapse includes a lesion that requires excision, or if the prolapse has lost viability, a complete rectal prolapse excision is considered. The dog or cat is placed in ventral recumbency with the rear legs draped over a padded end of the surgery table. The tail is taped forward, and perineal region is prepared aseptically for surgery. Lubricated surgery sponges may be placed well cranial to the prolapse within the rectal lumen to help keep fecal material from obscuring the surgical site. Four, full-thickness stay sutures separated at 90° intervals are placed in healthy rectal tissue at least 1 cm orad to the proposed rectal resection level, to include both prolapsed bowel walls. It is helpful to insert an appropriately-sized syringe casing into the rectum prior to stay suture placement. The syringe casing helps guide the needle through *both* prolapsed rectal walls without accidentally incorporating the opposing rectal wall, and the casing can be used to cut against during sharp rectal prolapse excision. These stay sutures also help keep the inside rectal segment (that is under considerable tension) from retracting back into the pelvic canal after resection of the prolapsed region.

The dorsal aspect of the prolapse just proximal to the diseased area is sharply incised 180° directly against the inserted syringe casing. The two rectal wall layers are closed with 4-0 monofilament absorbable suture in an interrupted or continuous pattern to form a single-layer anastomosis. Sutures should incorporate 3 mm of rectal submucosa and are placed approximately 3 mm apart. The remaining portion of the rectum is excised circumferentially and closed similarly. After the anastomosis is finished, the stay sutures are removed, and the remaining viable rectal repair section is gently reduced.

33.2.1.5 Transanal Rectal Pull-Through Technique and Hand Suture

This technique can be used successfully for limited mid to terminal rectal resections involving generally 6 cm or less of the rectum, depending on the size of the patient (Morello et al. 2008). When planning on resecting more

extensive rectal lesions or masses spreading further orad, a combined transabdominal-transanal technique is used (see 33.2.2). Epidural anesthesia is considered to provide an extra level of analgesia, and to help relax structures in and around the anorectal region. The perineal region and proximal portion of the tail are clipped, and the rectum and anal sacs are digitally evacuated. The dog is positioned in sternal recumbency with the tail secured cranially and dorsally. The region is prepared for aseptic surgery. The surgery table is tilted head down, and the abdomen and limbs are padded at the caudal edge of the surgery table. A Lone Star retractor (or a series of stay sutures) is used to dilate the anus at the mucocutaneous junction.

For lesions encroaching the anorectal junction, a series of rectal wall stay sutures are placed just inside the anorectal junction. For lesions found more than 1.5 cm cranial to the anorectal junction, the rectal wall is everted digitally and held in place with four to six stay sutures to help expose the terminal aspect of the lesion. An additional series of six or more stay sutures are placed in the caudal rectal margin that is to be removed. These stay sutures help to mobilize and prevent the involved segment from accidentally retracting deep within the pelvic canal during dissection. While placing caudal retraction and tension between the two sets of stay sutures, a full-thickness 360° incision is made (Figure 33.3). Incision in this area will not affect the more caudal-situated anal sphincter or caudal rectal nerves. Starting at this incision, the involved rectal segment (with help from tension on the stay sutures) is carefully mobilized by dissecting as close to the rectal wall as possible, particularly near the region of the peritoneal reflections. The rectococcygeus muscle will be transected on the dorsal aspect of the rectum in the

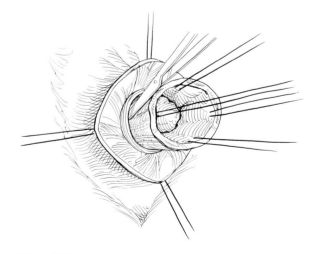

Figure 33.3

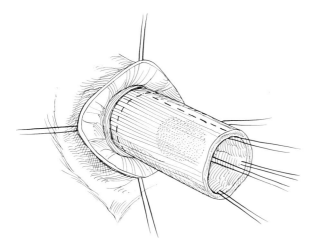

Figure 33.4

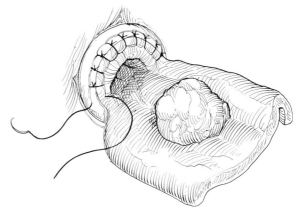

Figure 33.6

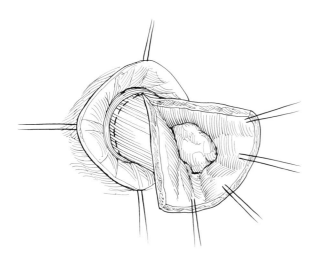

Figure 33.5

process of dissection and mobilization. Once the involved segment has been adequately exposed (Figure 33.4), a series of stay sutures are placed proximal (orad) to the proposed excision site (not shown on figure).

The rectal segment containing the mass is either palpated or incised longitudinally to establish the level of proximal transection (Figure 33.5). Depending on the disease process, the level of transection can be made within 0.5 cm of a benign lesion (for example a stricture), or at least 2–3 cm of normal-appearing rectal wall should be removed for more invasive rectal masses. The normal cranial rectal margin is anastomosed to the healthy distal rectal stump (or anorectal junction for lesions close to the anorectal line) with 3-0 simple interrupted, prolonged absorbable, monofilament sutures taking care to grasp at least 3 mm of sub-

mucosa with each needle purchase (Figure 33.6). It is best to circumferentially resect then suture in 90° increments (cut and sew technique), rather than excising the entire involved rectal tube at one time, to help control tension and provide proper alignment during repair. Afterwards, the anastomosis is carefully inspected for gaps, stay sutures are removed, and the rectum is allowed to retract back into the pelvic cavity (Figures 33.7 and 33.8).

For some dogs with rectal lesions that are terminal and not circumferential, a partial transanal pull-through is performed. The procedure is similar to what has just-been described, except that the initial terminal incision is extended only as far as necessary around the circumference of the anus or terminal rectum to achieve appropriate margins. Dissection is carried out just deep to the rectal wall as far proximally as necessary to expose the focal lesion. The remainder of the procedure is completed as previously described (Tobias and Johnston

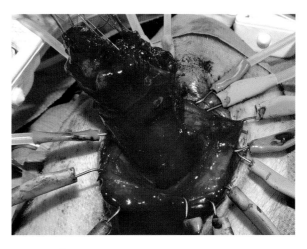

Figure 33.7

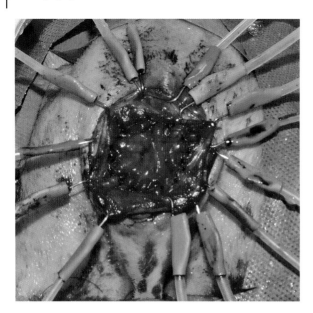

Figure 33.8

2012). Unless the perirectal area was grossly contaminated during the procedure, there is usually no need to provide active suction drainage.

33.2.1.6 Transanal Pull-Through Technique with Circular Stapler

A circular stapler can also be used for anastomosis during a rectal pull-through procedure. However, a 1.5 cm healthy cuff of distal rectum is required to complete the procedure with the circular stapler. After exteriorization of the part of the rectum that needs to be resected (as described previously) a purse-string suture is applied with a Furness clamp proximal to the segment containing the lesion. A purse-string suture is also applied to the distal margin of healthy rectum, but without the aid of a Furness clamp. A simple continuous, full-thickness suture is hand-applied 360° around the distal part of the rectum to form a 1 cm cuff. The purse string applied to the proximal and distal segments of the rectum are released once the circular stapler is introduced transanally. The extended anvil (exposing the anvil shaft) is inserted through the purse string on the proximal rectal segment. The purse string is then tied firmly around the shaft of the extended anvil. The purse string applied to distal cuff of rectum is also tied firmly around the shaft of the anvil. The anvil is compressed against the circular stapler base. It is important to ensure that the entire circumference of the proximal and the distal ends of the rectum are included within the circular stapler. Staples are fired and the blade in the circular stapler is activated. The

anvil is partially released and the circular stapler is removed.

33.2.2 Combined Transanal and Abdominal Techniques

When more extensive infiltrative lesions are located in the mid to caudal third of the rectum and extending into or close to the descending colon, a combined transabdominal-transanal approach can be used. The anastomosis is then completed with hand suture or with a circular stapling device as described below.

33.2.2.1 Combined Transabdominal-Transanal Pull-Through Technique, Hand-Sutured

When more extensive infiltrative lesions are located in the distal third of the rectum and extending into the descending colon or proximal rectum, a combined transabdominal-transanal approach can be used. Another surgical option for removal of a mid-rectal lesion extending proximally into the colon is a celiotomy/pubic osteotomy technique with transanal circular stapling (see 33.2.2.2). Through a ventral midline celiotomy, a complete abdominal exploration is performed first, and regional lymph nodes draining the rectal area are examined and biopsied. Medial iliac lymph nodes are sampled for biopsy regardless of whether they are grossly abnormal or not. The involved colorectal segment is examined to determine the cranial colonic resection site (at least 2–3 cm orad to the lesion). After grossly measuring the feasibility of an end-to-end anastomosis, the involved colorectal segment is isolated and corresponding vasculature are double ligated and divided. If the caudal mesenteric pedicle joining the distal colon severely limits advancement of the proximal stump into the pelvic canal or increases tension on the terminal anastomosis, it can be ligated and divided. The colon is divided at the appropriate predetermined resection site and the stumps are oversewn with separate continuous Parker–Kerr inverting suture lines using 3-0 monofilament suture. The two closed stumps are connected using four interrupted 2-0 monofilament sutures, leaving a gap of 1–2 cm between the stumps (Figure 33.9a). Alternately, the end tags from the Parker–Kerr lines are tied to the respective mesenteric and antimesentic sides exiting each stump. The celiotomy is then closed and the dog is repositioned in ventral recumbency. A transanal pull-through technique is used to isolate the terminal rectal segment as described previously. The distal portion of the involved rectal segment is isolated by incising circumferentially between preplaced stay sutures (Figure 33.9b). The affected rectal segment is dissected free from its attachments

(a)

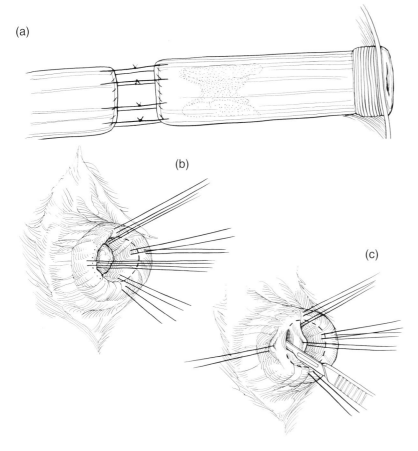

(b)

(c)

Figure 33.9

(Figure 33.9c). After excision of the distal colorectal stump containing the lesion, the oversewn segment on the colonic side is pulled externally by the attached sutures between the two inverted rectal cuffs (Figure 33.10a). The proximal Parker–Kerr suture cuff is excised on the dashed line (Figure 33.10b), and the incised colonic margin is anastomosed to the remaining preserved distal rectum cuff (or anorectal line depending on the terminal extent of the lesion) with full-thickness interrupted monofilament 3-0 absorbable suture (Figure 33.11a and b).

33.2.2.2 Rectal Resection with Transanal Circular Stapled Anastomosis Technique via Pubic Osteotomy Approach

Another option to remove colorectal to mid-rectal lesions is rectal resection and circular stapled anastomosis via a midline celiotomy with or without a pubic osteotomy approach, depending on the caudal extent of the rectal lesion (Chapter 32) (Banz et al. 2008). End-to-end circular anastomosis requires less exposure than hand-sewn anastomosis, so this technique is particularly useful when anastomosis is confined to the intrapelvic region. The animal is positioned in dorsal

(a)

(b)

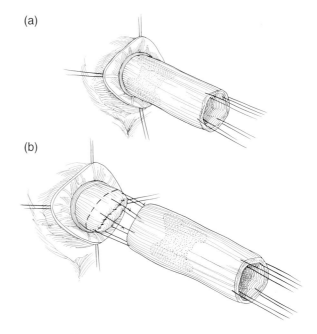

Figure 33.10

recumbency with the perineum positioned at the edge of the operating table and the tail fixed in extension to facilitate insertion of the stapler through the anus.

(a)

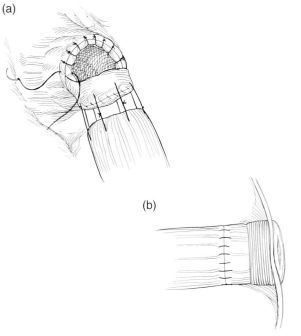

(b)

Figure 33.11

(a)

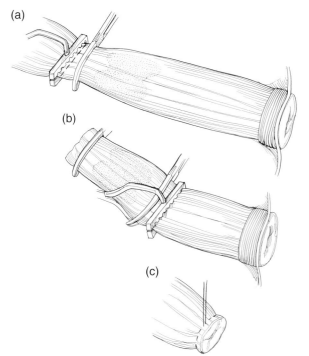

(b)

(c)

Figure 33.12

After the caudal ventral midline approach and a thorough abdominal exploration are completed, the involved colorectal segment is carefully examined and palpated to determine the region to be excised. It is very important to extend the linea alba incision to the level of the pubic symphysis to facilitate cranial intrapelvic exposure during the anastomosis. Both ureters are identified and preserved, and the remaining abdominal contents are retracted with malleable retractors. All connecting soft tissue is meticulously removed from the surface of the involved colorectal segment while avoiding damage to the intrapelvic peritoneal reflections. The vascular supply is ligated to the involved segment. Colonic contents are milked 5–7 cm proximal to the area to be resected and feces are contained with Doyen forceps. A purse-string suture is placed on the proximal colorectal resection site using a Furness clamp. The segment of rectum between the Carmalt clamp and Furness clamp (dashed line) is incised using the Furness clamp edge as a cutting guide (Figure 33.12a). The Furness clamp is applied to the proposed distal site and another purse-string suture is applied. A second Carmalt clamp is placed next to the distal Furness clamp to prevent contamination as the entire affected segment is excised (Figure 33.12b). A similar sharp incision is performed on the distal side of the involved rectal segment and the affected segment is removed. The purse-string suture and rectal cuff

extending from the purse-string sutures should be uniform (Figure 33.12c). Depending on the size of the patient (approximate diameter of the rectum) and thickness of the bowel at the anastomosis site, a 21–25 mm circular stapling device is chosen for the anastomosis with either 3.5 or 4.8 mm staples. Unless the colorectal region is grossly dilated (when a larger size may be considered), generally the 21 mm size staple device will fit medium-sized dogs, while the 25 mm device will suffice for larger dogs. If any serosal tearing is observed during introduction of the larger diameter EEA device into the rectum or colon, circular stapling is not chosen, and a hand-sutured anastomosis is undertaken. Forcing the circular stapler into a narrow diameter intestinal segment will cause staple misfiring or result in catastrophic rectal wall tears. A nonsterile surgeon outside the aseptic field introduces an appropriate-size lubricated EEA instrument through the anus into the caudal rectal segment to the level of the purse string (Figure 33.13a). The EEA stapler is opened exposing the shaft and loosed anvil to protrude from the distal rectal segment through the loosened purse-string suture line. The distal rectal purse-string suture is tied firmly around the anvil shaft (Figure 33.13b). The proximal purse string is loosened, and the anvil is placed within the proximal segment. The purse string is tightened firmly around the shaft of the anvil

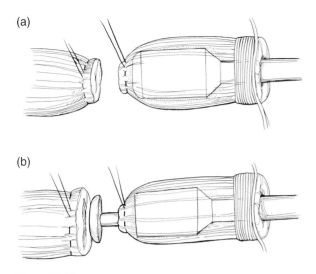

Figure 33.13

(Figure 33.14a). For both purse-string suture ends, the tissue within the purse string should be snug against the EEA cartridge and anvil shafts to reduce the possibility of bunching or overlapping of tissue as the instrument is closed. This can result in poor staple engagement in the opposing segment. The wing nut on the stapler is turned until the reference markers on the device are aligned indicating the two bowel ends are properly compressed. As the device is engaged, a circular, double, staggered row of staples joins the bowel and a circular blade in the instrument cuts a stoma (Figure 33.14b). The stapling device is opened slightly, and a set of traction sutures is placed at the staple line to help lift the staple line over the anvil for device removal. The EEA instrument is withdrawn under the staple line and removed from the rectum by slow rotation and traction. The two circular tissue rings that were cut when the device was fired are inspected as the

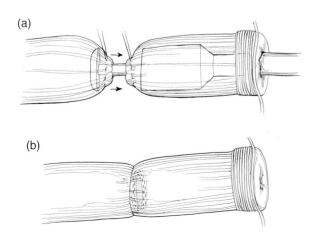

Figure 33.14

stapling device is fully opened. The two cut "donut cores" of rectal wall should each have an equal margin around the circumference. These circular pieces are submitted for histological examination. This circular stapler forms a true inverted anastomosis. The inverted cuff of tissue from this stapling technique has the potential to cause luminal stenosis just as other sutured inverting anastomoses, so under-sizing the circular stapler device should not be considered. If the surgeon chooses to check for gaps and leaks, the region is flooded with sterile saline and an appropriate-size Foley catheter is placed through an anal purse-string suture. With the Doyen remaining on the proximal segment, the rectum is slowly inflated and observed for bubbles around the staple line to determine whether any gaps in the line need additional suture reinforcement.

33.3 Tips

Preoperative preparation of the patient undergoing rectal surgery may be necessary to reduce the risk of complications (Zelhart et al. 2014). Administration of intraoperative parenteral antibiotics is particularly important since there is a higher risk of significant bacterial contamination during procedures that involve rectal resection (Nelson et al. 2014). When gross contamination in the region of a rectal surgery occurs, this can dramatically increase the risk of dehiscence. Perioperative antibiotics are administered parenterally an hour before the operation and repeated every 90 minutes until the procedure is completed. Cefoxitin is the author's antibiotic of choice since it achieves good tissue penetration and is effective against gram – bacteria such as *Escherichia coli*, with activity against gram + bacteria and anaerobes (Cuchural et al. 1990). There appears to be little value in continuing parenteral antibiotic use past the immediate post-operative period in an otherwise uncomplicated rectal repair (Scher 1997). For aggressive resections of the rectum, bowel cleansing and enteral antibiotics should also be considered, although this practice remains controversial (Bucher et al. 2004; Guenaga et al. 2011). Administration of enteral antibiotics without first cleansing the bowel may not significantly alter infection risk after rectal surgery (Lewis 1979; Niebauer 1990; Walshaw 1990). Oral neomycin and metronidazole administration may be elected one to two days before surgery once bowel cleansing has been initiated (Baines and Aronson 2018).

There are two schools of thought about mechanical intestinal preparation before rectal surgery. Firm compact stool at the surgery site is easier to contain and remove without spillage, however, the contamination that does manage to leak into the surrounding region is highly concentrated. Removal of solid feces makes sense to help reduce bacterial numbers, improve intraoperative exposure, reduce post-operative discomfort stemming from posturing and passing stool through a painful surgery region, and it helps reduce stresses on the operative site (Baines and Aronson 2018). If bowel preparation is elected, the patient is fasted for 48 hours before surgery if tolerable. Oral administration of GoLYTELY (polyethylene glycol and electrolytes) is very effective at cleaning the bowel in preparation for aggressive open rectal procedures. Two doses of GoLYTELY (40 ml/kg) are administered with a nasogastric tube. One dose is given the night before planned colonoscopy and surgery, and the second dose is given four to six hours before surgery. Some surgeons also give an enema with GoLYTELY to ensure the bowel is free of all debris at the time of anesthesia (Baines and Aronson 2018). Enemas are contraindicated in patients with suspected rectal perforations, and many surgeons do not recommend enemas in small animals with obstructive lesions (Baines and Aronson 2018). The author prefers to administer intravenous fluids during the bowel preparation process to be sure the patient is well hydrated before anesthesia. In all patients undergoing rectoanal procedures, digital evacuation of the terminal rectum and anal sacs should be performed. When appropriate, a purse-string suture in the anus is placed before aseptic preparation of the surgical site. Epidural or sacrococcygeal regional nerve blocks with longer duration local anesthetics should be considered.

Particularly for extensive intrapelvic approaches and transanal techniques, epidural analgesia should be elected to provide an extra level of analgesia, and to help relax structures in and around the anorectal region during the procedure (Otero and Campoy 2013).

The Lone star retractor seems to provide better exposure than four or five stay sutures placed at the anocutaneous junction for transanal approaches (Figure 33.15). In addition, the Lone Star retractor facilitates the procedure if limited assistance is available.

Circular stapling is technically demanding to use, and improper use can result in severe complications, including dehiscence and death. When performed by experienced surgeons, circular stapled rectal anastomosis has been demonstrated to be a rapid and effective method of colorectal anastomosis with low leakage rates, accurate alignment of tissues, and rapid healing in animals and humans (Ravitch and Steichen 1979; Bellenger 1982; Kudisch and Pavletic 1993; Kudisch 1994; Docherty et al. 1995).

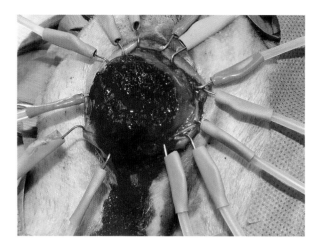

Figure 33.15

33.4 Post-Operative Care and Complications

Since rectal surgeries are classified as clean-contaminated, most surgeons do not continue antibiotic administration past the immediate post-operative period. For patients that have undergone aggressive rectal resections, stool softeners such as lactulose, and low residue diets are usually continued for several weeks to decrease tension on the repair and improve patient comfort after surgery. Intravenous fluids and electrolyte supplementation are given when appropriate until the patient is showing interest in food and is drinking. The incision sites are protected from self-trauma with an Elizabethan collar.

Vital signs are carefully monitored after surgery to detect signs indicative of dehiscence and peritonitis. Any evidence of infection or rectal dehiscence should be early and aggressively diagnosed and managed. Generalized sepsis and peritonitis from a rectal dehiscence will advance quickly if not diagnosed early. Abdominal and intrapelvic ultrasound with fine needle aspiration of perirectal fluid should be attempted if there are early signs of infection.

Animals that are incontinent after surgery are managed with routine perianal cleaning and surface skin protectants. The animal is re-evaluated in two weeks, and gentle digital rectal examination is performed to rule out significant stricture formation. For patients undergoing malignant rectal mass excision, monitoring for local recurrence and distant metastasis is recommended every three months up to one year, and six-month intervals thereafter.

Numerous complications are possible after rectal surgery. Post-operative tenesmus, hematochezia, and fecal incontinence are not uncommon. Increased frequency of defecation and loose stool can be expected over a variable period of time (weeks to months). Owners should be warned that many dogs experience transient fecal incontinence that generally begins to subside in less than two weeks. Rectal prolapse, perirectal abscessation, dehiscence, and stenosis are other less common complications.

For partial rectal wall resections to remove benign lesions, recovery is generally uncomplicated. The literature states, however, that aggressive rectal resections hold considerable risk of post-operative complications. The risk of dehiscence is greater for full rectal segment resections greater than 6 cm (Anderson et al. 1987; Phillips 2001).

In one report, nearly 80% of dogs undergoing rectal pull-through developed at least one complication after surgery. Incontinence (up to 50%), transient diarrhea (55%), tenesmus (40%), stricture formation (27%), rectal bleeding (14%), constipation (12%), dehiscence (10%), and wound infection (6%) were reported (Nucci et al. 2014). In another retrospective study of 11 patients undergoing extensive transanal rectal pull-through or combined abdominal-transanal procedures for extensive benign and malignant rectal tumor excision, all dogs developed rectal bleeding and tenesmus, which resolved in most cases by two weeks. Two dogs died within four days of surgery. Three developed rectal stricture, and two dogs developed incontinence that resolved spontaneously as long as five months after surgery. Local recurrence of rectal masses was detected in 18% of the dogs. Of the dogs that survived the early postoperative period with clean excisions, long-term survival was reported. Rectal carcinomas removed with the combined abdominal-transanal approach carry a guarded prognosis (50% early mortality rate) (Morello et al. 2008; Baines and Aronson 2018). More details about prognosis after rectal tumor excision can be found elsewhere (Baines and Aronson 2018).

Two major contributing factors for fecal continence include external anal sphincter function, or the integrity of both the muscular and nerve components of the anal sphincter, and reservoir continence (Nucci et al. 2014; Baines and Aronson 2018). Sphincteric continence involves the ability to sufficiently contract the external anal sphincter to resist pressure during peristalsis of the rectum and colon. Afferent and efferent fibers of the caudal rectal nerve, a branch of the pudendal nerve, govern sphincteric function. Reservoir continence involves the ability of the descending colon and rectum to expand and store fecal matter until an appropriate time for elimination. Innervation of the rectum originates from the pelvic plexus which is largely contained within the peritoneal reflections (Nucci et al. 2014). Preservation of a minimum of 1.5 cm of the terminal rectal tube along with the anal sphincter is thought to be necessary in most cases to safeguard fecal incontinence after circumferential rectal resection (Anson et al. 1988; Morello et al. 2008). The terminal rectal mucosa and internal anal sphincter have a primary role in differentiating between solids, liquids and gases (Guilford 1990). Loss of the terminal internal anal sphincter may result in a dog being unaware of the contents of the distal rectum and subsequently developing fecal incontinence (Nucci et al. 2014). In the past, rectal segment amputations greater than 4–6 cm in length (which necessitates division of the peritoneal reflection) was thought to consistently cause incontinence (Anson et al. 1988; Morello et al. 2008). In a more recent study, it appears that resections of this magnitude may not cause incontinence provided the perirectal dissection is meticulous and is not carried away from the rectal wall (to prevent damage to the pelvic plexus within the peritoneal reflection) (Morello et al. 2008; Nucci et al. 2014). More extensive colorectal resections risk reservoir fecal incontinence, resulting in signs of frequent and unconscious defecation (Morello et al. 2008).

References

Aly, E.H. (2014). SILS TEM: the new armamentarium in transanal endoscopic surgery. *J. Min. Access Surg.* 10 (2): 102–103.

Anderson, G.I., McKeown, D.B., Partlow, G.D. et al. (1987). Rectal resection in the dog: a new surgical approach and the evaluation of its effect on fecal continence. *Vet. Surg.* 16: 119–125.

Anson, L.W., Betts, C.W. et al. (1988). A retrospective evaluation of the rectal pull-through technique. *Vet. Surg.* 17: 141–146.

Baines, S.J. and Aronson, L.R. (2018). Rectum, anus, and perineum. In: *Veterinary Surgery Small Animal* (eds. S.A. Johnston and K.M. Tobias), 1783–1827. St. Louis: Elsevier.

Banz, W.J., Jackson, J., Richter, K. et al. (2008). Transrectal stapling for colonic resection and anastomosis (10 cases). *J. Am. Anim. Hosp. Assoc.* 44: 198–204.

Bellenger, C.R. (1982). Comparison of inverting and appositional methods for anastomosis of the small intestine in cats. *Vet. Rec.* 12: 265–268.

Bucher, P., Mermillod, B., Gervaz, P. et al. (2004). Mechanical bowel preparation for elective colorectal surgery: a meta-analysis. *Arch. Surg.* 139: 1359–1364.

Cuchural, G.J., Tally, F.P., Jacobus, N.V. et al. (1990). Comparative activities of newer beta-lactam agents against members of the Bacteroides fragilis group. *Antimicrob. Agents Chemother.* 343: 479–480.

Docherty, J.G., McGregor, J.R., Akyol, A.M. et al. (1995). Comparison of manually constructed and stapled anastomoses in colorectal surgery. West of Scotland and Highland anastomosis study group. *Ann. Surg.* 22: 176–184.

Gerlach, K.F., Rocken, F.E. et al. (1992). The transanal proctectomy (rectal pull-through technique) in dog. *Kleintierpraxis* 37: 617–628.

Guenaga, K.F., Matos, D., and Wille-Jorgensen, P. (2011). Mechanical bowel preparation for elective colorectal surgery. *Cochrane Database Syst. Rev.* 9 (9): CD001544. https://doi.org/10.1002/14651858. CD001544.

Guilford, W.G. (1990). Fecal incontinence in dogs and cats. *Compend. Contin. Educ. Pract. Vet.* 12: 313–324.

Holt, P.E. and Durdey, P. (1999). Transanal endoscopic treatment of benign canine rectal tumours: preliminary results in six cases (1992–1996). *J. Small Anim. Pract.* 40: 423–427.

Kudisch, M. (1994). Surgical stapling of large intestines. *Vet. Clin. N. Am. Small Anim. Pract.* 24: 323–333.

Kudisch, M. and Pavletic, M. (1993). Subtotal colectomy with surgical stapling instruments via a trans-cecal approach for treatment of acquired megacolon in cats. *Vet. Surg.* 22: 457–463.

Lewis, R.T. (1979). Advances in antibiotic prophylaxis in gastrointestinal surgery. *Can. Med. Assoc. J.* 121: 265–266.

Morello, E., Martano, M., Squassino, C. et al. (2008). Transanal pull-through rectal amputation for treatment of colorectal carcinoma in 11 dogs. *Vet. Surg.* 37: 420–426.

Nelson, R.L., Gladman, E., and Barbateskovic, M. (2014). Antimicrobial prophylaxis in colorectal surgery. *Cochrane Database Syst. Rev.* 2014 (5): CD001181. https://doi.org/10.1002/14651858.CD001181.

Niebauer, G.W. (1990). Rectum, anus, and perianal and perineal regions. In: *Small Animal Surgery* (eds. C.E.

Harvey, C.D. Newton and A. Schwartz), 381–402. Philadelphia: JB Lippincott.

Nucci, D.J., Liptak, J.M. et al. (2014). Complications and outcomes following rectal pull-through surgery in dogs with rectal masses: 74 cases (2000–2013). *J. Am. Vet. Med. Assoc.* 245: 684–695.

Otero, P.E. and Campoy, L. (2013). Epidural and spinal anesthesia. In: *Small Animal Regional Anesthesia and Analgesia* (eds. L. Campoy and M. Read), 227–260. New York: Wiley Blackwell.

Palminteri, A. (1966). The surgical management of polyps of the rectum and colon of the dog. *J. Am. Vet. Med. Assoc.* 148: 771–778.

Phillips, B.S. (2001). Tumors of the intestinal tract. In: *Small Animal Oncology* (eds. S.J. Withrow and G.E. MacEwen), 335–346. Philadelphia: Saunders.

Ravitch, M.M. and Steichen, F.M. (1979). A stapling instrument of end-to-end inverting anastomoses in the gastrointestinal tract. *Ann. Surg.* 189: 791–797.

Scher, K.S. (1997). Studies on the duration of antibiotic administration for surgical prophylaxis. *Am. Surg.* 63: 59–62.

Shelley, B.A. (2002). Use of the carbon dioxide laser for perianal and rectal surgery. *Vet. Clin. North Am. Small Anim. Pract.* 32: 621–637.

Swiderski, J. and Withrow, S. (2009). A novel surgical technique for rectal mass removal: a retrospective analysis. *J. Am. Anim. Hosp. Assoc.* 45: 67–71.

Tobias, K.M. and Johnston, S.A. (2012). Rectum, anus, and perineum. In: *Veterinary Surgery Small Animal*, 1564–1571. St Louis: Elsevier.

Valerius, K.D., Powers, B.E., Hutchison, J.M. et al. (1997). Adenomatous polyps and carcinoma in situ of the canine colon and rectum: 34 cases (1982–1994). *J. Am. Anim. Hosp. Assoc.* 33: 156–160.

van den Boezem, P.B. et al. (2011). Transanal single-port surgery for the resection of large polyps. *Dig. Surg.* 28 (5–6): 412–416.

Walshaw, R. (1990). Removal of rectoanal neoplasms. In: *Current Techniques in Small Animal Surgery* (eds. M.J. Bojrab, S.T. Birchard and J.L. Tomlinson), 274–290. Philadelphia: Lea & Febiger.

Zelhart, M.D., Hauch, A.T., Slakey, D.P. et al. (2014). Preoperative antibiotic colon preparation: have we had the answer all along? *J. Am. Coll. Surg.* 219: 1070–1077.

34

Anal Sac Resection
Daniel D. Smeak

Department of Clinical Sciences, College of Veterinary Medicine and Biomedical Sciences, Colorado State University, Fort Collins, CO, USA

34.1 Indications

Anal sac diseases in dogs are relatively common in small animal practice but are less frequently observed in cats (Halnan 1976a,b,c). Three of the most common non-neoplastic anal sac conditions are impaction, sacculitis, and abscessation (Washabau and Brockman 1994; Baines and Aronson 2018). These anal sac conditions are generally associated with a generalized dermatological condition, so both anal sacs can be expected to be involved to some degree. For this reason, when a dog has a history of bilateral anal sac disease, even if it is admitted with only one gland obviously affected at the time, a bilateral anal sacculectomy is generally recommended.

A variety of neoplastic diseases of the anal sacs have been reported in the dog and cat, the most common being apocrine gland adenocarcinoma (Berrocal and Vos 1989; Turek and Withrow 2007; Skorupski et al. 2018). This tumor is typically not highly infiltrative, but it tends to be metastatic, with over half of affected dogs showing signs of involvement of the median iliac lymph nodes on presentation (Turek and Withrow 2007). Anal sac carcinomas behave somewhat differently in cats. They should be considered more infiltrative but have less risk of metastasis compared to the dog. Over one quarter of dogs affected with apocrine gland adenocarcinoma will have paraneoplastic hypercalcemia of malignancy. This primary anal sac tumor is often quite small measuring 0.5–1 cm but invaded regional lymph nodes may be greatly enlarged. The anal sacs should be carefully palpated during routine digital rectal examination. A firm, well-circumscribed mass in the region is suspect for an anal sac malignancy. Surgical resection of the involved anal sac mass, and removal of the enlarged regional lymph nodes via midline laparotomy or laparoscopy is indicated. En bloc excision of the mass including a portion of the surrounding anal sphincter is recommended with larger more infiltrative anal sac tumors (Turek and Withrow 2007).

34.2 Surgical Techniques

Various procedures for anal sacculectomy can be subdivided into three categories, open, modified open, and closed techniques (Greiner et al. 1975; Johnston 1985; Matthiesen and Manfra Marretta 1993; Manfra Marretta 1998; Hill and Smeak 2002; Aronson 2003). All three techniques can be utilized successfully for benign anal sac diseases.

Open techniques should not be used for neoplastic processes since these techniques risk incising directly through the mass. The closed anal sacculectomy technique is particularly indicated when the anal sac orifice or neck cannot be identified or cannulated, or when a neoplastic condition is diagnosed (Baines and Aronson 2018).

34.2.1 Preparation and Positioning of the Patient

Patients are positioned in ventral recumbency with the head of the table tilted down slightly to elevate the perineum. Adequate padding is placed, such as a bundled soft towel beneath the caudal abdomen and thighs over the edge of the surgery table. The tail up is pulled up and forward and secured to the table with tape. The animal's legs should hang freely and directly down from the edge of the surgery table. To avoid fecal soilage of

Gastrointestinal Surgical Techniques in Small Animals, First Edition. Edited by Eric Monnet and Daniel D. Smeak.
© 2020 John Wiley & Sons, Inc. Published 2020 by John Wiley & Sons, Inc.
Companion website: www.wiley.com/go/monnet/gastrointestinal

the sterile field, a lubricated tampon is inserted in the terminal rectum and a purse-string suture (3-0 nylon) is placed around the mucocutaneous junction at the anal opening. Incorporation of the anal sac neck or orifice with the purse-string needle bites is avoided so there is access to the anal sac orifice during surgery. A patent orifice may be required to permit insertion of a hemostat when the surgeon needs help locating the anal sac or neck during dissection. The purse-string and the tampon are noted on the surgery checklist to be removed at the end of surgery.

Before sterile preparation of the region, the involved anal sac(s) are gently expressed and flushed with dilute antiseptic solution. A sacral-caudal nerve block is helpful to reduce pain in the early stages of patient recovery. The author prefers to intravenously administer a single dose of a second-generation cephalosporin antibiotic at anesthetic induction.

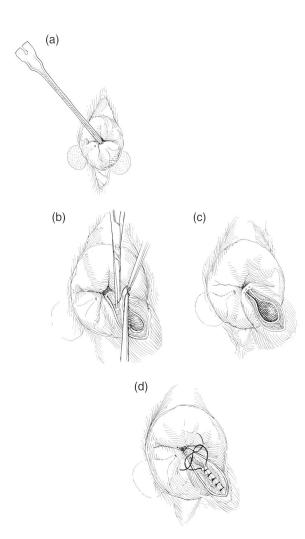

Figure 34.1

34.2.2 Open Technique

34.2.2.1 Standard Open Technique

A probe (grooved director) or curved hemostatic forceps is fully inserted though the orifice into the anal sac (Figure 34.1a). An initial skin incision is made radially from the orifice to the base of the sac over the hemostat or groove director with a scalpel blade or electroscalpel. The incision is continued radially just past the gland such that the lumen of the anal sac neck and grayish-brown sac lining are fully exposed. The cut edges of incised anal sac and neck are grasped with hemostatic forceps, and the sac and neck are removed from the underlying tissue. Dissection is extended on the deep and lateral sides of the neck and sac to free up the remaining sac wall. The rectal wall near the medial side of the dissection plane is avoided. Dissection is kept close to the sac wall to avoid damage to the sphincter muscle or underlying caudal rectal nerve. After anal sac removal, the sac is inspected carefully to ensure that no residual epithelial tissue is left in the wound. The wound bed is lavaged with saline and the gland is submitted for biopsy. The incised anal sphincter muscle is closed with interrupted monofilament absorbable suture. The skin wound can be closed with intradermal sutures, skin adhesive, or percutaneous sutures. If percutaneous sutures are used, the knot ear facing the anus is cut short and the opposite ear is left about 1 cm in length to reduce local irritation.

34.2.2.2 Modified Open

Similar to the open technique, a probe or forceps is placed into the sac (Figure 34.1a). The incision, however, can be made from the anal sac orifice to only the proximal portion of the anal sac (preferred) or it can be extended to the base of the gland. A shorter incision and exposure may reduce damage to the deeper lateral sphincter muscle fibers. In addition, with the modified technique, dissection begins at the anal sac neck directed toward the sac, which helps expose the dissection plane during deep dissection of the sac.

A skin incision is made from the anal sac orifice to the proximal portion of the anal sac exposing the lumen of the neck and a portion of the sac. Next, a 2 mm fringe of anal skin is incised around and medial to the incised anal sac orifice on the dotted line (Figure 34.1c), so the opening is isolated from surrounding tissue.

Straight hemostatic forceps are used to grasp the cut edges of the skin surrounding the sac orifice on either side of the incision. While placing caudolateral tension on the hemostats with the less dominant hand, the more firmly adherent tissue is dissected sharply from the medial side of the anal sac neck (Figure 34.1b). Applying caudolateral traction on the anal sac neck and sac as dissection continues helps avoid damage to the rectal wall medially and the deeper caudal rectal nerve. This helps protect these important structures during further medial dissection. Sharp dissection is continued with a scalpel, electroscalpel, or tenotomy scissors on looser muscle attachments at the medial aspect of the sac as caudolateral traction is maintained. The exposed surface of the anal sac is "draped" over the less dominant index finger to help stretch the remaining sac wall so the dissection plane can be kept close to the external surface of the sac. Any remaining attachments to the sac are dissected free, and the tissue is submitted for biopsy. The wound closure is similar to the description above for the open technique (Figure 34.1d).

34.2.3 Closed Technique for Benign Anal Sac Disease

If the anal sac neck and orifice are patent (and the anal sac does not contain a mass) identification and dissection of the anal sac and neck from surrounding tissue

can be facilitated by filling and distending the sac first with a self-hardening gel or resin, colored yarn, umbilical tape, or dental acrylic. The author prefers using a #6 French Foley catheter fully inserted in the anal sac with the balloon inflated to distend the sac (mentioned later). It should be noted that filling the anal sac with material should only be performed for benign anal sac processes.

34.2.3.1 Closed Technique Without Filling the Anal Sac

A small forceps can be introduced in the anal sac to help locate the apex of the sac. A curved skin incision is made centered over the apex of the anal sac (Figure 34.2a).

Dissection is started from the apex margin of the anal sac. The sac is dissected out of the anal sphincter fibers with a combination of blunt and sharp dissection. Electroscalpel dissection is preferred by the author to minimize bleeding during the procedure. The surgical field is kept free of blood to help visualize the rectal wall and the caudal rectal nerve. The freed apex of the anal sac is grasped with an Allis tissue forceps to help pull the anal sac caudally and medially (Figure 34.2b). This maneuver

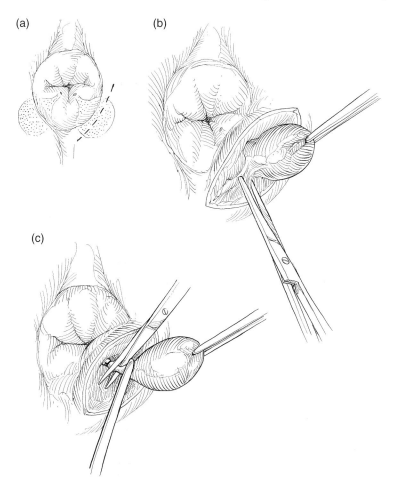

(a) (b)

(c)

Figure 34.2

helps separate the wall of the rectum from the medial dissection plane. Dissection is continued entirely around the anal sac toward the proximal portion of the neck. The neck is ligated with an encircling 4-0 monofilament absorbable suture just deep to the anal sac orifice (Figure 34.2c).

After inspecting the wall of the rectum and the integrity of the wall of the anal sac, the surgical field is flushed and closed in a routine fashion. An intradermal suture is often used to close the skin.

34.2.3.2 Foley Catheter Closed Technique

The Foley catheter technique is particularly useful for anal sacculectomy when the surgeon has no assistance. A #6 French silicone or latex Foley catheter bulb is fully inserted into the anal sac (Figure 34.3a). Since the silicone Foley catheter has a shorter tip, it fits inside smaller anal sacs without backing out as the bulb is inflated, so it is preferred for smaller dogs and cats. The Foley bulb is slowly filled with saline until the distended sac can be readily palpated beneath the skin (Figure 34.3a). About 1–3 ml of saline is usually sufficient. If the inflated bulb tends to back out of the sac before it is fully distended, an offset stitch is placed partially across the anal sac orifice to hold the bulb in place. The distended sac is then easily identified and palpated throughout the procedure. The merit of this technique is the protruding catheter

tube can be used as a "handle" to manipulate the gland during dissection. During the entire procedure, the catheter is placed under traction in a caudolateral direction to hold the gland and dissection plane away from the deeper rectal wall and caudal rectal nerve.

The anal sac orifice is incised and isolated for 360° leaving a 2 mm rim of anal skin around the protruding catheter (Figure 34.3b). Using blunt-tipped tenotomy scissors or electroscalpel, the anal sac neck is sharply dissected out until the sac wall begins to be exposed. Caudal traction on the catheter is continued while the remaining sphincter muscle is dissected from the sac (Figure 34.3c). An attempt is made to stay as close to the anal sac wall as comfortably possible to reduce bleeding and damage to the sphincter muscle. Once the sac is dissected free, it is inspected to be sure the excision was complete. The pocket that remains after sac removal is thoroughly flushed. The underlying muscle and skin defect are closed as described previously.

34.2.4 Closed Technique for Anal Sac Neoplasia

A 3–4 cm curvilinear skin incision is made centered adjacent to the mass, about 1–1.5 cm lateral to the cutaneous junction of the anus. Subcutaneous tissue is incised with electrotomy or scissors to expose the underlying brick-red colored anal sphincter. The mass is located with digital palpation, and using either tenotomy scissors or electroscalpel, adjacent muscle tissue is dissected 3–5 mm from the mass/sac being careful to avoid exposing these structures. While retracting the partially isolated anal sac caudolaterally, dissection is carried medial to the sac being careful not to damage the nearby rectal wall or deeper caudal rectal nerve. After the entire anal sac and neck are dissected free, the anal sac neck is ligated and transected close to the orifice. The margins of the excised tissue are "inked" first (for excision margin analysis) then submitted for biopsy. The surgical site is lavaged thoroughly with sterile saline. The incised fibers of the external anal sphincter are reapposed with interrupted synthetic monofilament absorbable sutures. The subcutaneous layer is closed with similar suture material. An intradermal pattern or percutaneous skin sutures are used to close the skin.

34.3 Tips

Before surgery, resolution of inflammation or infection of the affected anal gland(s) is attempted to reduce the potential for post-operative complications. The region

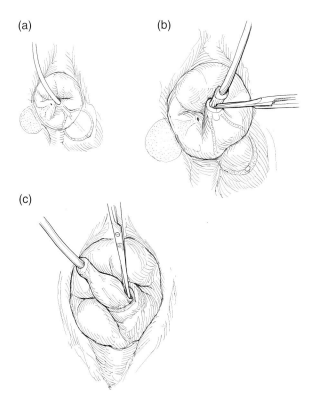

(a)

(b)

(c)

Figure 34.3

of the anal glands is highly vascular, and coupled with inflammation or infection, bleeding can be brisk. Bleeding obscures the surgeon's dissection plane, and this increases the risk of incomplete excision of the sac or collateral damage to the sphincter muscle or nerves. Dogs with paraneoplastic hypercalcemia may require medical therapy and diuresis to help reduce the calcium concentrations before anesthesia.

For the open and modified open techniques, a portion of the anal sac neck and sac are incised (modified open), or the entire neck and sac are opened (open) to expose the lumen (Hill and Smeak 2002). The anal sac can be readily visualized and dissected away from surrounding tissues while ensuring complete removal of the sac since the lining of the opened sac is clearly exposed and identified. Open techniques, however, potentially expose the surgical field to contaminated anal sac contents.

One important surgical goal for anal sacculectomy is complete removal of the sac and neck, since any remnant of these epithelialized structures left after surgery will result in long-standing draining perianal fistulas.

Anal sacs are supplied by a rich network of blood vessels arising from the caudal hemorrhoidal, perineal, and caudal gluteal arteries. As previously mentioned, careful hemostasis throughout the procedure is critical to allow identification of the sac and surrounding structures. The author prefers electrosurgical dissection to help reduce bleeding during surgery.

The external anal sphincter surrounding the anal sacs is supplied by paired caudal rectal nerves originating from the pudendal nerves. These nerves enter the anal sphincter on the ventromedial aspect of the external anal sphincter and are solely responsible for innervation to the external anal sphincter. Surgeons should avoid "stray" dissection along the deep wall of the anal sacs to avoid inadvertent damage to these nerves which can result in incontinence. Removal of the most diseased gland should be planned first. If there are complications during the dissection of the first anal gland, the second sac removal is delayed until the wound has healed. Active anal sphincter contraction (positive perineal reflex) is assessed on the side of the first surgery before progressing with the second side. If there is negative perineal reflex on the first side, warn the owner of an increased possibility of anal sphincteric incontinence after the second surgery.

According to the author's experience, if resection involves less than one-half of the anal sphincter on one side, most dogs can be expected to retain tolerable continence after surgery, provided neurological function of the anal sphincter is preserved.

34.4 Post-Operative Care and Complications

Acute complications associated with anal sacculectomy include pain and self-trauma, with infection/dehiscence not commonly reported (Hill and Smeak 2002; Charlesworth 2014). The incision is monitored carefully post-operatively for discharge, progressive swelling and pain. An Elizabethan collar should be placed, and animals should be discouraged from scooting. Appropriate analgesic therapy is recommended for three to five days.

In one retrospective study, 15% of dogs undergoing bilateral anal sacculectomy for benign disease had long-term complications. Fecal incontinence occurred in 3% of the dogs and all were performed as open (not modified open) anal sacculectomies (Hill and Smeak 2002). Fistulation occurred in 4% of the dogs, and this was due to retained anal sac epithelium (incomplete anal sac excision). All dogs exhibiting fistulation had their anal sacs removed by the closed technique in that study. In the author's experience, damage to one caudal rectal nerve does not cause overt fecal incontinence provided the sphincter muscle and nerve on the opposite side are unaffected. If the wound becomes infected, the incision is opened and the wound is left to heal by second intention. Fecal incontinence is rare when this procedure is performed by experienced surgeons. Occasionally, signs resembling mild fecal incontinence occurs within the first one to two weeks post-operatively, but these signs usually resolve spontaneously (Hill and Smeak 2002; Charlesworth 2014). Stool softeners are not routinely prescribed unless the stools are firm and painful to void.

Bibliography

Aronson, L. (2003). Rectum and anus. In: *Textbook of Small Animal Surgery*, 3e (ed. D.H. Slatter), 682–706. Philadelphia: Saunders.

Baines, J.S. and Aronson, L.R. (2018). Rectum, anus, and perineum. In: *Veterinary Surgery Small Animal*, 2e (eds. S.J. Johnston and K.M. Tobias), 1783–1827. St. Louis: Elsevier.

Berrocal, A. and Vos, J.H. (1989). Canine perineal tumors. *Zentralbl Veterinarmed A* 36: 739–749.

Charlesworth, T.M. (2014). Risk factors for postoperative complications following bilateral closed anal sacculectomy in the dog. *J. Small Anim. Pract.* 55: 350–354.

Downs, M.O. and Stampley, A.R. (1998). Use of a Foley catheter to facilitate anal sac removal in the dog. *J Am Anim Hosp Assoc.* 34 (5): 395–397.

Greiner, T.P., Johnson, R.G., and Betts, C.W. (1975). Diseases of the rectum and anus. In: *Textbook of Veterinary Internal Medicine*, 2e (ed. S.J. Ettinger), 1505–1508. Philadelphia: Saunders.

Halnan, C.R.E. (1976a). Diagnosis of anal sacculitis in the dog. *J. Small Anim. Pract.* 17: 527–535.

Halnan, C.R.E. (1976b). Frequency of occurrence of anal sacculitis in the dog. *J. Small Anim. Pract.* 17: 537–541.

Halnan, C.R.E. (1976c). Therapy of anal sacculitis in the dog. *J. Small Anim. Pract.* 17: 685–691.

Han, T.-S., Lee, H.Y., Cho, K.R. et al. (2007). Use of a Foley catheter for anal sacculectomy in dogs. *J Vet Clin.* 24: 35–37.

Hill, L.N. and Smeak, D.D. (2002). Open versus closed bilateral anal sacculectomy for treatment of non-neoplastic anal sac disease in dogs: 95 cases (1969–1994). *J Am Vet Med Assoc* 221: 662–665.

Johnston, D.E. (1985). Surgical diseases-rectum and anus. In: *Textbook of Small Animal Surgery* (ed. D. Slatter), 770–794. Philadelphia: Saunders.

Manfra Marretta, S. (1998). Anal sac disease and removal. In: *Current Techniques in Small Animal Surgery* (ed. M.J. Bojrab), 283–286. Baltimore: Williams & Wilkins.

Matthiesen, D.T. and Manfra Marretta, S. (1993). Diseases of the anus and rectum. In: *Textbook of Small Animal Surgery*, 2e (ed. D.H. Slatter), 627–645. Philadelphia: Saunders.

Skorupski, K.A. et al. (2018). Outcome and clinical, pathological, and immunohistochemical factors associated with prognosis for dogs with early-stage anal sac adenocarcinoma treated with surgery alone: 34 cases (2002–2013). *J Am Vet Med Assoc* 253 (1): 84–91.

Turek, M.M. and Withrow, S.J. (2007). Perianal tumors. In: *Withrow and MacEwen's Small Animal Oncology*, 4e (eds. S.J. Withrow and D.M. Vail), 503–510. St. Louis: Elsevier.

Washabau, R.J. and Brockman, D.J. (1994). Recto-anal disease. In: *Textbook of Veterinary Internal Medicine*, 4e (eds. S.J. Ettinger and E.C. Feldman), 1398–1409. Philadelphia: Saunders.

Section VIII

Liver and Gall Bladder

35

Liver Lobectomy

Eric Monnet

Department of Clinical Sciences, College of Veterinary Medicine and Biomedical Sciences, Colorado State University, Fort Collins, CO, USA

35.1 Indications

Liver lobectomies are most commonly performed in dogs and cats for removal of primary liver tumors or neoplasia of the biliary system. Hepatocellular carcinoma, hemangiosarcoma, and biliary carcinoma are the most common tumors to resect in dogs (Liptak 2004, 2013; Liptak et al. 2004). Large liver masses can occupy a significant portion of the abdominal cavity and patients are presented with lethargy and a distended abdomen. In older cats, large benign cysts are found and resected because of their volume.

Liver lobe abscess and liver lobe torsion are the other two common indications for liver lobe resection (Downs et al. 1998; Schwarz et al. 1998; von Pfeil et al. 2006; Bhandal et al. 2008). Liver lobectomy after trauma is very rare in dogs and cats.

Most of the time complete liver lobectomy is performed, but partial liver lobectomy is indicated if the lesion is localized at the tip or on the margins of the liver lobe.

Liver lobectomy requires ligation of the branch of the portal vein and the hepatic artery perfusing the liver lobe resected, the hepatic vein draining the liver lobe, and the bile duct draining the liver lobe resected.

35.2 Technique

35.2.1 Liver Biopsy

A liver biopsy is collected on the periphery of the liver lobe if there is no obvious lesion present in the liver parenchyma (Monnet and Twedt 2003; Twedt and Monnet 2005; Vasanjee et al. 2006; McDevitt et al. 2016; Kimbrell et al. 2018).

Liver biopsies can be collected with open abdominal surgery or with laparoscopy. When a liver biopsy is collected a complete abdominal exploration is performed.

35.2.1.1 Laparotomy

After a midline incision of the skin and the abdominal wall, the liver lobes are exposed with caudal retraction of the stomach.

A loop of absorbable suture size 3-0 is placed around the tip of a liver lobe. The suture is tightened to crush the liver parenchyma and compress the blood vessels present within it (Figure 35.1). Metzembaum scissors or a #15 blade are used to collect the biopsy without cutting the suture.

If a mass is present in the middle of a liver lobe, a punch biopsy can be used to collect a biopsy. Hemostatic material is then packed in the biopsy site to provide hemostasis.

Usually three biopsies are taken. One biopsy is used for histology, one for culture, and one for heavy metal testing.

35.2.1.2 Laparoscopy

Liver biopsies can be collected during laparoscopy (Monnet and Twedt 2003; Twedt and Monnet 2005; McDevitt et al. 2016; Kimbrell et al. 2018). The patient can be placed in left lateral recumbency or dorsal recumbency. If the patient is placed in left lateral recumbency, the right limb of the pancreas, the gall bladder, the cystic duct, and the common bile duct are visible for inspection, biopsy, or aspiration (Monnet and Twedt 2003).

Gastrointestinal Surgical Techniques in Small Animals, First Edition. Edited by Eric Monnet and Daniel D. Smeak.
© 2020 John Wiley & Sons, Inc. Published 2020 by John Wiley & Sons, Inc.
Companion website: www.wiley.com/go/monnet/gastrointestinal

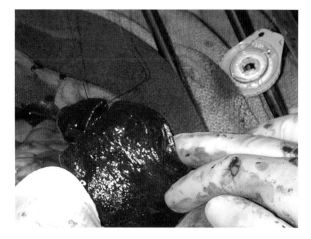

Figure 35.1

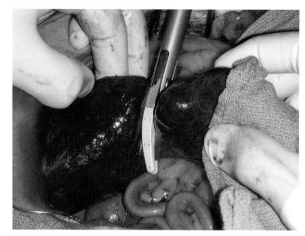

Figure 35.3

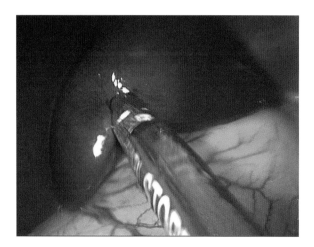

Figure 35.2

Two 5 mm cannulas are placed either in the right caudal abdomen or on midline after insufflation with carbon dioxide to 8–10 mmHg. An endoscope is introduced in the abdominal cavity through one of the cannulas. Through the other cannula, a 3 or 5 mm cup biopsy forceps is introduced. Biopsies are taken on the edge of the liver lobe (Figure 35.2). The biopsy forceps is used to compress the liver parenchyma for 20 seconds to provide hemostasis before the biopsy is removed. If bleeding occurs, a palpation probe is used to provide tamponade for 5 minutes on the biopsy site. Also hemostatic absorbable material can be applied on the biopsy site to control bleeding.

35.2.2 Partial Liver Lobectomy

Partial liver lobectomy is performed when lesions are small and peripheral.

Partial liver lobectomy can be performed with hand sutures, loop ligatures, staples, or a vessel sealant device (De Weese and Lewis 1951; Lewis et al. 1987; Risselada et al. 2010). The liver parenchyma is finger fractured or crushed, depending on whether sutures or staples are used. Partial liver lobectomies have a tendency to bleed because a large surface of the liver parenchyma is left exposed. When a vessel sealant device is used the device is activated while the jaws of the device are crushing the liver parenchyma (Figure 35.3). When the clamp is closed the device is activated a second time. The blade in the device is activated to separate the resected portion of liver lobe.

If sutures are used, the liver parenchyma is finger fractured where the resection is going to be performed. Blood vessels and intrahepatic bile ducts are spared during the finger fracturing and are ligated with a 4-0 monofilament absorbable suture or clips. Mattress sutures placed across the liver parenchyma have been used instead of finger fracturing. It is better to use a straight needle to place the mattress sutures across the parenchyma. Monofilament absorbable suture size 2-0 or 3-0 is used. The sutures are tightened to crush the parenchyma and provide hemostasis.

A loop ligature has also been used to perform a partial liver lobectomy in dog with minimal blood loss (Risselada et al. 2010; Goodman and Casale 2014).

Thoraco-abdominal staples are another alternative to perform a partial liver lobectomy (Figure 35.4) (Lewis et al. 1987; Bellah 1994). The stapler is applied across the liver lobe. If the liver lobe is larger than the length of the stapler, a second cartridge of staples is used. The stapler is closed crushing the liver parenchyma and the staples are then applied. A #15 blade is used to severe the portion of the liver lobe resected. This technique has a

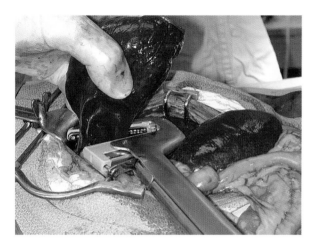

Figure 35.4

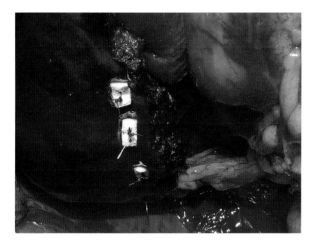

Figure 35.5

tendency to be associated with excessive bleeding from the raw edges of the liver parenchyma.

After the partial resection is completed with hand sutures or staples, mattress sutures mounted on pledgets can be used to provide further hemostasis if needed. Those sutures are placed across the liver parenchyma on the edge of the resection to provide compression of the blood vessels (Figure 35.5).

35.2.3 Complete Liver Lobectomy

A complete liver lobectomy can be performed with hand suture or with stapling equipment (Lewis et al. 1990; Martin et al. 2003; Tobias 2007; Covey et al. 2009; Risselada et al. 2010; Goodman and Casale 2014). Hand suture requires dissection and isolation of the portal vein, the hepatic vein, the hepatic artery, and the hepatic duct of the liver lobe being resected. If the quadrate lobe is removed, a cholecystectomy is also performed because

the gall bladder is not supported and the cystic duct can become kinked.

35.2.3.1 Liver Lobectomy with Sutures

After a midline approach, the stomach is retracted caudally to expose the hilus of the liver. If a right liver lobe is resected, the duodenum is also retracted medially and caudally.

35.2.3.1.1 *Lobectomy of the Left Lateral Liver Lobe, Left Medial Liver Lobe, and Quadrate Liver Lobe*   The lobectomy of the left medial and lateral lobe, and the quadrate lobe are performed with the same technique since their hepatic vein is visible from the diaphragmatic side of the liver. The triangular ligaments and the coronary ligaments are transected first.

The dissection starts by dissecting the branch of the portal vein feeding the liver lobe being resected. Very often the hepatic artery perfusing the liver lobe is seen traveling across or along the portal vein. The hepatic artery is ligated when seen. The portal vein is dissected with a right-angle forceps. The peritoneum covering the branch of the portal vein is sharply dissected with electrocautery to minimize bleeding from the liver parenchyma. A right-angle forceps is then used to dissect the branch of the portal vein. The dissection is performed on both sides of the branch of the portal vein until both sides communicate dorsally. The dissection should be extended over 1 cm to be able to apply two encircling sutures. A 3-0 monofilament absorbable suture with slow resorption is used. Metzembaum scissors are used to cut the portal vein between the two sutures.

The bile duct draining the liver lobe is ligated when identified with two encircling sutures.

The liver lobe is then finger fractured at the level of the hilus in a direction parallel to the caudal vena cava until the hepatic vein draining the liver lobe is identified. The hepatic vein is then dissected with right-angle forceps. The vein should be exposed over 1 cm to be able to place two encircling sutures. If the hepatic vein cannot be exposed over 1 cm, an encircling suture might not stay on the hepatic vein and major hemorrhage could occur. A tangential vascular clamp is placed on the hepatic vein at the junction with the caudal vena cava and a second one against the liver parenchyma (Figure 35.6a). The hepatic vein is then transected as far as possible from the vena cava to leave at least 0.5 cm of the vein distal to the clamp on the caudal vena cava (Figure 35.6b). The hepatic vein is then closed with two simple continuous sutures. A 5-0 monofilament nonabsorbable suture is used. One suture is placed at each end of the

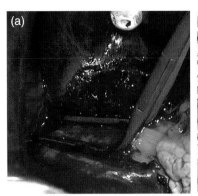 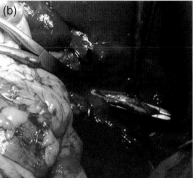 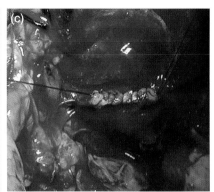

Figure 35.6

vein. Those sutures are placed as stay sutures and also used to close the vein with a double, simple continuous suture pattern. First, the suture closest to the diaphragm is used to perform a simple continuous suture pattern. When the suture is completed it is tightened to the second suture. Then a second simple continuous pattern is applied backward with the second stay suture. It is then tightened to the first stay suture tag. The tangential vascular clamp is removed (Figure 35.6c). If some bleeding is observed, it is controlled by placement of a mattress suture with 5-0 monofilament nonabsorbable suture. Pledgets of Teflon can be used to help provide better hemostasis.

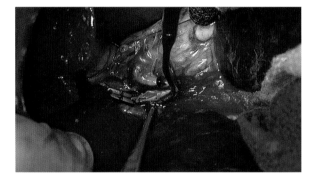

Figure 35.7

35.2.3.1.2 Lobectomy of the Right Medial and Lateral Liver Lobes

The hepatic vein and the branch of the portal vein of the right liver lobes are very short and buried in the liver parenchyma. The connection of the hepatic vein with the caudal vena cava is usually very wide, which makes placement of an encircling suture difficult and dangerous. Not only can the suture slide off the stump of the hepatic vein, it can also bend the caudal vena cava and partially occlude caudal vena cava flow. Therefore, it requires finger fracturing of the parenchyma from caudal to cranial along the caudal vena cava to expose, first, the branch of the portal vein. The vein is clamped with a tangential vascular clamp and sutured as described above for the hepatic vein of the left liver lobes (Figure 35.7). The hepatic vein is then exposed and clamped with a tangential vascular clamp. It is then sutured as described above for the hepatic vein of the liver lobes. The hepatic artery and the bile ducts from those liver lobes are ligated when identified.

35.2.3.2 Liver Lobectomy with Staples

A liver lobectomy can also be performed with staples. Usually a thoraco-abdominal stapler is used (Lewis et al. 1990; Risselada et al. 2010). It is recommended to use the vascular staples since they close down to 1 mm and

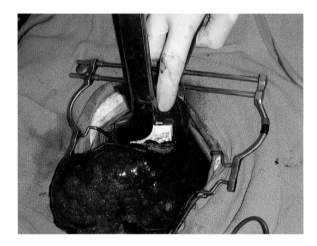

Figure 35.8

three rows of staples are staggered to provide better hemostasis. If other staples are used, there is a significant risk of hemorrhage after surgery and it is recommended to oversew the staple line with 4-0 monofilament absorbable suture in a simple continuous pattern.

The left lateral and medial liver lobes are easily removed with staples because the thoraco-abdominal staplers can be applied to the base of the hilus without too many problems (Figure 35.8). The triangle ligaments are transected first to facilitate the placement of the thoraco-abdominal stapler. The stapler is closed at the hilus of the liver, making sure the caudal vena cava is not partially occluded. The arterial blood pressure will decrease if the caudal vena cava is partially occluded. The staples are then applied. A #15 blade is used to cut the liver parenchyma along the cartridge of staples.

The quadrate lobe is usually too thick to be able to apply the stapling equipment to its base. Therefore this lobe is commonly removed with sutures.

The right medial and lateral liver lobes can be removed with staples if the stapler can be slid along the caudal vena cava. The parenchyma is sometime too thick to be able to place the stapler appropriately. Also even if the stapler can be placed properly it crushes a lot of liver parenchyma, which might partially occlude the caudal vena cava or might result in bleeding on the raw surface. Absorbable hemostatic agent is then applied on the surface of the liver. The electrocautery can be used in a fulguration mode to provide hemostasis.

35.3 Tips

Providing excellent hemostasis is paramount during liver lobectomy (Risselada et al. 2010; Haley et al. 2015; Hanson et al. 2017). It has been shown that anatomical dissection at the hilus of the liver results in less blood loss during liver lobectomy (Covey et al. 2009). Skeletonization of the lobar vessel is associated with more blood loss than any other technique used for partial liver lobectomy.

When a tumor is present the hilus may not be easily exposed, especially if a massive hepatocellular carcinoma is present. If not enough space is present at the hilus of the left liver lobes to place a thoraco-abdominal stapler, a feeding tube can be used to facilitate the placement of the stapler. The thoraco-abdominal stapler is inserted in the distal tip of the feeding tube. The proximal tip of the tube is placed around the hilus of the liver lobes after incising the triangular ligaments (Figure 35.9). The feeding tube is then pulled and it drags the thoraco-abdominal staplers around the hilus of the liver lobe. If a stapler cannot be applied then finger fracturing of the liver parenchyma is used to isolate any vascular structures present. Large tumors usually have a lot of collateral circulation that needs to be controlled. Massive hepatocellular carcinomas have a very good long-term prognosis even if the margins are dirty (Liptak et al. 2004).

A partial median sternotomy of the caudal part of the sternum may be required to resect large liver tumor. Opening the sternum allows cranial exposure of the liver mass and the hilus.

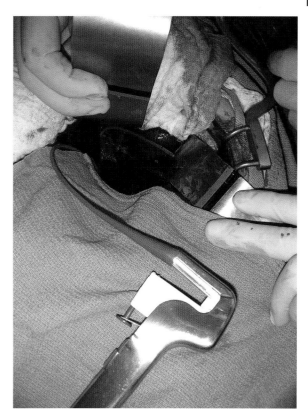

Figure 35.9

35.4 Complications

After a partial or complete liver lobectomy, the patients are monitored with continuous electrocardiogram, and arterial pressure measurement. In addition, blood work including complete blood count and biochemistry should be performed 24 hours after surgery. Venous blood gas should also be monitored every six hours to monitor lactate levels, and blood glucose. Sixty percent of the liver can be resected in dogs without consequences for survival (Ogata et al. 1997).

Hemorrhage, hypoglycemia, hyperbilirubinemia, and elevation of liver enzymes are potential complications after liver lobectomy. Liver enzymes are usually elevated after liver lobectomy because of the manipulation of the liver lobe and local ischemia. It should improve within one week after surgery (Stone et al. 1969).

Hemorrhage occurs after partial or complete liver lobectomy. With partial lobectomy the hemorrhage is coming from the fragmented liver parenchyma. After complete liver lobectomy the hemorrhage is coming from either the portal vein, the hepatic vein, or a branch of the hepatic artery. Hypotension and tachycardia are characteristic of hypovolemia. Heart rate and blood pressure improve after intravenous boluses of crystalloids in patients with hemorrhage after liver lobectomy.

Whole blood and plasma should be delivered to patients with hemorrhage (Risselada et al. 2010; Haley et al. 2015; Hanson et al. 2017). If more than two units of blood or plasma are needed to stabilize the patients, an abdominal exploration is required to see if the source of the bleeding can be identified and corrected. If the source is identified, a mattress suture is used over the bleeding blood vessel. If the source cannot be identified, simple continuous sutures are placed over the staple lines or the previous suture lines. A 4-0 or 5-0 monofilament nonabsorbable suture is used.

Hypoglycemia occurs after a liver lobectomy without sepsis. The hypoglycemia is a function of the amount of liver resected since the liver is responsible for maintenance of the concentration of glucose in blood (Stone et al. 1969). If hypoglycemia is occurring, septic peritonitis should be ruled out first then 2.5% dextrose is added to the crystalloids delivered intravenously. Usually the hypoglycemia is very transient over 24 hours (Stone et al. 1969).

Hyperbilirubinemia can happen after liver lobectomy. It results from an increased bilirubin load presented to the reduced number of hepatocytes (Stone et al. 1969). However, it can be due to a ligation of the common bile duct or a bile peritonitis. The risk of ligation of the common bile duct is higher during resection of large tumor on the right side of the liver. An ultrasound should be performed if the elevated bilirubin is getting worse over 48 hours. If the biliary system is becoming distended on ultrasound, the surgical site should be explored to correct the problem.

Bile peritonitis occurs if a bile duct was not identified and/or not ligated properly. Bile peritonitis is associated with large amount of abdominal effusion and elevated concentration of bile in the abdominal effusion. If a bile peritonitis is present, an abdominal exploration is required to identify and ligate the source of the leakage. If the source is not obvious and the duodenum is open, the common bile duct is catheterized with a 3.5 or 5 Fr feeding tube. Sterile saline is then injected in the feeding tube to help identify the leakage. Methylene blue can also be used to help identify the leakage. After identification of the leakage the leaking duct is repaired with a 6-0 monofilament absorbable suture.

Septic peritonitis or septic shock can develop after liver lobectomy for a liver abscess (Schwarz et al. 1998). It is not unusual to have dogs in early septic shock with a liver lobe abscess or torsion. If peritonitis is already present at the time of surgery because the abscess already ruptured, an abdominal drain is required to drain the abdominal cavity after surgery.

Disseminated intravascular coagulation is another potential complication of liver lobectomy, mostly when a liver lobe abscess is present.

Prognosis after liver lobectomy is a function of the histological nature of the disease resected. Liver lobe abscess usually carries a good long-term prognosis if the patient is not in septic shock at the time of surgery. Massive hepatocellular carcinoma carries an excellent prognosis even if the margins are not clean because the tumor is slow-growing and rarely metastasizes (Liptak 2004; Liptak et al. 2004). Hemangiosarcoma carries a very poor prognosis. Dogs with a large liver tumor are very often presented with a hemoabdomen because the tumor has ruptured.

References

Bellah, J.R. (1994). Surgical stapling of the spleen, pancreas, liver, and urogenital tract. *Vet. Clin. North Am. Small Anim. Pract.* 24 (2): 375–394.

Bhandal, J. et al. (2008). Spontaneous left medial liver lobe torsion and left lateral lobe infarction in a rottweiler. *Can. Vet. J.* 49 (10): 1002–1004.

Covey, J.L. et al. (2009). Hilar liver resection in dogs. *Vet. Surg.* 38 (1): 104–111.

De Weese, M.S. and Lewis, C. Jr. (1951). Partial hepatectomy in the dog; an experimental study. *Surgery* 30 (4): 642–651.

Downs, M.O. et al. (1998). Liver lobe torsion and liver abscess in a dog. *J. Am. Vet. Med. Assoc.* 212 (5): 678–680.

Goodman, A.R. and Casale, S.A. (2014). Short-term outcome following partial or complete liver lobectomy with a commercially prepared self-ligating loop in companion animals: 29 cases (2009–2012). *J. Am. Vet. Med. Assoc.* 244 (6): 693–698.

Haley, A.L. et al. (2015). Perioperative red blood cell transfusion requirement for various surgical procedures in dogs: 207 cases (2004–2013). *J. Am. Vet. Med. Assoc.* 247 (1): 85–91.

Hanson, K.R. et al. (2017). Incidence of blood transfusion requirement and factors associated with transfusion following liver lobectomy in dogs and cats: 72 cases (2007–2015). *J. Am. Vet. Med. Assoc.* 251 (8): 929–934.

Kimbrell, T.L. et al. (2018). Comparison of diagnostic accuracy of laparoscopic 3 mm and 5 mm cup biopsies to wedge biopsies of canine livers. *J. Vet. Intern. Med.* 32 (2): 701–706.

Lewis, D.D. et al. (1987). Partial hepatectomy using stapling instruments. *J. Am. Anim. Hosp. Assoc.* 23: 597–602.

Lewis, D.D. et al. (1990). Hepatic lobectomy in the dog. A comparison of stapling and ligation techniques. *Vet. Surg.* 19 (3): 221–225.

Liptak, J.M. (2004). Liver tumors in cats and dogs. *Compend. Contin. Educ. Pract. Vet.* 26 (1): 50–57.

Liptak, J.M. (2013). Hepatobiliary tumors. In: Withrow & macewen's Small Animal Clinical Oncology (eds. S.J. Withrow et al.), 405–412. St Louis: Elsevier.

Liptak, J.M. et al. (2004). Massive hepatocellular carcinoma in dogs: 48 cases (1992–2002). *J. Am. Vet. Med. Assoc.* 225 (8): 1225–1230.

Martin, R.A. et al. (2003). Liver and biliary system. In: Textbook of Small Animal Surgery, 3e (ed. D. Slatter), 708–726. Philadelphia: Saunders.

McDevitt, H.L. et al. (2016). Short-term clinical outcome of laparoscopic liver biopsy in dogs: 106 cases (2003–2013). *J. Am. Vet. Med. Assoc.* 248 (1): 83–90.

Monnet, E. and Twedt, D.C. (2003). Laparoscopy. *Vet. Clin. North Am. Small Anim. Pract.* 33 (5): 1147–1163.

Ogata, A. et al. (1997). Short-term effect of portal vein arterialization on hepatic protein synthesis and endotoxaemia after extended hepatectomy in dogs. *J. Gastroenterol. Hepatol.* 12 (9–10): 633–638.

Risselada, M. et al. (2010). Comparison of 5 surgical techniques for partial liver lobectomy in the dog for intraoperative blood loss and surgical time. *Vet. Surg.* 39 (7): 856–862.

Schwarz, L.A. et al. (1998). Hepatic abscesses in 13 dogs: a review of the ultrasonographic findings, clinical data and therapeutic options. *Vet. Radiol. Ultrasound* 39 (4): 357–365.

Stone, H.H. et al. (1969). Physiologic considerations in major hepatic resections. *Am. J. Surg.* 117 (1): 78–84.

Tobias, K.M. (2007). Surgical stapling devices in veterinary medicine: a review. *Vet. Surg.* 36 (4): 341–349.

Twedt, D.C. and Monnet, E. (2005). Laparoscopy: technique and clinical experience. In: Veterinary Endoscopy for Small Animal Practitioner (ed. T.C. McCarthy), 357–386. Philadelphia: Elsevier.

Vasanjee, S.C. et al. (2006). Evaluation of hemorrhage, sample size, and collateral damage for five hepatic biopsy methods in dogs. *Vet. Surg.* 35 (1): 86–93.

von Pfeil, D.J.F. et al. (2006). Left lateral and left middle liver lobe torsion in a Saint Bernard puppy. *J. Am. Anim. Hosp. Assoc.* 42 (5): 381–385.

36

Surgery of the Gallbladder
Eric Monnet

Department of Clinical Sciences, College of Veterinary Medicine and Biomedical Sciences, Colorado State University, Fort Collins, CO, USA

36.1   Indications

Cholecystotomy, cholecystectomy, and cholecystostomy are the possible procedures involving the gallbladder. Cholecystoduodenostomy and cholecystojejunostomy are also procedures related to the gallbladder already described in Chapter 37. Biliary stones can be removed via a cholecystotomy if the gallbladder is viable and not contributing to the formation of the biliary stones.

Cholecystostomy is recommended for a temporary decompression of the biliary system. This procedure is further described in a subsequent chapter related to biliary diversion (Chapter 37).

Gallbladder mucocele, necrotic cholangiohepatitis, and neoplasia of the gallbladder represent the most common indications for a cholecystectomy (Pike et al. 2004; Worley et al. 2004; Cornejo 2005; Amsellem et al. 2006; Aguirre et al. 2007). Cholecystectomy may also be indicated when the condition of the gallbladder can affect the recurrence of cholelithiasis. Traumatic rupture of the gallbladder is rare and may require a cholecystectomy if the gallbladder cannot be repaired.

Before a cholecystectomy it is important to confirm the patency of the common bile duct because after a cholecystectomy it is very difficult to provide biliary diversion if an occlusion of the common bile duct is present.

36.2   Techniques

36.2.1   Cholecystostomy

Techniques for cholecystostomy have been described in Chapter 37.

36.2.2   Cholecystotomy

Cholecystotomy is very rarely performed in veterinary surgery. The most common indication would be for a biopsy or retrieval of a stone in the gallbladder.

After a midline approach, the liver and the gallbladder are exposed with laparotomy sponges and malleable retractors. A stay suture is placed at the apex of the gallbladder and another one toward the cystic duct. A #11 blade is used to puncture the gallbladder next to the stay suture at the apex. Suction is used to aspirate the bile before it contaminates the peritoneal cavity. Metzembaum scissors are then used to extend the incision toward the cystic duct and the second stay suture. The length is adjusted to the size of the stones to be removed, or the size of the biopsy to be collected.

After completion of the procedure, the wall of the gallbladder is closed with a simple apposition continuous pattern with a 5-0 monofilament absorbable suture. A second layer with an inverting pattern can be applied.

36.2.3   Cholecystectomy

36.2.3.1   Laparotomy
After a midline incision the quadrate lobe is isolated with laparotomy sponges.

Before the gallbladder can be removed it is important to confirm the patency of the common bile duct. The duodenum is opened on the antimesenteric side at the level of the papilla of the bile duct. A 3 or 5 Fr catheter is then advanced in a retrograde fashion up the common bile duct. The bile duct is flushed with warm sterile saline. The catheter is then removed and the duodenum closed with a simple apposition continuous suture pattern with 4-0 monofilament absorbable suture.

Gastrointestinal Surgical Techniques in Small Animals, First Edition. Edited by Eric Monnet and Daniel D. Smeak.
Companion website: www.wiley.com/go/monnet/gastrointestinal

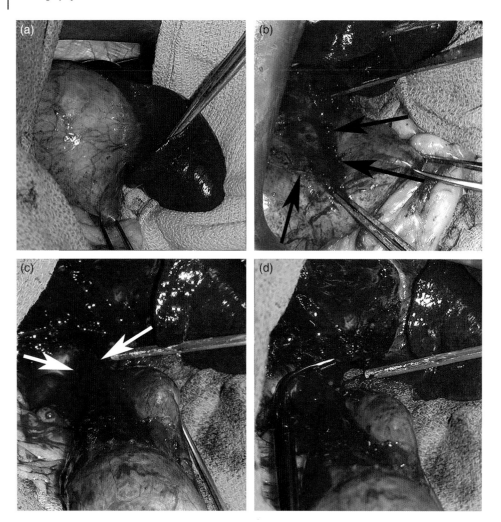

Figure 36.1

As an alternative to avoid opening the duodenum, a cholecystotomy is performed and the gallbladder is drained. A catheter can then be advanced into the cystic duct and further down the common bile duct and the duodenum in a normograde fashion. The catheter is then removed while flushing the common bile duct and the cholecystectomy completed.

If the common bile duct is not patent the cholecystectomy cannot be performed. A surgery on the bile duct is performed to correct the obstruction (Chapter 38).

The cholecystectomy is performed starting at the apex and moving toward the cystic duct. A plane of dissection is established between the gallbladder and the liver parenchyma by first incising the peritoneal attachment. Electrocautery is recommended to facilitate the dissection and minimize blood loss during the procedure. It is important to avoid penetrating the liver parenchyma in order to minimize bleeding. If severe cholangiohepatitis has been present, the plane of dissection is difficult to establish because of the many adhesions that can form between the wall of the gallbladder and the liver.

After starting the dissection, it is possible to grasp the apex of the gallbladder with an Allis tissue forceps to facilitate handling of the gallbladder (Figure 36.1a). The dissection is conducted toward the cystic duct. The peritoneal attachment (black arrows) of the gallbladder to the liver parenchyma are dissected (Figure 36.1b). Sometimes a branch of the portal vein is very superficial. It is then important to identify this branch and avoid any iatrogenic trauma to the vessel. If the branch of the portal vein is damaged, either a simple interrupted suture can be placed with a 6-0 prolene suture to repair the blood vessel, or a liver lobectomy is required if the bleeding cannot be controlled.

When the cystic duct (white arrows) is reached (Figure 36.1c) it is ligated with 4-0 monofilament absorbable suture. To facilitate the placement of the encircling suture, one or two right-angle forceps are

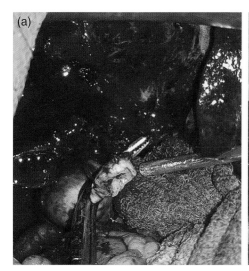 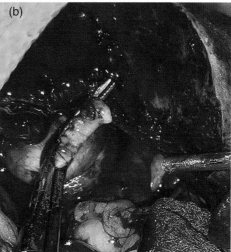

Figure 36.2

applied to the cystic duct (Figure 36.1d). If two right-angle forceps have been placed, the cystic duct is transected between the two forceps. An encircling suture is placed distal to the clamp left on the cystic duct. If only one right-angle forceps has been used, the encircling suture is placed before transecting the cystic duct. If the cystic duct is friable, it can be oversewn with a simple continuous suture with 5-0 monofilament absorbable suture (Figure 36.2). One or two simple continuous sutures can be placed. Usually the cystic artery is ligated with the cystic duct because it usually follows the cystic duct very closely. After ligation of the cystic duct and artery they can be transected. The gallbladder is then removed. The fossa of the gallbladder in the quadrate lobe is inspected for bleeding. If bleeding is present, tamponade can be applied for five minutes. If the bleeding persists, gel foam cube is applied or electrocautery can be applied with a fulguration technique.

The abdominal cavity is then flushed with warm sterile saline and closed routinely.

If a bile peritonitis is present at the time of surgery because of a rupture of the gallbladder, the abdominal cavity is copiously lavaged with warm saline. Usually 4–5 l of warm saline for a 20 kg dog is used to lavage the peritoneal cavity. Either a closed suction drain is placed to drain the abdominal cavity or the abdomen can be left open for 24 hours if the bile peritonitis is very severe. Also, a gastrostomy and a jejunostomy tube should be placed to support the patient in the post-operative period.

36.2.3.2 Laparoscopy

Laparoscopic cholecystectomy is possible in dogs. Dogs without any indication of obstruction of the biliary system on ultrasound and biochemistry are considered good candidates for a laparoscopic cholecystectomy (Mayhew et al. 2008; Scott et al. 2016). If the gallbladder is too distended, it will make the surgery more difficult.

The dog is placed on dorsal recumbency with a slight tilt toward the left to move the falciform ligament away from the surgical field.

Usually four portals are required to complete a cholecystectomy. It could be four separate portals or one single-incision laparoscopic port, plus an extra cannula on the left side of the abdomen.

If separate portals are used, three 5 mm and one 10 mm portals are required. The larger portal is needed for endoclip placement and retrieval of the gallbladder. One 5 mm portal is placed caudal to the umbilicus on midline for the camera. The 10 mm portal is placed cranial to the umbilicus on midline. Then the two other 5 mm portals are placed in each site of the abdominal cavity at the level of the umbilicus.

If a single-incision laparoscopy port is used, it is placed caudal to the umbilicus on midline. Another 5 mm portal is placed in the left side of the abdomen at the level of the umbilicus.

The dissection usually starts at the level of the cystic duct with a right-angle forceps. A fine-toothed grasping forcep is used to grasp the apex of the gallbladder and pull it ventrally toward the diaphragm. Another fine-toothed grasping forcep is used to grasp the gallbladder at the infundibulum to pull the cystic duct in a ventral and caudal direction (Deveney 2006; Katkhouda 2011).

A right-angle forcep from the left side of the of the abdominal cavity is used to dissect around the cystic duct without traumatizing the common big duct or any hepatic ducts (Figure 36.3). It is important to not traumatize the liver parenchyma to minimize bleeding that

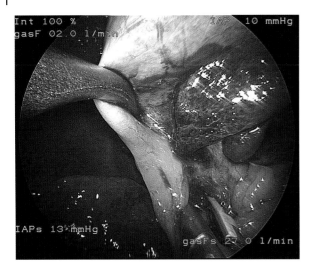

Figure 36.3

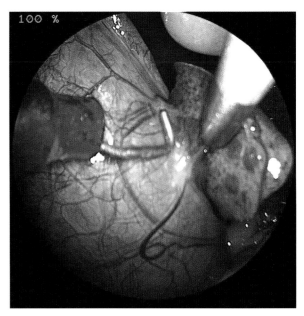

Figure 36.5

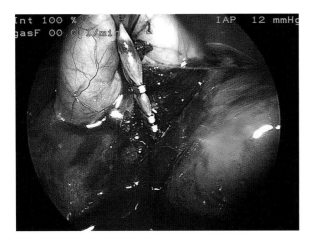

Figure 36.4

would obscure the surgical field. Suction and irrigation devices are used to keep the surgical field clean.

After dissection of the cystic duct over 1.5 cm, three 10 mm large endoclips are placed on the cystic duct (Marvel and Monnet 2014). Two clips are placed close to the junction with the common bile duct, and a third closer to the infundibulum (Figure 36.4). The cystic duct is transected between the endoclips, leaving two clips on the cystic duct. Usually the cystic artery is ligated at the same time.

After transection of the cystic duct, the gallbladder is detached from the fossa of the quadrate lobe with electrocautery or a 5 mm vessel sealant device (Figure 36.5). The cystic duct is pulled ventrally to expose the fossa of the quadrate lobe. Very often stronger attachments are present at the apex of the gallbladder and they are transected with a vessel sealant device or electrocautery.

If the cystic duct cannot be visualized because of the size of the gallbladder, the dissection is started at the level of the apex of the gall gladder. A palpation probe and a fine-toothed grasping forceps are then used to expose the plan of dissection. Electrocautery with a J hook is used to dissect the gallbladder from the fossa of the quadrate lobe (Figure 36.5). The cystic duct is ligated last, as described above after complete dissection of the gallbladder.

The fossa of the quadrate lobe is explored for signs of bleeding. Electrocautery in the fulguration mode is used to control the bleeding. Tamponade can also be applied with a cherry applicator.

The gallbladder is then placed in a retrieving bag and removed from the abdominal cavity either by enlarging one of the portals on midline or by removing the single-incision access port.

Each portal is removed and blocked with a local anesthetic for pain control. Each portal is then closed appropriately, with abdominal wall closure for the 10 mm portal or the single-access port, and subcutaneous and skin closure for all the portals.

36.3 Tips

It is paramount to establish a plan of dissection between the wall of the gallbladder and the liver parenchyma. If the liver parenchyma is traumatized, it can generate lot of intraoperative and post-operative

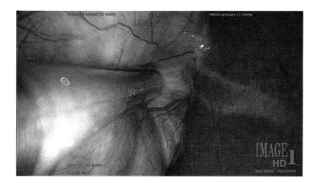

Figure 36.6

bleeding. At the apex of the gallbladder the peritoneal layers can be incised with electrocautery to start the cholecystectomy.

A severely distended cystic duct with a concurrent gallbladder mucocele can be very friable. The author prefers to oversew the end of the cystic duct with one or two simple continuous sutures with 5-0 monofilament absorbable suture.

During the dissection of the gallbladder from the hepatic fossa it is possible to encounter small bile ducts penetrating in the gallbladder. They need to be ligated separately. If not identified at the time of surgery, they might induce bile peritonitis in the post-operative period.

Branches of the portal vein can be very superficial in the hepatic fossa. Therefore it is important to recognize those branches to avoid iatrogenic damage and hemorrhage. If a branch of the portal vein is seen during the laparoscopy dissection, a conversion is recommended (Figure 36.6).

Placement of a gastrostomy and a jejunostomy tube is recommended at the time of surgery, especially if the patient has been vomiting or is anorexic.

If peritonitis was present or minor leakage of bile occurs before surgery or at the time of surgery, a closed suction drain should be applied at the time of closure. Open abdominal drainage has been attempted to treat bile peritonitis with limited success (Ludwig et al. 1997; Staatz et al. 2002).

If the gallbladder is punctured during laparoscopic cholecystectomy, the site of the perforation can be grasped with a 5 mm grasping forceps and rolled like spaghetti to stop the leakage (Frantzides et al. 2009; Katkhouda 2011). Therefore a perforation of the gallbladder is not necessarily a conversion. The peritoneal cavity is copiously lavaged with warmed saline at the end of the procedure.

During laparoscopic cholecystectomy, the dissection around the cystic duct is greatly facilitated by an articulated instrument. Laparoscopic right-angle forceps are not always long enough to go around the cystic duct.

The cystic duct is more effectively closed with large 10 mm endoclips. However, it has been shown in a canine cadaveric model that a vessel sealant device can be used (Marvel and Monnet 2014). However, a vessel sealant device has not been tested in a diseased bile duct. Extracorporeal sutures have been used to ligate the cystic duct (Mayhew et al. 2008; Scott et al. 2016). Also endoscopic staples can be applied if the cystic duct is very distended or does not taper down to a smaller diameter before getting to the common bile duct.

When applying clips to the cystic duct during laparoscopy it is important not to include the common bile duct. Utilization of forceps on the infundibulum and applying traction caudally retracts the cystic duct away from the common bile duct.

36.4 Complications and Post-Operative Care

Bile peritonitis or septic bile peritonitis are the most serious complications that can occur after a surgery of the gallbladder. Post-operative monitoring with continuous ECG and arterial blood pressure measurement may help early diagnosis of complications. Measurement of blood glucose and lactate are also indicated.

If an abdominal drain has been placed at the time of surgery because peritonitis was already present, sampling of the fluid for daily cytology and biochemistry is appropriate to monitor the progression of the peritonitis. Bile peritonitis is very effusive because bile salts are very caustic (Ackerman et al. 1985; Ludwig et al. 1997). Therefore it is important to maintain an appropriate fluid rate of crystalloids in the post-operative period. Also the addition of fresh frozen plasma is indicated as the abdominal effusion has a high protein content (Ludwig et al. 1997; Staatz et al. 2002).

If there is a biliary obstruction, a mortality rate between 20 and 30% has been reported after cholecystectomy (Pike et al. 2004; Worley et al. 2004; Amsellem et al. 2006; Mehler 2011). Age, γ-glutamyltransferase activity, elevated BUN, bilirubin concentrations, and the use of biliary diversion procedures were risk factors for long-term survival (Amsellem et al. 2006).

If the biliary system is not obstructive and the cholecystectomy is performed on an elective basis, the mortality rate is 2% (Youn et al. 2018).

References

Ackerman, N.B. et al. (1985). Consequences of intraperitoneal bile: bile ascites versus bile peritonitis. *Am. J. Surg.* 149 (2): 244–246.

Aguirre, A.L. et al. (2007). Gallbladder disease in Shetland sheepdogs: 38 cases (1995–2005). *J. Am. Vet. Med. Assoc.* 231 (1): 79–88.

Amsellem, P.M. et al. (2006). Long-term survival and risk factors associated with biliary surgery in dogs: 34 cases (1994–2004). *J. Am. Vet. Med. Assoc.* 229 (9): 1451–1457.

Cornejo, L. (2005). Canine gallbladder mucoceles. *Compend. Contin. Educ. Pract. Vet.* 27 (12): 912–930.

Deveney, K. (2006). Laparoscopic cholecystectomy. In: *The Sages Manual: Fundamentals of Laparoscopy, Thoracoscopy, and Gi Endoscopy*, 2e (ed. C.E.H. Scott-Conner), 147–155. New York: Springer.

Frantzides, C.T. et al. (2009). Laparoscopic cholecystectomy. In: *Atlas of Minimally Invasive Surgery* (eds. C.T. Frantzides and M.A. Carlson), 155–160. Philadelphia: Saunders Elsevier.

Katkhouda, N. (2011). Cholecystectomy. In: *Advanced Laparoscopic Surgery* (ed. N. Katkhouda), 21–39. Berlin: Springer-Verlag.

Ludwig, L.L. et al. (1997). Surgical treatment of bile peritonitis in 24 dogs and 2 cats: a retrospective study (1987–1994). *Vet. Surg.* 26 (2): 90–98.

Marvel, S. and Monnet, E. (2014). Use of a vessel sealant device for cystic duct ligation in the dog. *Vet. Surg.* 43 (8): 983–987.

Mayhew, P.D. et al. (2008). Laparoscopic cholecystectomy for management of uncomplicated gall bladder mucocele in six dogs. *Vet. Surg.* 37 (7): 625–630.

Mehler, S.J. (2011). Complications of the extrahepatic biliary surgery in companion animals. *Vet. Clin. North Am. Small Anim. Pract.* 41 (5): 949–967.

Pike, F.S. et al. (2004). Gallbladder mucocele in dogs: 30 cases (2000–2002). *J. Am. Vet. Med. Assoc.* 224 (10): 1615–1622.

Scott, J. et al. (2016). Perioperative complications and outcome of laparoscopic cholecystectomy in 20 dogs. *Vet. Surg.* 45 (S1): O49–O59.

Staatz, A.J. et al. (2002). Open peritoneal drainage versus primary closure for the treatment of septic peritonitis in dogs and cats: 42 cases (1993–1999). *Vet. Surg.* 31 (2): 174–180.

Worley, D.R. et al. (2004). Surgical management of gallbladder mucoceles in dogs: 22 cases (1999–2003). *J. Am. Vet. Med. Assoc.* 225 (9): 1418–1422.

Youn, G. et al. (2018). Outcome of elective cholecystectomy for the treatment of gallbladder disease in dogs. *J. Am. Vet. Med. Assoc.* 252 (8): 970–975.

37

Biliary Diversion

Eric Monnet

Department of Clinical Sciences, College of Veterinary Medicine and Biomedical Sciences, Colorado State University, Fort Collins, CO, USA

37.1 Indications

Biliary diversion is required to re-establish flow of bile when the common bile duct is obstructed by either an extraluminal mass, biliary lithiasis, acute or chronic pancreatitis, or neoplasia of the common bile duct. The diversion is either temporary or permanent depending upon the nature of the obstruction and if the obstruction is surgically correctible.

37.2 Surgical Techniques

37.2.1 Temporary Biliary Diversion

Biliary diversion can be temporarily performed while waiting for resolution of an obstruction, for example with an acute pancreatitis.

It requires placement of a temporary cholecystostomy tube. This procedure can be performed during a laparotomy or with laparoscopy. If the surgery is performed with a laparotomy, a pexy of the gallbladder is added to provide a better seal around the stoma to reduce the risk of bile peritonitis.

Another option for temporary decompression of the biliary system is the placement of a temporary stent in the duodenal papilla. This requires a duodenotomy, which contaminates the abdominal cavity. If the wall of the gallbladder is not intact or viable, a temporary diversion will likely not be possible and a temporary stent should be placed in the common bile duct at the level of the duodenal papilla.

37.2.1.1 Temporary Cholecystostomy Tube During Laparotomy

At the end of the laparotomy the gallbladder is evaluated for its integrity and mobility toward the abdominal wall on the right side of the abdominal cavity.

Usually the gallbladder does not need to be mobilized from the quadrate lobe. A purse-string suture with 4-0 monofilament absorbable suture is placed at the apex of the gallbladder (Figure 37.1a). The suture is placed full thickness. A 5 or 8 Fr infant feeding tube is placed percutaneously in the right side of the abdominal cavity caudal to the last rib where the gallbladder will be pexied (Figure 37.1b). A #11 blade is used to puncture the apex of the gallbladder in the middle of the purse-string suture. Suction is used to reduce the amount of bile leaking into the abdominal cavity. The infant feeding tube is advanced into the gallbladder and the purse-string suture closed. Four pexy sutures are then placed between the apex of the gallbladder and the abdominal wall around the entry site of the infant feeding tube (Figure 37.1b). The tube is secured to the skin with a Chinese finger trap with 3-0 or 2-0 nylon suture. The infant feeding tube is connected to a closed collection system.

37.2.1.2 Temporary Cholecystostomy Tube with Laparoscopy

If a laparotomy is not required the temporary biliary diversion can be established with laparoscopy (Murphy et al. 2007). A pig-tail catheter is used. Ultrasound has also been used to place a catheter in the gallbladder. However, the success rate of placement of the catheter

(a)

(b)

(a)

(b)

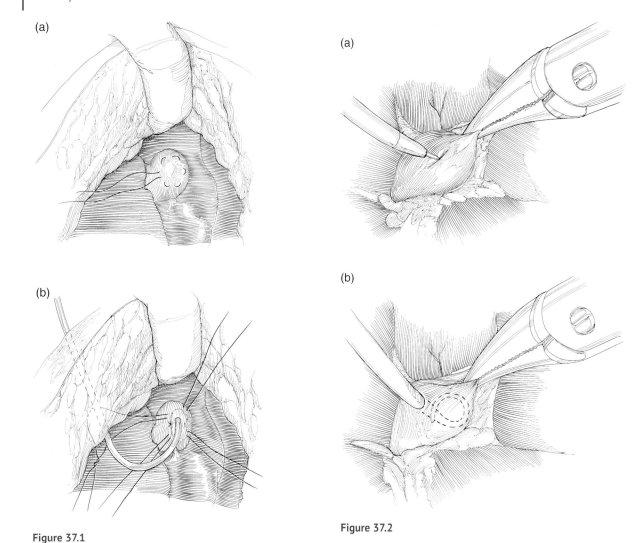

Figure 37.1

Figure 37.2

was 0% with ultrasound while it was 100% with laparoscopy (Murphy et al. 2007).

After insufflation of the abdominal cavity with carbon dioxide to a pressure of 8 mmHg, a 5 mm cannula is placed on midline 1–2 cm caudal to the umbilicus. The telescope is introduced into this cannula to visualize the gallbladder. Another 5 mm cannula is placed 1–2 cm cranial to the umbilicus. A 5 mm fine-toothed grasping forceps is introduced through this cannula to stabilize the gallbladder while the catheter is introduced in the lumen.

After making a skin incision, a 5–8 Fr pig-tail catheter mounted on a trocar is introduced percutaneously caudal to the last rib on the right side of the abdomen. Under laparoscopic visualization the catheter is directed toward the gallbladder. While the pig-tail catheter is advanced toward the apex of the gallbladder the 5 mm fine-toothed grasping forceps is stabilizing the gallbladder to provide

counter-traction (Figure 37.2a). The trocar of the pig-tail catheter is removed and the pig tail locked in placed with the locking mechanism provided (Figure 37.2b). The pig-tail catheter seems very safe since none of the catheters have leaked in a cadaveric study when tested at 20 cm of H_2O. Leakage happened at 75 ± 20 cm H_2O (Murphy et al. 2007). Four pexy sutures can be placed with intracorporeal suturing.

The catheter placed with laparotomy or laparoscopy has to be maintained for a minimum of 10 days to allow strong adhesions to form between the abdominal wall and the gallbladder. The catheter can be used to perform a cholangiogram to evaluate the status of the biliary system. Also, samples of bile can be collected for cytology and culture as needed. When the catheter is removed, the Chinese finger-trap suture is cut and the catheter pulled. The patient is then monitored for signs of peritonitis. Laparoscopy can also be performed when

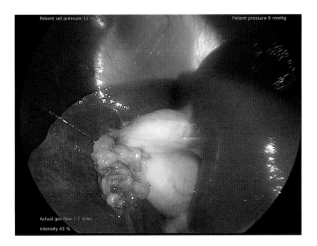

Figure 37.3

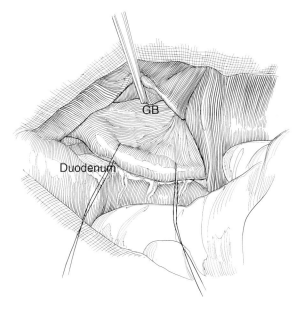

Figure 37.4

the pig-tail catheter is removed and a suture can be placed over the stoma if adhesions are not sufficient to provide a good seal to prevent leakage (Figure 37.3).

37.2.2 Permanent Biliary Diversion

Permanent diversion of bile from the biliary tree to the intestinal tract can be accomplished with an anastomosis of the gallbladder to either the duodenum or jejunum, or by transposing the common bile duct outside the pancreas into the duodenum or the jejunum. This last option is most commonly used in cases with chronic pancreatitis and fibrosis around the common bile duct.

37.2.2.1 Cholecystoduodenostomy

The gallbladder is mobilized from its fossa in the quadrate lobe to reduce tension on the cholecystoduodenostomy. The duodenum is then brought against the gallbladder to complete the side-to-side anastomosis. The surgical site is well isolated with laparotomy sponges.

First, two stay sutures are preplaced between the wall of the gallbladder and the antimesenteric side the duodenum (Figure 37.4). If possible, the two stay sutures should be placed 4 cm apart. The anastomosis will be performed between the two stay sutures. It is paramount to maintain the gallbladder in an anatomical orientation to minimize the risk of twisting the cystic duct.

The gallbladder and the duodenum are incised between the two stay sutures (Figure 37.5a). It has been recommended to make an incision 4 cm long if possible (Blass and Seim 1985; Martin et al. 1985; Matthiesen and Rosin 1986). During the healing process and with reflux of intestinal contents in the hepatobiliary system, fibrosis develops and reduces the diameter of the stoma. A stoma of 4 cm should be created at the time of surgery,

if possible. After healing, a stoma of 2.5 cm might then be maintained. With a simple continuous pattern using 4-0 monofilament absorbable suture, the walls of the gallbladder and the duodenum are then sutured together along the dorsal surface (Figure 37.5b). It is paramount to carefully place the sutures in the corners of the incision to prevent leakage. The same suture patterns are repeated on the ventral side (Figure 37.5c).

37.2.2.2 Roux-en-Y Diversion

With a cholecystoduodenostomy, ascending infection can occur, resulting in cholangiohepatitis (Martin et al. 1985). Chronic antibiotic therapy is usually needed to control the associated clinical signs. To prevent this ascending infection into the biliary system, a Roux-en-Y diversion is possible. Two options exist. The first option is to create a cholecystojejunoduodenostomy with the interposition of a loop of jejunum between the apex of the gallbladder and the duodenum. The second option is to perform a cholecystojejunojejunostomy with the interposition of a loop of jejunum between the apex of the gallbladder and the proximal jejunum. With either technique, the gallbladder does not need to be dissected from the hepatic fossa.

37.2.2.2.1 Cholecystojejunoduodenostomy A loop of jejunum, based on two jejunal arteries, is isolated on its own blood supply from the rest of the jejunum. Arcadial vessels are ligated with 4-0 monofilament absorbable sutures (Figure 37.6). Doyen clamps are used to prevent

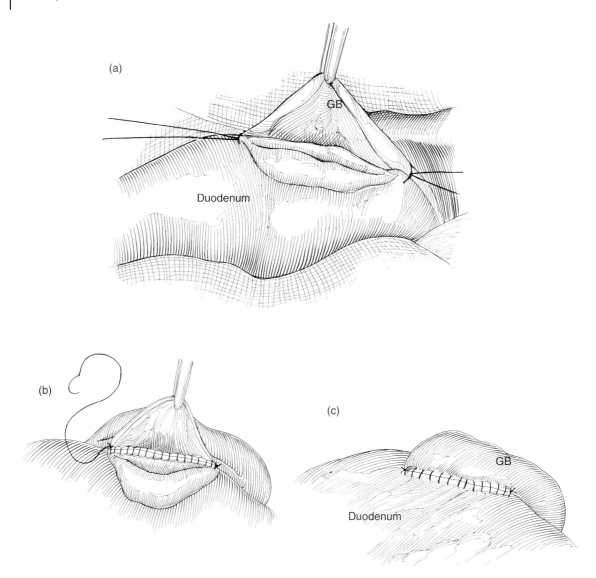

Figure 37.5

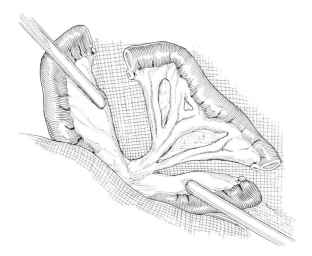

Figure 37.6

contamination of the peritoneal cavity from the isolated loop of bowel. The integrity of the jejunum is restored by creating an end-to-end anastomosis with 4-0 monofilament absorbable suture.

The proximal open end of the isolated loop of jejunum is sutured to the apex of the gallbladder with a two-layer suture, as described in the cholecystoduodenostomy (Figure 37.7a and b). To achieve a stoma 4 cm long it is necessary to incise the antimesenteric border of the proximal end of the loop of jejunum to create a stoma 4 cm long, including the proximal open end of the loop of jejunum.

A gastrointestinal anastomosis (GIA) stapling device can be used to create this stoma. The stoma is completed with 4-0 monofilament absorbable suture to close the

(a)

(b)

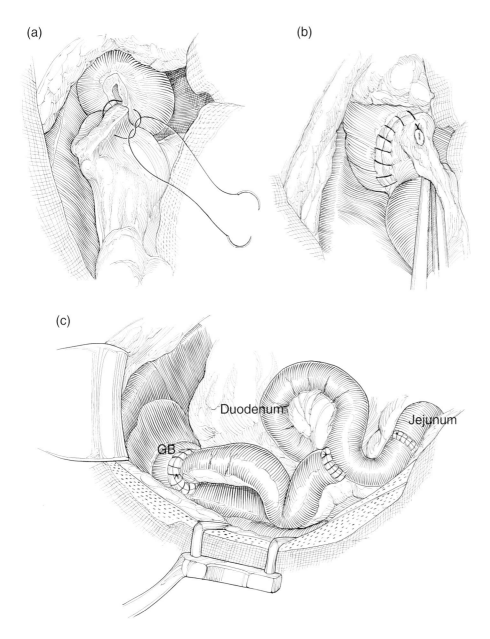

(c)

Duodenum

Jejunum

GB

Figure 37.7

open end of the jejunum and the point of introduction of the GIA stapler in the gallbladder.

The distal end of the isolated loop of jejunum is then anastomosed with an end-to-side anastomosis to the distal duodenum with two simple continuous apposition suture pattens (Figure 37.7c). Monofilament absorbable suture size 4-0 is used for the anastomosis.

37.2.2.2.2 Cholecystojejunojejunostomy The procedure is similar to the cholecystojejunoduodeostomy but this time the distal part of the segment of jejunum is anastomosed to the jejunum instead to the duodenum.

37.2.2.3 Cholecystojejunostomy
To simplify the cholecystojejunojejunostomy and eliminate an enterotomy, a cholecystojejunostomy can be performed with a Roux-en-Y limb.

The proximal jejunum is transected after ligation of the arcadial vessels. Doyen clamps are used to prevent contamination of the peritoneal cavity. The distal part of the jejunum is brought toward the apex of the gallbladder and anastomosed. Two stay sutures are first placed to maintain the distal part of jejunum against the wall of the gallbladder. A #11 blade is used to open the gallbladder between the two stay sutures. The bile is

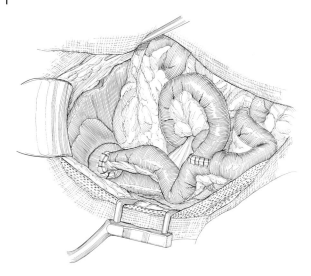

Figure 37.8

aspirated. The anastomosis between the gallbladder and the jejunum is completed with two simple continuous appositional patterns as described in Figure 37.7 for the cholecystojejunoduodenostomy. Monofilament absorbable suture size 4-0 is used. The proximal jejunum is then anastomosed to the rest of the jejunum 10–15 cm from the cholecystojejunostomy, with an end-to-side anastomosis with 4-0 monofilament absorbable suture (Figure 37.8).

37.2.2.4 Choledochoduodenostomy or Choledochojejunostomy

If a chronic pancreatitis is the cause of the obstruction of the bile duct, a transposition of the common bile duct to the duodenum outside the pancreas or to the jejunum is indicated.

To facilitate this procedure it is beneficial to have a dilated common bile duct, which is very frequently the case.

The common bile duct is dissected out of the pancreas and ligated as close as possible to the duodenum. The common bile duct is spatulated if the diameter is not sufficient to safely perform the anastomosis.

The common bile duct is then implanted in either the duodenum or the jejunum as described in Chapter 39. If it is implanted in the duodenum, the anastomosis is close to the pylorus, which might increase the risk of bile reflux.

37.3 Tips

It might be helpful to place a laparotomy sponge between the diaphragm and the quadrate lobe to improve exposure of the apex of the gallbladder during the anastomosis. It will help reduce the tension on the sutures during the procedure.

The gallbladder should be maintained in the hepatic fossa as much as possible to minimize the risk of kinking the cystic duct. The distal duodenum can usually be brought to the gallbladder without mobilizing the gallbladder. If too much tension is present then the gallbladder is mobilized. It is paramount to keep the cystic artery intact during the mobilization of the gallbladder. If the cystic artery is damaged, the gallbladder will undergo necrosis.

Placement of a gastrostomy tube and a jejunostomy tube, or a J through G tube, is indicated to support the patient in the immediate post-operative period. The gastrostomy tube is used to suction the stomach content to prevent vomiting and aspiration pneumonia. The jejunostomy tube is used to feed the patient in the immediate post-operative period.

37.4 Complications

Post-operatively the patient is monitored for signs of septic and bile peritonitis. Sampling of the abdominal fluid post-operatively might be indicated for an early detection of a septic bile peritonitis.

Long-term patients with a cholecystoduodenostomy or cholecystojejunostomy are at risk of cholangiohepatitis because of the reflux of intestinal content into the gallbladder. It has been assumed that a large stoma should allow for a better drainage of the content of the gallbladder. Martin et al. in a study of three dogs showed significant reflux of intestinal content into the gallbladder and severe histologic changes to the biliary system. Also *Escherichia coli* and *Klebsiella* were the organisms commonly identified in the biliary system. Patients with a cholecystoduodenostomy or a cholecystojejunostomy required regular treatment for cholangiohepatits. Denamarin, ursodial, and enrofloxacin are commonly administered in the long term to support these patients.

The creation of a Roux-en-Y limb should help prevent reflux. In human patients it is recommended to have a limb of jejunum 40–60 cm long (Chojnacki and Yeo 2019).

Martin et al. (1985) used a 15 cm limb to create a cholecystojejunostomy. Intestinal reflux was still present with the Roux-en-Y limb. The histopathologic changes observed in the cases with the Roux-en-Y limb were similar to the changes observed in the dogs that received a cholecystoduodenostomy. It has been shown that the Roux-en-Y limb has a peristaltic activity toward the proximal part of the limb instead of the aborad part (Cullen and Kelly 1993). This may explain why a limb that is only 15 cm is not sufficient to palliate intestinal reflux in the gallbladder.

References

Blass, C.E. and Seim, H.B. 3rd (1985). Surgical techniques for the liver and biliary tract. *Vet. Clin. North Am. Small Anim. Pract.* 15 (1): 257–275.

Chojnacki, K.A. and Yeo, C.J. (2019). Operative management of bile duct stricture. In: Shackelford's Surgery of the Alimentary Tract, 8e (eds. C.J. Yeo et al.), 1352–1360. Philadelphia: Elsevier.

Cullen, J.J. and Kelly, K.A. (1993). Gastric motor physiology and pathophysiology. *Surg. Clin. North Am.* 73 (6): 1145–1160.

Martin, R.A. et al. (1985). Effect of intestinal reflux into the hepatobiliary ducts following biliary enteric anastomosis in the dog. *Vet. Surg.* 14 (1): 59.

Matthiesen, D.T. and Rosin, E. (1986). Common bile duct obstruction secondary to chronic fibrosing pancreatitis: treatment by use of cholecystoduodenostomy in the dog. *J. Am. Vet. Med. Assoc.* 189 (11): 1443–1446.

Murphy, S.M. et al. (2007). Minimally invasive cholecystostomy in the dog: evaluation of placement techniques and use in extrahepatic biliary obstruction. *Vet. Surg.* 36 (7): 675–683.

38

Surgery of the Bile Duct

Eric Monnet

Department of Clinical Sciences, College of Veterinary Medicine and Biomedical Sciences, Colorado State University, Fort Collins, CO, USA

38.1 Indications

Surgery of the bile duct is rare in dogs and cats. Chronic pancreatitis and neoplasia in the wall of the duodenum are the most common causes of obstruction of the distal segment of the common bile duct (Mehler et al. 2004; Amsellem et al. 2006; Mayhew et al. 2006; Mehler and Bennett 2006; Baker et al. 2011; Mehler 2011). Other indications include an obstruction of the distal part of the common bile duct requiring the transposition outside of the pancreas, an obstruction secondary to stones or the repair of the bile duct after traumatic rupture or iatrogenic transection.

38.2 Techniques

38.2.1 Choledochotomy

Choledochotomy is indicated for removal of biliary stones wedged in the common bile duct or for the repair of a ruptured common bile duct (Baker et al. 2011). Usually, the stones are wedged in the distal segment of the common bile duct just proximal to the duodenal papilla. Since the common bile duct is distended, a choledochotomy is possible.

After localization of the stones, the obstruction or the rupture, the common bile duct is isolated from the hepato-duodenal ligament and the pancreas if needed. Two stay sutures with 5-0 monofilament sutures are placed on the common bile duct where the incision will be performed (Figure 38.1). An #11 blade is used to incise the common bile duct over the stone. The

choledochotomy should be long enough to retrieve the stones without tearing the wall of the common bile duct (Figure 38.2a). Bile is aspirated from the proximal part of the common bile duct to minimize the risk of bile peritonitis. After removal of the stones (Figure 38.3), the common bile duct is flushed proximally and distally with a 3 or 5 Fr catheter. The distal part of the common bile duct is catheterized to make sure it is patent into the duodenum.

The bile duct is then closed with a simple continuous suture pattern (Figure 38.2b). A 5-0 monofilament absorbable suture is used. The sutures are placed full thickness through the wall of the common bile duct. A temporary stent made of a short segment (3–5 cm) of a 3 Fr infant feeding tube can be placed in the lumen of the common bile duct exiting in the duodenum (Mayhew et al. 2006). The stent facilitates the closure of the bile duct because it outlines the lumen of the common bile duct. The stent is not sutured in place and will be eliminated later by the peristaltic waves in the duodenum.

38.2.2 Resection and Anastomosis of the Common Bile Duct

If a tumor is present or if a segment of the common bile duct is necrotic because of the presence of stones, a resection and anastomosis of the common bile duct can be performed. If the common bile duct is ruptured after trauma or iatrogenically, it can be repaired and anastomosed (Baker et al. 2011; Ball and Lillemoe 2019).

After isolation of the common bile duct at the level of the neoplasia or the necrosis, two stay sutures are placed

Gastrointestinal Surgical Techniques in Small Animals, First Edition. Edited by Eric Monnet and Daniel D. Smeak.
© 2020 John Wiley & Sons, Inc. Published 2020 by John Wiley & Sons, Inc.
Companion website: www.wiley.com/go/monnet/gastrointestinal

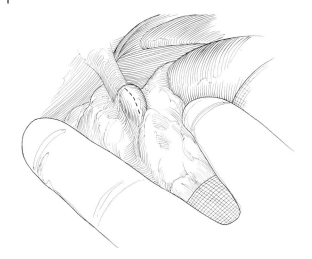

Figure 38.1

(a)

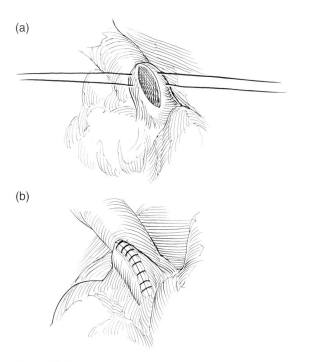

(b)

Figure 38.2

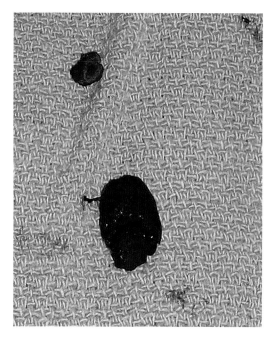

Figure 38.3

continuous suture pattern is started on the dorsal side first with one strand of suture and the anastomosis is completed on the ventral side by tying both strands together (Figure 38.4c).

The duodenum is mobile enough in dogs and cats to complete the anastomosis with minimal tension. If the resection is close to the connection of the cystic duct with the common bile duct, the proximal and distal segments of the common bile duct are ligated and a cholecystoduodenostomy or a cholecystojejunostomy should be performed (Chapter 37).

38.2.3 Choledochoduodenostomy or Choledochojejunostomy

An obstruction of the distal part of the common bile duct at the level of the duodenal papilla and pancreas can be treated with a choledochoduodenostomy or a choledochojejunostomy instead of doing a cholecystoduodenostomy or a cholecystojejunostomy. It should help prevent reflux of intestinal content into the biliary system and reduce the risk of cholangiohepatitis.

After isolation of the common bile duct distally as it enters the pancreas, it is dissected from the mesentery and the hepatoduodenal ligament (Figure 38.5). The dissection should not extend too far cranially to maintain blood supply to the distal part of the common bile duct. The common bile duct is ligated with 4-0 monofilament absorbable suture as distally as possible (Figure 38.5b) and transected with Metzembaum scissors. The proximal

in the cranial and caudal segments of the common bile duct before it is transected (Figure 38.4a). Bile is aspirated from the proximal part of the common bile duct to minimize the risk of bile peritonitis.

After resection of the neoplasia or the necrotic tissue, the anastomosis is completed with 5-0 double armed monofilament absorbable suture. A 5 Fr infant feeding tube is placed in the lumen of the common duct as a temporary stent to help visualize the lumen during the anastomosis (Figure 38.4b). Two simple appositional continuous suture patterns are used to complete the anastomosis. The sutures are placed full thickness. The

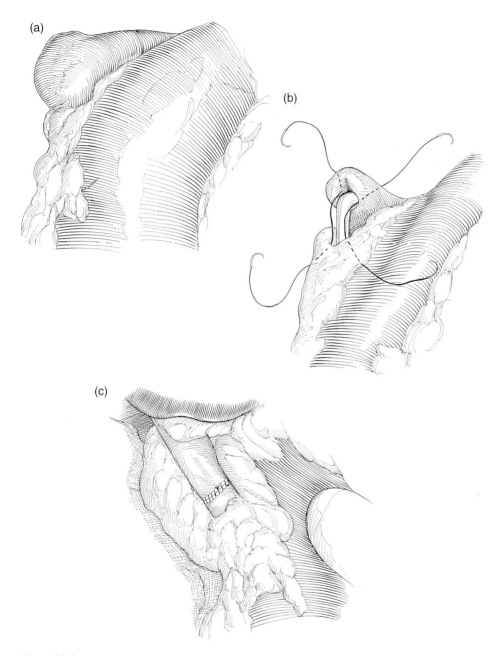

(a)

(b)

(c)

Figure 38.4

part of the common bile duct is then catheterized with a 5–8 Fr feeding tube to collect bile (Figure 38.6a).

The common bile duct is spatulated with an incision on its ventral part. The length of the incision should be equal to the diameter of the bile duct. The common bile duct is then anastomosed either to the proximal duodenum or the jejunum. The surgical technique is similar for a choledochoduodenostomy or a choledochojejunostomy.

A full-thickness incision is made with a #11 blade through the wall of the duodenum or jejunum. The length of the incision should match the length of the diameter of the bile duct after spatulation (Figure 38.7a). Two stay sutures are then placed between the wall of the duodenum or jejunum and the common bile duct to bring the common bile duct to the incision of the duodenum or the jejunum. A 5-0 double armed monofilament absorbable suture is used for the stay sutures. The stay sutures are then used to complete the anastomosis (Figure 38.7a). Two simple continuous suture patterns are used. The sutures are placed full thickness through the wall of the duodenum or jejunum and the bile duct.

(a)

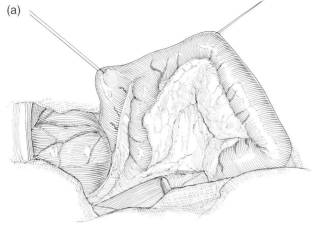

(b)

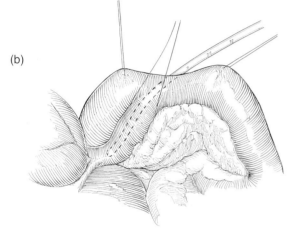

Figure 38.5

(a)

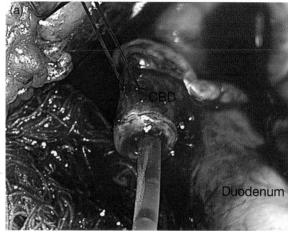

(b)

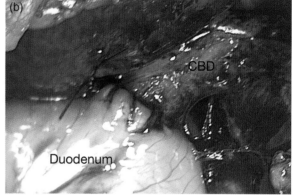

Figure 38.6

The dorsal side of the anastomosis is completed first before completing the ventral side (Figures 38.6b and 38.7b).

A gastrostomy and a jejunostomy feeding tubes are placed at the end of the surgery. The gastrostomy tube is aspirated four times a day to limit the risk of esophageal reflux and vomiting and the jejunostomy tube is used to feed the patient. If a choledochojejunostomy was performed, the jejunostomy feeding tube is placed distal the surgical site.

38.3 Tips

Since the bile duct is usually distended after an obstruction, the surgery should be facilitated. However, magnification is recommended during the surgery of the bile duct.

A stricture can develop after resection and anastomosis of the bile duct. However, there is no data reported in the veterinary literature about the incidence of stricture following bile duct surgery. Nonetheless, the risk of stricture and obstruction is judged to be low given the local bile duct distension. If a stenosis develops, a cholecystojejunostomy is required.

To prevent a stricture of the bile duct after a resection and anastomosis, it is important to spatulate both ends of the bile duct. Also, placement of a 5 Fr infant feeding tube should reduce the risk of stenosis at the time of surgery. The tube also prevents placement of a suture across the lumen of the bile duct, inducing an obstruction (Ball and Lillemoe 2019). A stricture has been reported in 37% of human patients after bile duct resection and anastomosis, with only 22% of patients experiencing a good outcome. The choledocojejunostomy with a Roux-en-Y procedure is associated with a good outcome in 54% of human patients (Ball and Lillemoe 2019).

The author prefers to perform choledochojejunostomy to minimize the risk of bile reflux in the stomach. When the bile duct is transposed in the proximal duodenum, it is very close to the pyloric antrum which may result in biliary gastric reflux.

(a)

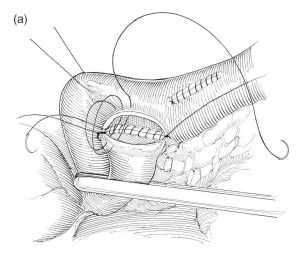

(b)

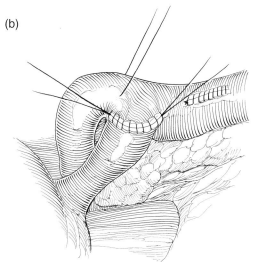

Figure 38.7

If a choledochojejunostomy has been performed, it is the author's impression that the jejunum proximal to the anastomosis should be pexied to the cranial part of the abdomen along the last rib. Pexying the jejunum cranially allows the proximal jejunum to line up parallel to the common bile duct, which seems to reduce or prevent reflux of jejunal content in the common bile duct.

In human surgery, a Roux-en-Y is preferred with an end-to-side anastomosis of the common bile duct to a loop of jejunum (Chojnacki and Yeo 2019). In human patients if a resection of more than 1 cm of the bile duct is necessary, a primary repair is not warranted because tension might increase the risk of stricture formation. A choledochojejunostomy with a Roux-en-Y procedure is recommended (Ball and Lillemoe 2019).

During the choledochoduodenostomy or the choledochojejunostomy, diversion of bile can be accomplished with a temporary stent as described above or with a percutaneous cholecystotomy drain as described in Chapter 37. It is also possible to place a percutaneous drain in the distal duodenum or proximal jejunum like a duodenostomy or jejunostomy feeding tube, and advance it to the level of the choledochoduodenostomy or the choledochojejunostomy and into the common bile duct as described in Section 39.2.1. The drain is connected to a closed collection system. Usually the peristaltic waves move the drain out of the bile duct into the duodenum or the jejunum within three days. It can then be used as a feeding tube. The drain cannot be removed until seven days after surgery to prevent leakage into the abdominal cavity.

38.4 Complications

Bile peritonitis or septic bile peritonitis are the most serious complications after bile duct surgery. Postoperative monitoring with continuous ECG and arterial pressure measurement may help early diagnosis of shock and bile peritonitis. Measurement of blood glucose and lactate are important also.

It is important to monitor the bilirubin concentration during the first 48 hours after surgery to evaluate the patency of the biliary system. An elevation of the bilirubin level can be due to an obstruction of the biliary system or leakage of the surgery site. An ultrasound of the liver and biliary tree is then recommended. If the hepatic bile ducts are distended, the surgical site is obstructed by either edema or narrowing at the surgical site. Placement of a temporary stent or drainage system allows the prevention of obstruction due to edema. Usually, the edema is resorbed in 24 or 48 hours. If abdominal effusion is identified on abdominal ultrasound, an abdominocentesis is required to measure the bilirubin concentration. If bile peritonitis is confirmed, an abdominal exploration is required to evaluate the surgical site.

Patients should be monitored for signs of cholangiohepatitis even if a choledochoduodenostomy or choledochojejunostomy were performed. Medical therapy of cholangiohepatitis may include antibiotics, Ursodiol and Denamarin.

To prevent stricture formation, it is important to have a good apposition of the duodenal or jejunal mucosa with the bile duct. If a stricture develops, a cholecystojejunostomy is recommended.

References

Amsellem, P.M. et al. (2006). Long-term survival and risk factors associated with biliary surgery in dogs: 34 cases (1994–2004). *J. Am. Vet. Med. Assoc.* 229 (9): 1451–1457.

Baker, S.G. et al. (2011). Choledochotomy and primary repair of extrahepatic biliary duct rupture in seven dogs and two cats. *J. Small Anim. Pract.* 52 (1): 32–37.

Ball, C.G. and Lillemoe, K.D. (2019). Prevention and management of bile duct injury. In: *Shackelford's Surgery of the Alimentary Tract* (eds. C.J. Yeo et al.), 1340–1351. Philadelphia: Elsevier.

Chojnacki, K.A. and Yeo, C.J. (2019). Operative management of bile duct stricture. In: *Shackelford's Surgery of the Alimentary Tract*, 8e (eds. C.J. Yeo et al.), 1352–1360. Philadelphia: Elsevier.

Mayhew, P.D. et al. (2006). Choledochal tube stenting for decompression of the extrahepatic portion of the biliary tract in dogs: 13 cases (2002–2005). *J. Am. Vet. Med. Assoc.* 228 (8): 1209–1214.

Mehler, S.J. (2011). Complications of the extrahepatic biliary surgery in companion animals. *Vet. Clin. North Am. Small Anim. Pract.* 41 (5): 949–967.

Mehler, S.J. and Bennett, R.A. (2006). A review of canine extrahepatic biliary tract disease and surgery. *Compend. Contin. Educ. Pract. Vet.* 28 (2): 302–315.

Mehler, S.J. et al. (2004). Variables associated with outcome in dogs undergoing extrahepatic biliary surgery: 60 cases (1988–2002). *Vet. Surg.* 33 (6): 644–649.

39

Biliary Stenting

Eric Monnet

Department of Clinical Sciences, College of Veterinary Medicine and Biomedical Sciences, Colorado State University, Fort Collins, CO, USA

39.1 Indications

Stenting of the biliary system, and mostly the common duct, is indicated to palliate either a permanent or a temporary obstruction of the common bile duct or to support the biliary system while a tear is healing by second intention. It has also been used in human surgery to treat bile leakage after cholecystectomy. The stent allows a reduction of the pressure in the biliary system.

Acute pancreatitis and acute cholangiohepatitis can induce a temporary obstruction of either the distal part of the common bile duct at the level of the duodenal papilla or in the more proximal part of the common bile duct. In these circumstances, patients will benefit from temporary stenting of their common bile duct to palliate their clinical signs.

Chronic pancreatitis with fibrosis around the duodenal papilla, stricture of the common bile duct, neoplasia of the common bile duct or extrahepatic neoplasm can induce a permanent obstruction of the common bile duct. If a biliary diversion procedure cannot be performed, a permanent stent can be considered to palliate the clinical signs.

39.2 Technique

39.2.1 Short-Term Temporary Stenting

After performing an abdominal exploration and evaluation of the biliary system, the duodenum is exposed for placement of a short-term temporary stent.

A 5 Fr infant feeding tube for cats and small breed dogs and an 8 Fr infant feeding tube for medium- to large-breed dogs is introduced percutaneously in the right side of the abdominal cavity at the level of the duodenocolic curvature (Figure 39.1a). A purse-string suture with a 4-0 monofilament absorbable suture is placed on the antimesenteric border of the distal duodenum. After making a stab incision in the center of the purse-string, the infant feeding tube is then introduced in the distal duodenum in a retrograde fashion toward the major duodenal papilla. The duodenum is then incised on the antimesenteric border at the level of the duodenal papilla. The feeding tube is advanced retrograde through the duodenal papilla in the common bile duct (Figure 39.1b). It is important to choose a tube that is not too large for the bile duct. The tube should not be snug against the wall of the common bile duct to allow for the bile to drain around the tube. A 6-0 simple interrupted suture can be placed around the tube to secure it to the mucosa of the duodenum. This suture should not engage the submucosa because when the tube is pulled after four to five days, it will only tear the mucosa (Figure 39.1c). The duodenum is then closed with a simple continuous pattern with 4-0 monofilament absorbable suture material. The distal duodenum is pexied to the abdominal wall where the feeding tube has been introduced with four simple interrupted sutures with 4-0 monofilament absorbable suture. The feeding tube is secured to the skin with a Chinese finger-trap suture with 4-0 nylon. The feeding tube is connected to a closed collection system. The tube is left in place for four to five days.

39.2.2 Long-Term Temporary Stenting

After performing an abdominal exploration and evaluation of the biliary system, the duodenum is incised on the antimesenteric border at the level of the duodenal papilla.

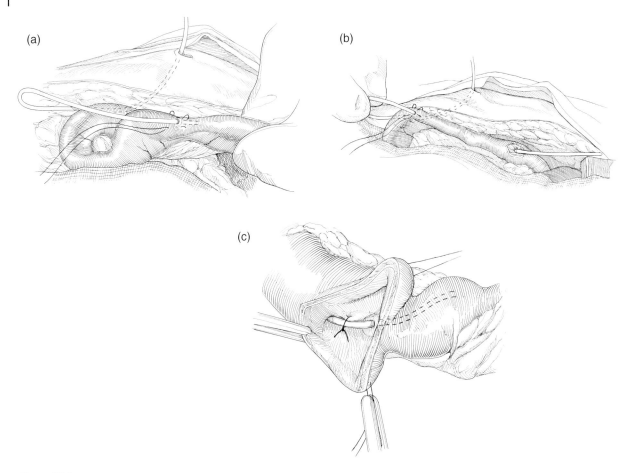

Figure 39.1

After identification of the papilla, an infant feeding tube is introduced in the common bile through the duodenal papilla. Usually, a 5 Fr infant feeding tube is used for cats and small dogs and an 8 Fr infant feeding tube is used for medium- and large-breed dogs. If a small tube cannot be introduced in the common bile duct, a biliary diversion should be performed. If the common bile duct can be catheterized, an infant feeding tube with additional fenestration is introduced in a retrograde fashion from the major duodenal papilla into the common bile duct proximal to the obstruction. The tube should be left to extend in the duodenum for 2–3 cm. The diameter of the tube should be such that it fills in the bile duct without stretching it. One or two simple interrupted sutures are placed to secure the stent to the mucosa/submucosa of the duodenum with a 4-0 monofilament absorbable suture, as in Figure 39.1c. In a study on 10 dogs with extrahepatic biliary obstruction, the stent passed in the feces 1–11 months after surgery (Mayhew et al. 2006). In a study on six cats with chronic pancreatitis, two cats had re-obstruction of their bile duct five to six days after stent placement (Mayhew and Weisse 2008). Sludge from the biliary system apparently occluded the stent in another cat. When the stent is not dislodged naturally with the peristaltic wave and passage of a food bolus in the duodenum, an endoscope can be used to release the stent.

39.2.3 Permanent Stenting

Permanent stenting can be accomplished by placing a covered or non-covered self-expanding stent in the common bile duct and the duodenal papilla in dogs (Vorwerk et al. 1993; Yasumori et al. 1993). Hyperplasia of the mucosa happened either within the lumen of the stent or at the ends of the stent. In one study, all covered stents were occluded within four months after implantation (Vorwerk et al. 1993). The covered stents with polytetrafluoroethylene seem to be better tolerated in dogs (Zografakis et al. 2003). Six months after implantation, all stents were patent.

Permanent stenting can be performed with a laparotomy, percutaneously, or endoscopically (Vorwerk et al. 1993; Yasumori et al. 1993; Youngelman et al. 1997; Marks et al. 1998; Berent et al. 2015).

After a laparotomy, the apex of the gallbladder is exposed. After placing a purse-string at the apex of the gallbladder, a catheter is introduced in the middle of the purse-string suture into the gallbladder and a cholangiogram is performed to localize the stricture.

A guide is advanced through the catheter into the gallbladder, through the cystic duct, the common bile duct, and out the duodenal papilla. The catheter is removed and the stent delivery system is advanced over the wire. After confirming appropriate placement of the delivery system with fluoroscopy, the stent is delivered at the level of the stricture. The delivery system is removed and a cholangiogram is performed to confirm patency of the common bile duct. The puncture site at the level of the gallbladder is sutured with a simple interrupted suture.

The percutaneous placement of a biliary stent requires ultrasonography to localize the gallbladder in the abdominal cavity and to insert the device. Bile is aspirated from the gallbladder for sample collection (cytology, culture and sensitivity) and decompression. The steps described previously for wire passage, stent delivery system placement and stent deployment are performed with fluoroscopy guidance.

The endoscopic placement of a stent requires a sideview duodenoscope. The major duodenal papilla is visualized and cannulated. A retrograde cholangiogram can be performed. After a sphincterotomy, a self-expanding stent can be delivered (Berent et al. 2015).

39.3   Tips

When a temporary stent is placed surgically, it is important to choose a catheter of smaller diameter than the common bile to allow bile to drain around the stent in case it gets obstructed. Also, fenestration in the drain should improve flow of the bile within the catheter.

The short-term temporary stents have a tendency to migrate in the duodenum when peristaltism is present. Usually, it takes three to four days for the peristaltic waves to dislodge the stent out of the common bile duct but the catheter should be left in until it is safe to pull out. Like a jejunostomy tube, it is recommended to wait six to eight days before it can be safely removed.

If the long-term temporary stent does not pass in the feces, it should be removed endoscopically after six months if the underlying disease is under control. Radiographs or ultrasound should allow visualization of the stent in the common bile duct. The infant feeding tubes have a radiodense line.

The self-expanding stents can be placed surgically with an access through the apex of the gallbladder.

39.4   Complications and Post-Operative Care

In the post-operative period, patients are watched for signs of septic bile peritonitis since the duodenum has been open. The biochemistry panel should show a rapid improvement in all measured liver and biliary parameters.

With a short-term temporary stent, it is not unusual to see a rapid decrease in bilirubin over the first 24–48 hours after surgery, followed by a slight increase in bilirubin if the stent has become obstructed by inspissated bile. A stent that is not snug along the wall of the common bile duct should allow bile to drain around the tube.

For permanent, self-expanding stents, proliferation and hyperplasia of the mucosa in the common bile duct can obstruct the stent even if it is a covered stent.

Temporary or permanent stents can migrate and pass in the feces. Recurrence of the biliary obstruction will happen if the underlying disease has not been controlled.

A stent may increase the risk of cholangiohepatitis by allowing duodenal content to migrate into the biliary system.

References

Berent, A. et al. (2015). Initial experience with endoscopic retrograde cholangiography and endoscopic retrograde biliary stenting for treatment of extrahepatic bile duct obstruction in dogs. *J. Am. Vet. Med. Assoc.* 246 (4): 436–446.

Marks, J.M. et al. (1998). Biliary stenting is more effective than sphincterotomy in the resolution of biliary leaks. *Surg. Endosc.* 12 (4): 327–330.

Mayhew, P.D. and Weisse, C.W. (2008). Treatment of pancreatitis-associated extrahepatic biliary tract obstruction by choledochal stenting in seven cats. *J. Small Anim. Pract.* 49 (3): 133–138.

Mayhew, P.D. et al. (2006). Choledochal tube stenting for decompression of the extrahepatic portion of the biliary tract in dogs: 13 cases (2002–2005). *J. Am. Vet. Med. Assoc.* 228 (8): 1209–1214.

Vorwerk, D. et al. (1993). Long-term patency of wallstent endoprostheses in benign biliary obstructions: experimental results. *J. Vasc. Interv. Radiol.* 4 (5): 625–634.

Yasumori, K. et al. (1993). Placement of covered self-expanding metallic stents in the common bile duct: a feasibility study. *J. Vasc. Interv. Radiol.* 4 (6): 773–778.

Youngelman, D.F. et al. (1997). Comparison of bile duct pressures following sphincterotomy and endobiliary stenting in a canine model. *Surg. Endosc.* 11 (2): 126–128.

Zografakis, J.G. et al. (2003). Endoluminal reconstruction of the canine common biliary duct. *Curr. Surg.* 60 (4): 437–441.

40

Arterio-Venous Fistula

Eric Monnet

Department of Clinical Sciences, College of Veterinary Medicine and Biomedical Sciences, Colorado State University, Fort Collins,ww0 CO, USA

40.1 Indications

Hepatic arterio-venous (AV) fistulas are the result of a congenital connection between a branch of the hepatic artery and a branch of the portal vein. They result in portal hypertension with hepatofugal flow. Acquired portosystemic shunts develop to palliate the portal hypertension. Dogs with AV fistula present with abdominal distension, ascites and signs of hepatic encephalopathy (Easley and Carpenter 1975; Legendre et al. 1976; Moore and Whiting 1986; Whiting et al. 1986; Schaeffer et al. 2001; Chanoit et al. 2007).

Patients with AV fistula will have hepatomegaly and abdominal effusion on preoperative abdominal radiographs and hepatofugal flow in the portal vein and acquired portosystemic shunt around the left kidney identified on abdominal ultrasound (Rogers et al. 1977; Bailey et al. 1988). A computed tomography angiogram is the most valuable imaging to identify the extent of the AV fistula (Figure 40.1). The arterial phase of the CT angiogram outlines the source of the AV fistula and the extent of the perfusion from the hepatic artery into the AV fistula. The delayed venous phase shows the drainage of the AV fistula into the portal vein and the hepatofugal flow into the acquired shunts (Figure 40.2).

40.2 Technique

AV fistulas are treated either with an open approach via a laparotomy or with a minimally-invasive approach via interventional radiology. The latter is recognized to be less invasive than surgery (Whiting et al. 1986; Chanoit et al. 2007).

40.2.1 Laparotomy

After a midline approach, an abdominal exploration is performed. A 20 G catheter is placed in a jejunal vein to measure the portal pressure with a water manometer. Usually, in patients with AV fistula and secondary portal hypertension, portal pressure is above 20 cm of water. The liver lobe affected by the AV fistula contains a lot of tortuous blood vessels (Figure 40.3).

The liver lobe including the arterio-venous fistula is resected while ligating all the blood vessels entering or exiting the liver lobe. The dissection is performed at the hilus of the liver lobe, with isolation of any major blood vessels. Hemostasis with either suture or clips is indicated, as a vessel sealant device may not be very efficient in sealing the very thin wall of the artery and vein. After isolation of the liver lobe at its hilus, the portal vein and the hepatic vein are clamped and ligated. Stapling equipment can be used to complete the liver lobectomy.

If possible, the branch of the portal vein draining the AV fistula is dissected and ligated at its connection with the main portal vein. A tangential vascular clamp is applied to the portal vein to isolate the connection of the portal and the branch draining the AV fistula (Figure 40.4). The portal vein is then closed with a simple continuous suture pattern with a 6-0 prolene (Figure 40.5). AV fistulas are associated with many fragile collateral blood vessels, therefore the manipulation of the entire liver lobe with the fistula has to be delicate to minimize hemorrhage. When the main source of arterial blood supply is ligated, the portal pressure is significantly reduced compared to baseline.

40.2.2 Interventional Radiology

Another approach to treat arterio-venous fistulas is to use interventional radiology. After placing an introducer in the femoral artery, a guide wire and a catheter

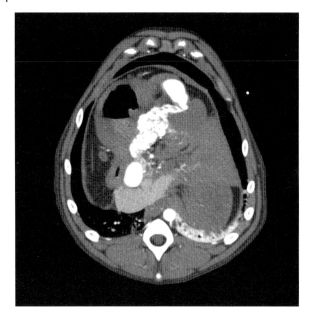

Figure 40.1

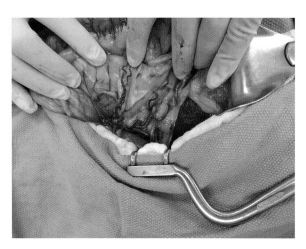

Figure 40.2

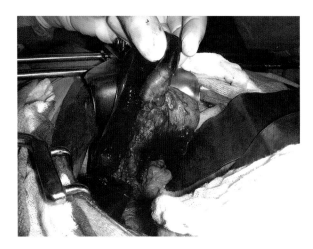

Figure 40.3

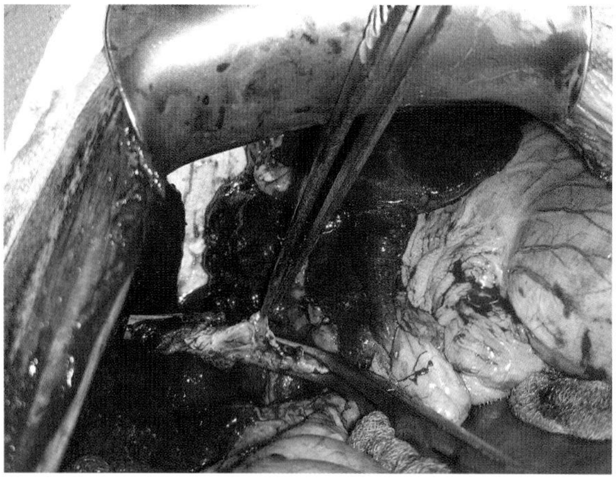

![Figure 40.4 photograph]

Figure 40.4

![Figure 40.5 photograph]

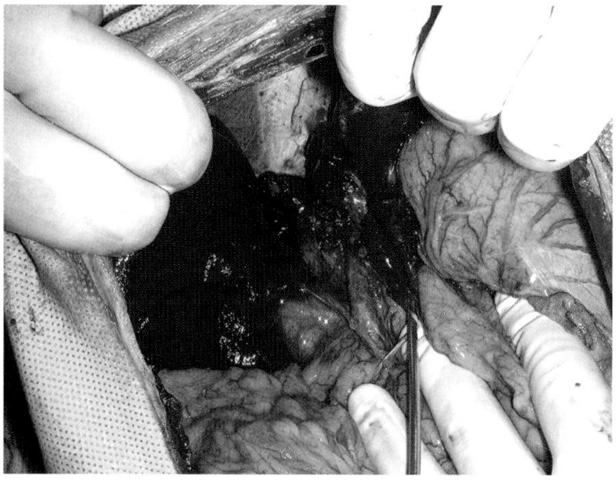

Figure 40.5

are advanced in the descending aorta. After injecting contrast medium, the celiac artery is identified and the guide wire is advanced into it. The catheter is advanced over the wire and more contrast is used to identify the hepatic artery and the branch perfusing the arterio-venous fistula. The catheter is advanced in that branch and the artery perfusing the fistula is embolized with glue (Chanoit et al. 2007). With a laparotomy, the vein draining the AV fistula is also ligated at its connection with the portal vein.

40.3 Tips

During the surgical treatment of an AV fistula, hemostasis is very important to avoid serious blood loss.

If the AV fistulas are in the quadrate lobe or the right medial liver lobe, a cholecystectomy is required.

Blood vessels are ligated around the hilus of the liver until the portal pressure is significantly reduced. It is the author's goal to reduce portal pressure below 20 cm of H_2O to try to reverse blood flow into the portal vein and limit the amount of blood shunting in the systemic circulation. Also, reducing the portal pressure will reduce the amount of ascites.

Banding of the caudal vena cava has been performed to help reverse the blood flow in the acquired shunts. This is performed by placing a larger suture around the caudal vena cava between the renal veins and the hilus of the liver. While monitoring the portal pressure and the pressure in the caudal vena cava, the suture is tightened until the pressure in the caudal vena cava equals the portal pressure (Breznock and Whiting 1985; Whiting et al. 1986). It is important not to raise the portal pressure.

40.4 Complications

The main complication from the surgery is intra-operative and immediate post-operative hemorrhage.

The main long-term complication is the recurrence of the hepatofugal blood flow, porto-caval shunting and development of ascites (Easley and Carpenter 1975; Whiting et al. 1986; Chanoit et al. 2007).

In a retrospective study on 20 dogs with AV fistula, 13 were treated by surgery alone while 4 were treated with embolization alone, and one with embolization and surgery (Chanoit et al. 2007). Two dogs were euthanized without treatment. Six dogs in the surgery group died or were euthanized because of lack of improvement. All of the dogs in the embolization group were alive at the time of follow-up between 9 and 17 months. Seventy-five percent of the dogs alive required medical treatment to control their clinical signs.

References

Bailey, M.Q. et al. (1988). Ultrasonographic findings associated with congenital hepatic arteriovenous fistulain three dogs. *J. Am. Vet. Med. Assoc.* 192 (8): 1099–1101.

Breznock, E.M. and Whiting, P.G. (1985). *Portacaval Shunts and Anomalies*. WB Saunders.

Chanoit, G. et al. (2007). Surgical and interventional radiographic treatment of dogs with hepatic arteriovenous fistulae. *Vet. Surg.* 36 (3): 199–209.

Easley, J.C. and Carpenter, J.L. (1975). Hepatic arteriovenous fistula in two saint Bernard pups. *J. Am. Vet. Med. Assoc.* 166 (2): 167–171.

Legendre, A.M. et al. (1976). Ascites associated with intrahepatic arteriovenous fistula in a cat. *J. Am. Vet. Med. Assoc.* 168: 589–591.

Moore, P.F. and Whiting, P.G. (1986). Hepatic lesions associated with intrahepatic arterioportal fistulae in dogs. *Vet. Pathol.* 23 (1): 57–62.

Rogers, W.A. et al. (1977). Intrahepatic arteriovenous fistulae in a dog resulting in portal hypertension, portacaval shunts, and reversal of portal blood flow. *J. Am. Anim. Hosp. Assoc.* 13: 470–475.

Schaeffer, I.G. et al. (2001). Hepatic arteriovenous fistulae and portal vein hypoplasia in a labrador retriever. *J. Small Anim. Pract.* 42 (3): 146–150.

41

Portosystemic Shunt

Eric Monnet

Department of Clinical Sciences, College of Veterinary Medicine and Biomedical Sciences, Colorado State University, Fort Collins, CO, USA

41.1   Indications

Congenital portosystemic shunts (PSS) are abnormal blood vessels that allow blood from the portal vein to bypass the liver parenchyma. Congenital PSS, unlike acquired shunts, are single shunts most of the time. They can be intrahepatic or extrahepatic depending on whether or not they enter the liver parenchyma.

Since the portal blood is not filtered by the liver, different toxins can reach the systemic vasculature and induce hepatic encephalopathy in dogs and cats (Maddison 1992; Butterworth 2002; Klopp et al. 2013). The most important toxins responsible for hepatic encephalopathy are ammonia, mercaptans, short-chain fatty acids, aromatic amino acids, benzodiazepin-like substances, GABA (gamma-aminobutyric acid), and false neurotransmitters synthesized in the brain (Maddison 1992; Butterworth 2002; Klopp et al. 2013).

Hepatic encephalopathy is characterized by abnormal behavior, cortical blindness, ataxia and seizures. The gastrointestinal tract and the urinary tract can be affected in dogs and cats with PSS. Ammonium biurate stones are common in dogs with PSS. Patients can be presented for stranguria, pollakiuria and hematuria.

Portal blood is important for the normal development of the liver. The hepatotrophic factors (insulin and glucagon) are mostly delivered to the liver by the portal vein. Liver atrophy occurs if portal blood flow is shunting away from the liver. Restoration of normal portal blood flow is important to prevent deterioration of liver function and liver atrophy. It has been shown that surgical attenuation of a PSS is associated with an increased liver parenchyma volume in the post-operative period (Kummeling et al. 2010).

It has been shown that dogs with complete occlusion of their PSS at the time of surgery have a better long-term outcome than dogs with partial occlusion (Hottinger et al. 1995). Therefore, restoration of a normal portal blood flow in the liver parenchyma is the goal of the surgical treatment. Complete occlusion of the PSS is desired to achieve this goal and to optimize long-term outcome. However, complete occlusion of the PSS at the time of surgery is not very common because the hepatic portal vasculature cannot accommodate an important increase in blood flow (Hottinger et al. 1995; Lee et al. 2006; Lipscomb et al. 2007). It would result in severe acute portal hypertension, which would be fatal for the patient. Therefore, a gradual shunt occlusion is ideal since it will give time to the hepatic portal vasculature to develop and to accommodate the progressive augmentation of blood flow. If the PSS is closing too quickly, there is a risk of chronic portal hypertension that will result in ascites and acquired shunting in the long-term.

Therefore, it is important to select a device or technique that induces a slow, progressive and complete shunt occlusion without inducing acute or chronic portal hypertension.

41.2   Technique

The surgical treatment of an intrahepatic or an extrahepatic PSS requires its identification and then its dissection. Finally, a device is used to induce a slow, progressive, and complete occlusion of the PSS.

Different imaging modalities have been used before surgery to collect information on the anatomy and the location of the PSS. Ultrasound, CT angiogram, and MRI are the modalities most commonly used (Frank et al. 2003; d'Anjou et al. 2004; Zwingenberger 2009; Kummeling et al. 2010). Ultrasound is a noninvasive technique that does not require general anesthesia but shunt localization is heavily dependent on the skills of the ultrasonographer. The anatomy and location of an intrahepatic shunt can be determined with ultrasound (d'Anjou et al. 2004) but extrahepatic shunts can be more difficult to visualize. Portovenogram and cranial mesenteric angiogram were used in the past and were the gold standard techniques. Now computed tomography angiogram and MRI allow accurate identification and localization of the shunt and are replacing the portovenogram and the cranial mesenteric angiogram but both require general anesthesia. Three-dimensional reconstruction can be made to further understand the anatomy of the shunts.

41.2.1 Identification and Dissection

41.2.1.1 Extrahepatic PSS

Extrahepatic PSS are either porto-caval or porto-azygous shunt depending if they are connecting a branch of the portal vein to the caudal vena cava (CVC) or the azygous vein respectively.

41.2.1.1.1 Identification

41.2.1.1.1.1 Porto-Caval Shunt
When searching for an extrahepatic PSS, the CVC should be evaluated first in the right side of the abdominal cavity after lifting the duodenum toward the midline.

Any vessel except the phrenico-abdominal vein connecting to the CVC between the renal vein and the hilus of the liver should be the shunt. Porto-caval PSS are usu-

ally coming from the gastro-splenic vein and connect to the CVC at the level of the epiploic foramen. Retraction ventrally and medially of the ventral border of the epiploic foramen (dotted line) is required to visualize the PSS (black arrow) as it enters the CVC (Figure 41.1).

If a PSS is not identified, then the omental bursa is opened to identify the tributaries of the portal vein. Usually the PSS vessel is large, red, and tortuous.

If a PSS is still not identified, then evaluation of the CVC between the liver and the diaphragm is performed. Some PSS (black arrows) travel around the lower esophageal sphincter and along the wall of the diaphragm toward the CVC (Figure 41.2).

If a PSS has not been identified, then the aortic hiatus should be evaluated for a porto-azygous shunt.

41.2.1.1.1.2 Porto-Azygous Shunt
The stomach is retracted ventrally toward the right to expose the left dorsal part of the abdominal cavity, the diaphragm, and the aortic hiatus. The azygous vein travels through the diaphragm in the aortic hiatus (white arrows) (Figure 41.3).

Usually a porto-azygous shunt (black arrow in Figure 41.3) is identified along the greater curvature of the stomach along the lower esophageal sphincter and then

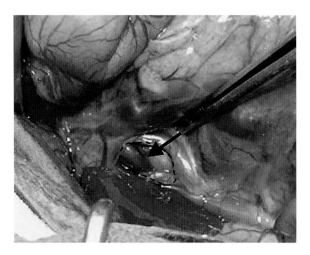

Figure 41.1

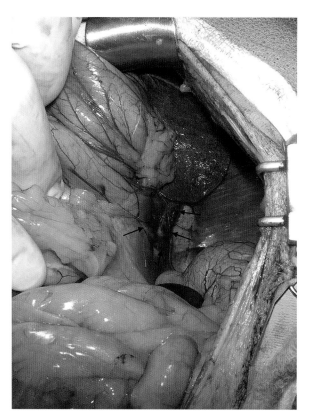

Figure 41.2

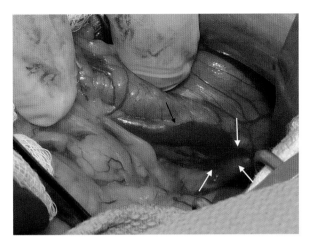

Figure 41.3

diving into the aortic hiatus to connect to the azygous vein. Very often, the PSS is the azygous vein by itself, with no clear connection between the shunt and azygous vein. The azygous vein is the continuation of the PSS. Therefore, there is no need to pursue the dissection through the diaphragm to find a connection with any intrathoracic vessel.

41.2.1.1.2 Dissection After the PSS has been identified, a right-angle forceps is used to dissect around the extrahepatic PSS. A window in the peritoneum on each side of the PSS can be sharply dissected first to help the dissection (Figure 41.4).

The dissection should be performed as close as possible to the CVC for a porto-caval shunt or against the aortic hiatus for a porto-azygous shunt to make sure that all the tributaries to the PSS are included (Figure 41.4). If a tributary is missed, shunting will persist in the long-term and clinical signs will not improve.

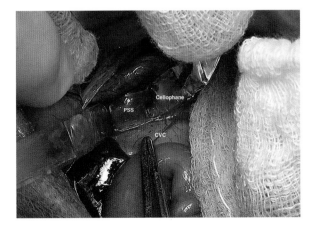

Figure 41.4

Extrahepatic PSS located along the diaphragm can be more difficult to dissect. Those shunts are coming from the left gastric vein and travel toward the cardia and along the diaphragm to connect with the CVC between the left lateral and medial liver lobes and the diaphragm. An incision is made in the peritoneum on the dorsal and ventral side of the shunt. A right-angle forceps is then used to complete the dissection and separate the shunt from the diaphragm. During the dissection, it is important not to damage the wall of the shunt.

41.2.1.2 Intrahepatic PSS
41.2.1.2.1 Identification
Intrahepatic PSS are located by visualization of the hepatic veins, the branches of the portal veins, palpation of the liver parenchyma, and detection of cavity or aneurysm. Also, measurement of portal pressure while occluding different vessels can give lot of information on the location of the intrahepatic PSS.

Portal pressure is measured with a catheter placed in a jejunal vein. A water manometer is connected to the catheter to measure the portal pressure in centimeters of water (Figure 41.5). A water manometer is more sensitive than an electronic pressure transducer to measure portal pressure and its variations. When the shunt, the hepatic vein draining the shunt, or the branch of the portal vein feeding the shunt is occluded, the portal pressure increases dramatically.

First, identification of an intrahepatic PSS is accomplished by evaluating the hepatic veins cranial to the liver as they enter the CVC. Incision of the triangular ligaments and the coronary ligament between the liver lobes and the diaphragm helps visualize the hepatic veins and the CVC. The hepatic vein draining the PSS is of a larger diameter (white arrows) than the other hepatic veins (Figure 41.6). It can be twice the diameter of the other hepatic veins or have a diameter similar to the CVC (black arrows).

Also, turbulent blood flow is visible within the hepatic vein and the CVC in front of the hepatic vein draining the PSS. Hepatic veins from the right middle and lateral liver lobes are difficult to visualize because they are very short and often buried in the liver parenchyma. However, since the liver lobes are atrophied, they can be visible.

Patent ductus venosus are usually seen in the left side of the liver, traveling in and out of the left lateral liver lobe, and entering the vena cava through one of the left hepatic veins.

If no difference is noticed in the hepatic veins, branches of the portal vein should be evaluated. The branch of the portal vein feeding into the shunt is of a

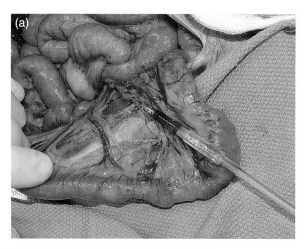

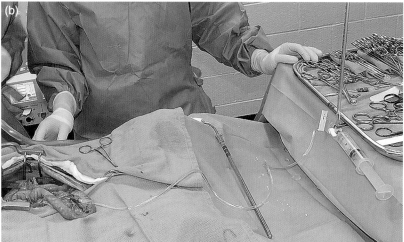

Figure 41.5

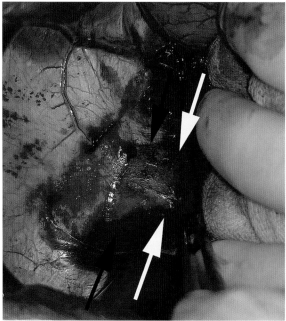

Figure 41.6

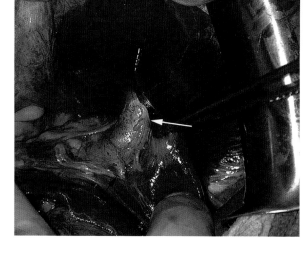

Figure 41.7

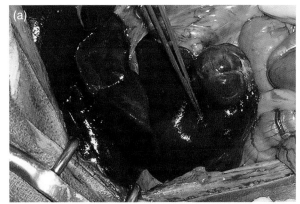

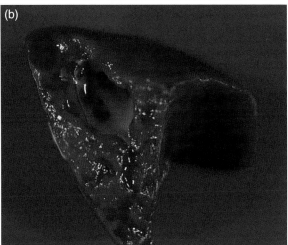

Figure 41.8

larger diameter (white arrows) than the other branches (black arrow) (Figure 41.7).

Finally, palpation of each liver lobe might help identify the aneurysm created by the shunt within the parenchyma (Figure 41.8).

41.2.1.2.2 Dissection

41.2.1.2.2.1 Extravascular Approach of the Hepatic Veins Inducing a complete, progressive occlusion of an

hepatic vein rather than a branch of the portal vein associated to a shunt is preferred because it maintains blood flow to the affected liver lobe. Therefore, it is important to identify the hepatic vein draining the intrahepatic PSS. Measuring portal pressure helps identify which vein is draining the shunt. Occlusion of an hepatic vein results in a transient congestion of the liver lobe drained by the hepatic vein.

The dissection of the hepatic vein draining the shunt requires the transection of the left triangular ligament, the coronary ligament for the left hepatic vein draining the left lateral and medial liver lobes and the quadrate lobe, or the right triangular ligament for the right hepatic veins (white arrows) (Figure 41.9). Retraction of the liver lobe caudally improves the exposure of the CVC and the hepatic vein.

The triangular ligaments and coronary ligament are an extension of the peritoneum and it surrounds the CVC and the hepatic veins. It can be peeled off the CVC and the hepatic veins to improve the dissection. It will help create a good plane of dissection around the hepatic vein to place a right-angle forceps (Figure 41.9b).

The largest hepatic vein drains the left lateral, the left medial, and the quadrate lobes of the liver. It enters the left ventral part of the CVC at the level of the caval foramen. This is the most cranial hepatic vein. In dogs with PSS, the different tributaries of the left hepatic vein can be visualized and isolated given the atrophy of their liver lobes. The tributary coming from the quadrate lobe is ventral to the CVC and it is usually large and short. On the right side of the CVC, there are two hepatic veins. The most cranial drains the right lateral and medial liver lobe whereas the most caudal drains the caudate lobe. Both are short and very often buried in the liver parenchyma.

Usually, an indentation between the hepatic vein and the CVC is visible (Figure 41.9). To start the dissection, the peritoneum covering the hepatic vein and vena cava

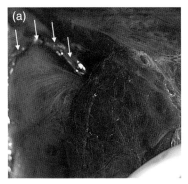
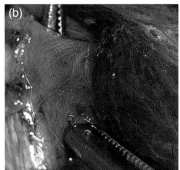
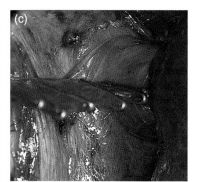

Figure 41.9

have to be sharply incised away from the wall of the vessels. The dissection is performed parallel to the wall of the vena cava on each side of the hepatic vein draining the PSS (Figure 41.9b). An incision of the diaphragm might be needed to get a better access to the CVC and the hepatic vein. A right-angle forceps is used to get around the caudal border of the hepatic vein and encircle the base of the vein. A combination of blunt and sharp dissection is required to be able to get around the larger hepatic vein (Figure 41.9b). It is important to keep in mind the shape of the connection of the hepatic vein with the CVC. It is not a cylinder and the caudal margin of the anastomosis is far caudal within the liver parenchyma. Blunt dissection or finger fracturing can be used in the liver parenchyma around the caudal border hepatic vein to complete the isolation of the vessel. Minor bleeding should be expected during this process. An ultrasound dissector has been used to separate the liver parenchyma and pursue the dissection. The dissection should be extended enough to place a band of cellophane, or an ameroid constrictor.

41.2.1.2.2.2 Extravascular Approach of the Portal Vein

If the dissection cannot be completed at the level of the hepatic vein, the branch of the portal vein feeding the shunt is dissected. The peritoneum is first opened on each side of the branch and a right-angle forceps is used to pursue the dissection around the dorsal side of the vein (white arrows) (Figure 41.10). For a branch from the right division of the portal vein, the dissection of the dorsal side might be very difficult and a technique has been described to pursue the dissection on each side of the branch toward the dorsal side of the portal vein. The suture is then pulled dorsal to the portal vein against the dorsal border of the branch of the right branch (Tobias et al. 2004).

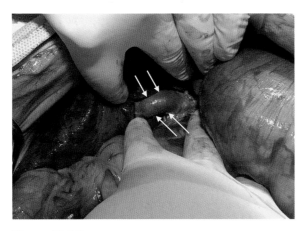

Figure 41.10

41.2.2 Techniques for Ligation or Progressive Occlusion of the Shunt

Different surgical techniques have been described for the treatment of PSS. Some techniques with sutures or coils result in a partial and fixed occlusion. Other techniques induce a slow, progressive, and complete occlusion of the shunt over time. Ameroid constrictors (Figure 41.11), a band of cellophane (Figure 41.12), a constrictor made of silicon-polyacrylic acid, and hydraulic occluders (Figure 41.13) have been recommended to induce a complete, progressive occlusion (Vogt et al. 1996; Kyles et al. 2002; Hunt et al. 2004; Adin et al. 2006; Bright et al. 2006; Wallace et al. 2016). Each of those techniques differ from each other by their rate of occlusion. The major advantage of the cellophane is that it does not require any extensive dissection around the shunt for its placement and it can be placed around the hepatic vein for the treatment of an intrahepatic shunt (Figure 41.12d).

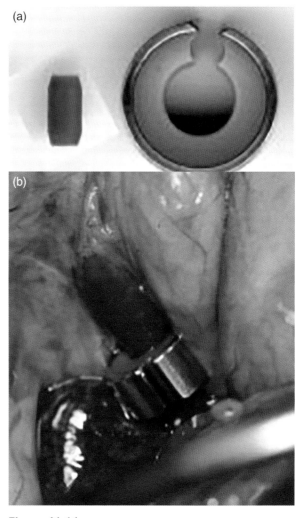

Figure 41.11

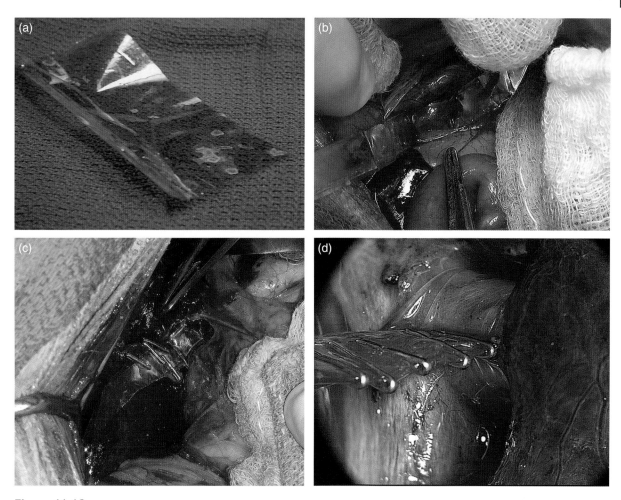

Figure 41.12

41.2.2.1 Techniques Resulting in Fixed Attenuation of a Shunt

41.2.2.1.1 *Attenuation with Sutures*

Originally, encircling sutures with silk or polypropylene have been used to attenuate either extrahepatic or intrahepatic shunts (Swalec and Smeak 1990; Hottinger et al. 1995; Hunt and Hughes 1999; Lee et al. 2006; Lipscomb et al. 2007; Bristow et al. 2017).

After complete dissection of the PSS, a suture is placed around the shunt. The suture is then tightened as much as possible, avoiding the induction of acute portal hypertension. Portal pressure is measured with a catheter placed in a jejunal vein and a water manometer zeroed at the level of the right atrium. Baseline portal pressure is measured. During attenuation of the shunt, the portal pressure should not increase more than 10 cm of water from baseline and should not be higher than 17 cm of water (Swalec and Smeak 1990). Also, if central venous pressure is measured, it should not decrease by more than 2 cm of water. If the central venous pressure decreases by more than 2 cm of water, this indicates that

the blood flow through the shunt is a significant contributor of preload and the suture around the shunt should be loosened.

41.2.2.1.2 *Attenuation with Mattress Sutures*

If the complete dissection of an intrahepatic shunt is not possible, mattress sutures with pledgets can be applied across the shunt (Figure 41.14). This technique is mostly used for intrahepatic shunt in the right side of the liver since the right hepatic veins are short and difficult to dissect. Double armed nonabsorbable monofilament suture size 4-0 is used for the mattress suture (Figure 41.15). Pledgets made of Teflon are used to prevent tearing the shunt wall. Pledgets exist in different sizes: small (3 mm), medium (7 mm), and large (9 mm) (Figure 41.14), although small pledgets are usually used. Pledgets are placed on both sides of the wall of the shunts. The mattress suture is tightened while the portal pressure is measured following the recommendations previously described. If one mattress suture is not sufficient to raise the portal pressure, a second mattress

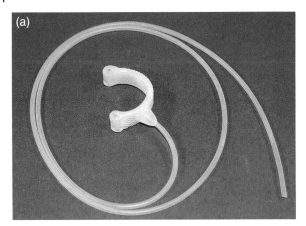

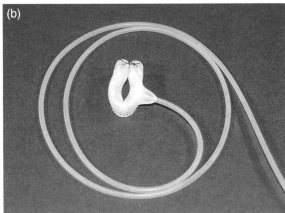

Figure 41.13

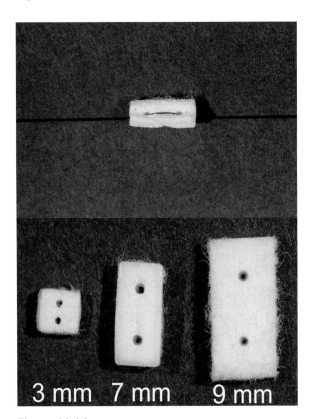

Figure 41.14

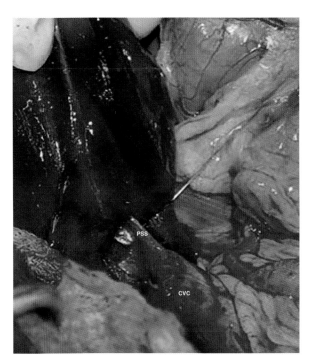

Figure 41.15

suture can be placed to occlude even further the shunt. This technique does not provide a slow, progressive occlusion of the shunt; however, it allows the attenuation of blood flow through an intrahepatic shunt with minimal risk for the patient.

41.2.2.1.3 Intravascular Approach of the Hepatic Vein or the Portal Vein

Intravascular approaches have been described to visualize an intrahepatic shunt (Breznock and Whiting 1985). It requires interruption of blood flow within the liver with temporary occlusion of the portal vein, the hepatic artery, and the CVC cranial and caudal to the liver. The Pringle maneuver is used to interrupt portal and arterial blood flow. The CVC is occluded with either tourniquets or vascular clamp cranial and caudal to the liver. The liver can tolerate 20 minutes of occlusion. After interrupting blood flow, either the post-hepatic CVC or the portal vein are incised longitudinally. A loose suture is then placed across the opening of the hepatic vein draining the shunt or the branch of the portal vein feeding the shunt. The venotomy is then closed with a 6-0 monofilament absorbable suture. After re-establishing blood flow, the suture across the shunt is tightened while the portal pressure is monitored as described above.

41.2.2.1.4 Percutaneous Transjugular Coil Embolization of Shunt with Interventional Radiology

Interventional radiology with the placement of a stent in the CVC and coils has been used for the occlusion of

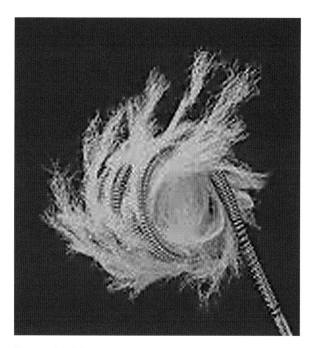

Figure 41.16

PSS (Bussadori et al. 2008; Weisse et al. 2014; Culp et al. 2017). With venous access from the jugular vein, a wire is advanced into the CVC across the right atrium.

The shunt is located with retrograde contrast injection. A marker catheter placed in the CVC is used to determine the diameter of the stent that will be placed at the level of the connection of the CVC and the hepatic vein draining the shunt. A stent is deployed in the CVC where the hepatic vein is connected with the vena cava. Thromboembolic coils (Figure 41.16) are then advanced through the stent and released in the intrahepatic shunt against the stent. The coils are deployed while portal pressure is monitored and measured with a catheter that is advanced through the stent in the vena cava into the shunt and the portal vein. A pressure gradient between the portal vein and the CVC is also measured.

41.2.2.2 Techniques Resulting in Slow Progressive and Complete Occlusion of a PSS

41.2.2.2.1 Ameroid Constrictor

Ameroid constrictors have been used to treat extrahepatic and intrahepatic shunts (Mehl et al. 2005, 2007; Bright et al. 2006; Traverson et al. 2018).

An ameroid constrictor consist of an outer ring of stainless steel and an inner ring of casein (Figure 41.11a). A key is placed to complete the constrictor after it has been placed around the PSS. The dissection

around the shunt has to be wide enough to allow for the placement of the ameroid constrictor. The constrictors exist in different internal diameters ranging from 3.5 to 9 mm. The ameroid constrictors of 3.5 and 5 mm are most commonly used. As the casein absorbs fluid, it expands concentrically to compress the shunt. It should close the abnormal blood vessel in 60 days (Vogt et al. 1996; Monnet and Rosenberg 2005; Bright et al. 2006). However, the shunt may occlude prematurely secondary to acute vessel thrombosis or fibrosis secondary to the inflammatory reaction to the foreign body (Besancon et al. 2004).

The dissection around the shunt should be sufficient to place the ameroid constrictor but no more to avoid movement of the constrictor and kinking of the shunt. Kinking of the shunt results in acute portal hypertension.

For an extrahepatic PSS, the constrictor should be placed against the wall of the CVC to improve its stability and prevent acute kinking of the vessel as it enters the CVC.

For an intrahepatic shunt, the placement of the ameroid constrictor can be difficult because the dissection required for its placement may not be possible, especially if the placement is attempted around the hepatic vein draining the shunt. For this reason, it has been mostly placed around the branch of the portal vein feeding the intrahepatic shunt (Mehl et al. 2007).

41.2.2.2.2 Cellophane Banding

Bands of cellophane have been used to induce complete, progressive occlusion of the shunt. There is no medical-grade cellophane (Figure 41.12a). Therefore, cellophane refers to a clear, thin film that can be sterilized. Cellophane triggers an inflammatory reaction that results in fibrosis of the shunt. A band of cellophane is more likely to induce closure of the shunt in six months (Youmans and Hunt 1998; Frankel et al. 2006). Usually, a 1 cm wide strip of cellophane is folded in three layers, resulting in a 3 mm-wide, three-layer-thick band of cellophane. The band of cellophane is placed around the shunt like a suture with minimal dissection. The band of cellophane is placed in contact with the wall of the shunt without decreasing the diameter of the shunt. Vascular clips are used to secure the cellophane in place (Figure 41.12d). The shunt should not be attenuated at the time of surgery when the band of cellophane is applied (Frankel et al. 2006). A partial attenuation at the time of surgery may result in chronic portal hypertension and opening of acquired shunts.

41.2.2.2.3 Silicon-Polyacrylic Acid Gradual Venous Occlusion Device

A constrictor made of silicon-polyacrylic acid can be placed around the shunt as a surrogate for the classic ameroid constrictor made with casein. This device does not require a key to prevent the shunt from slipping out of the ring. The inner part of the ring is made of silicone tube filled with a proprietary salt and polyacrylic acid. The outer ring is a polyether ether ketone encased in silicate. It has been shown to induce complete closure of an iliac vein after six weeks in dogs (Wallace et al. 2016).

41.2.2.2.4 Hydraulic Occluder

A hydraulic occluder placed around the shunt with a subcutaneous port under the skin has been used to induce a controlled, progressive, and complete occlusion of an intrahepatic shunt (Figure 41.13) (Adin et al. 2006). The hydraulic occluder could be placed around the hepatic vein draining the shunt or the branch of the portal vein feeding the shunt after complete dissection, similar to an ameroid constrictor. However, in a publication, the hydraulic occluders could only be placed around the branch of the portal vein feeding the shunt because the occluder was too bulky. The degree of occlusion of the shunt can be titrated to the improvement of the clinical signs and the return of the post-prandial bile acids toward normal.

41.3 Tips

It is paramount to have a good understanding of the anatomy of the portal vein and its tributaries as well as its branches in the liver parenchyma. The PSS should always be occluded as close as possible to its connection with the systemic circulation to include all branches of the portal vein feeding the shunt. If one branch is not included, shunting will persist in the long-term.

A combination of blunt and sharp dissection is used to dissect the PSS. Right-angle forceps of different sizes are very useful for the dissection of an intrahepatic shunt. The wall of a shunt can be very thin, and iatrogenic trauma to the shunt results in significant hemorrhage and the shunt should be repaired surgically with 6-0 suture without occluding it. An iatrogenic trauma to the shunt occurs mostly with an intrahepatic shunt during the dissection of the hepatic vein draining the shunt within the liver parenchyma. Computed tomography images and 3-D reconstructions give important information on the size and the anatomy of the connection between the hepatic vein and the CVC (Figure 41.17). During the dissection of the shunt, it is important to

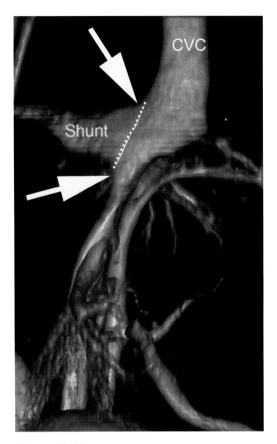

Figure 41.17

remember the oval shape of the connection between the hepatic vein/shunt and the vena cava, as demonstrated in Figure 41.17 (two white arrows). Therefore, it is paramount to extend the dissection caudally enough to be able go around the caudal border of the hepatic vein. It is also important to follow the wall of the CVC (dotted line on Figure 41.17) and not puncture its wall or incorporate the vena cava in the device used for attenuation.

The dissection of the hepatic vein can be greatly facilitated if the peritoneum is dissected away from the CVC between the liver and the diaphragm. Also, opening of the diaphragm may facilitate this approach and dissection.

Ameroid constrictors, bands of cellophane, a constrictor made of silicon-polyacrylic acid, and hydraulic occluders are going to occlude the PSS at different rates. An ameroid constrictor should close a shunt within 60 days, while the bands of cellophane can take up to 6 months to achieve complete occlusion (Vogt et al. 1996; Frankel et al. 2006). The constrictor made of silicon-polyacrylic acid should close the shunt in 6 weeks (Wallace et al. 2018). The slower the occlusion is, the better it is for the patient, allowing more time for the hepatic portal vasculature to develop and limit the risk of chronic portal hypertension and acquired shunting. The rate of acquired shunting has been as high as 25% with ameroid constrictors (Murphy et al. 2001) whereas it is around 5% with cellophane banding (Hunt et al. 2004; Frankel et al. 2006). A study reported residual shunting in 31% of the cases when cellophane was used; however, the follow-up period might have been too short in that study (Traverson et al. 2018).

If a technique inducing a fixed partial attenuation has been used, it might be recommended to perform a second procedure to further occlude the shunt while the hepatic portal vasculature develops, allowing a complete occlusion at the second surgery (Hottinger et al. 1995; Lee et al. 2006).

Even if the patient is normoglycemic, it is the author's preference to maintain patients on intravenous fluid with 2.5% glucose in the post-operative period to prevent any hypoglycemic episode that could trigger seizures.

The progression of the shunt occlusion can be followed with the measurement of post-prandial bile acids, ultrasound, and/or CT angiogram and the regression of the clinical signs.

41.4 Complications

41.4.1 Post-Operative Complications and Short-Term Outcome

41.4.1.1 Portal Hypertension

Acute and chronic portal hypertension are two complications that could happen during the treatment of a PSS. Acute portal hypertension happens in the immediate post-operative period while chronic portal hypertension happens in the long-term.

Even if the guidelines are followed, 14% of dogs and cats develop acute portal hypertension in the recovery period (Swalec and Smeak 1990; Hottinger et al. 1995; White et al. 1998; Hunt and Hughes 1999; Wolschrijn et al. 2000). Acute portal hypertension is less common when a band of cellophane or an ameroid constrictor are used (Vogt et al. 1996; Hunt et al. 2004; Frankel et al. 2006). Ameroid constrictors can induce acute portal hypertension if the constrictor acutely kinks the shunt because of its weight.

Acute portal hypertension induces congestion of the bowels, pancreas, and spleen. An acute, severe abdominal pain, bloody diarrhea, and septic shock develop quickly in patients with acute portal hypertension. The patients that develop mild acute portal hypertension mostly show signs of abdominal pain and should be

treated medically with pain medication, sedation, intravenous fluid, and gastrointestinal protectant. If severe acute portal hypertension develops, the only treatment is removal of the device used for the shunt attenuation.

41.4.1.2 Gastrointestinal Bleeding

Gastrointestinal bleeding has been documented in 13% of cases with an intrahepatic PSS that were treated with coil embolization and is suspected to be induced by acute portal hypertension (Weisse et al. 2014; Culp et al. 2018). This incidence of gastrointestinal bleeding has not been reported with other techniques used to occlude a PSS. Antacid therapy is recommended if gastrointestinal ulceration is present.

41.4.1.3 Hypoglycemia

Hypoglycemia is common in the post-operative period of shunt attenuation and can happen in 44% of cases (Holford et al. 2008). Most of the dogs or cats with a PSS are hypoglycemic before surgery and given the fasting period prior to surgery, their risk of post-operative hypoglycemia is increased until they are able to eat on their own.

Therefore, monitoring blood glucose in the post-operative period is paramount in order to prevent a hypoglycemic crisis that could trigger seizures. Some dogs may have hypoglycemia that is not responding to the addition of 2.5% glucose to their intravenous fluids. Those patients very often have a very slow recovery from anesthesia and may benefit from a physiological dose of dexamethasone. However, correlation between hypoglycemia and response to ACTH does not exist (Holford et al. 2008).

41.4.1.4 Hemorrhage

Since liver function is affected with a PSS, some dogs may have a deficit in some coagulation factors, resulting in hemorrhage after surgery (Hunt et al. 2004; Kummeling et al. 2006; Falls et al. 2013; Case et al. 2018). Blood transfusion is then needed to support the patient in the post-operative period. Hemorrhage after surgery has been seen in 1.8–4.5% of cases (Hunt et al. 2004; Kummeling et al. 2006; Falls et al. 2013; Case et al. 2018).

41.4.1.5 Neurological Complications

Neurological complications are the most devastating in the post-operative periods. Ataxia, facial twitching, muscle fasciculations, and blindness have been reported after surgery with any technique described above. Those clinical signs usually occur before the seizures start. Seizures can develop up to three days after surgery and are very difficult to control. Seizures have been reported in 3–18% of dogs after PSS manipulation and 8–22% of cats (Hardie et al. 1990; Heldmann et al. 1999; Hunt and Hughes 1999; Tisdall et al. 2000; Havig and Tobias 2002; Kyles et al. 2002; Yool and Kirby 2002; Winkler et al. 2003; Kummeling et al. 2004; Mehl et al. 2005; Frankel et al. 2006; Lee et al. 2006; Lipscomb et al. 2007; Worley and Holt 2008; Cabassu et al. 2011; Fryer et al. 2011). Phenobarbital, valium, flumazenil, propofol, and levetiracetam have been used with some very limited success (Hardie et al. 1990; Heldmann et al. 1999; Hunt and Hughes 1999; Tisdall et al. 2000; Havig and Tobias 2002; Kyles et al. 2002; Yool and Kirby 2002; Winkler et al. 2003; Kummeling et al. 2004; Mehl et al. 2005; Lee et al. 2006; Lipscomb et al. 2007; Worley and Holt 2008; Fryer et al. 2011).

Risk factors for the development of post-operative seizures have not been identified. However, it would seem that patients over two years of age are over-represented. Different strategies have been tested to reduce the risk of seizures, with very limited positive results. In one study, levetiracetam has been given before surgery to reduce the risk of post-operative seizures (Fryer et al. 2011).

41.4.1.6 Short-Term Outcome and Prognostic Indicators

The short-term outcome is highly variable. For dogs, the post-operative mortality rate reported from different retrospective studies varies from 0 to 12.5% (Hunt and Hughes 1999; Hunt 2004; Mehl et al. 2005, 2007; Adin et al. 2006; Frankel et al. 2006; Parker et al. 2008; Worley and Holt 2008; Falls et al. 2013; Greenhalgh et al. 2014; Weisse et al. 2014; Culp et al. 2017). For cats, the post-operative mortality rate reported from different retrospective studies varies from 0 to 22.2% (Havig and Tobias 2002; Kyles et al. 2002; Lipscomb et al. 2007; Cabassu et al. 2011).

Weight (HR: 0.80-0.99), total protein (HR: 0.18-0.87), albumin (HR: 0.14-0.91), and BUN (HR: 1.01-1.25) were risk factors for short-term complications in dogs with intrahepatic shunts (Papazoglou et al. 2002). The location of the intrahepatic shunt was not a risk factor for outcome (Papazoglou et al. 2002; Weisse et al. 2014). Risk factors have not been identified for the occurrence of seizures after surgery.

41.4.2 Long-Term Complications and Outcome

41.4.2.1 Portal Hypertension

In the long-term, chronic portal hypertension can develop if the shunt is closing too fast and the hepatic portal vasculature does not have time to develop. It can induce ascites and acquired shunting. The ascites can be controlled with diuretics but the acquired shunts will result in hepatic encephalopathy. If cellophane banding is used, partial attenuation of the shunt at the time of surgery is detrimental in the long-term and should not be attempted (Frankel et al. 2006). In the same study, a partial occlusion of the shunt resulted in elevation of post-prandial bile acids in the long-term, more likely because of acquired shunting. Therefore, loose application of the band of cellophane is recommended to prevent the development of acquired shunt.

Acquired shunting in the long-term have been reported as high as 17.5% with ameroid rings and 18% with cellophane banding (Hunt and Hughes 1999; Hunt et al. 2004; Mehl et al. 2005; Frankel et al. 2006; Landon et al. 2008; Falls et al. 2013).

Acute portal hypertension can also develop in the long-term if a partially attenuated intrahepatic shunt thrombosed (Roy et al. 1992). This complication has been described three weeks after surgery and it results in acute abdominal pain, bloody diarrhea, and septic shock.

41.4.2.2 Persistence of Shunting

Shunting of portal blood around the liver can persist in the long-term after surgical treatment. The persistence of shunting could be the result of different conditions: the original shunt remains partially or completely patent, a second shunt is present and was not identified at the time of the initial surgery, acquired shunts have opened because of portal hypertension, or the presence of portal vein hypoplasia.

The persistence of shunting may be diagnosed because of continued clinical signs with or without biochemical abnormalities. If clinical signs are still present, ultrasound or CT angiogram can be used to visualize the patency of the PSS. Usually, CT angiogram will be more sensitive because it is less operator-dependent than an ultrasound. Per-rectal scintigraphy with technetium pertechnetate 99 can also be used to determine if shunting is still present.

If the shunt is still patent and the patient has clinical signs, a second surgery is indicated to further close the shunt or identify and attenuate a second shunt. If there are no clinical signs, the persistent elevation of the post-prandial bile acids is more likely due to portal vein hypoplasia.

41.4.2.3 Long-Term Outcome and Prognostic Indicators

Long-term outcome is better evaluated with survival analysis. Survival analysis with Kaplan–Meier actuarial analysis is not common in dogs and cats treated for PSS.

Greenhalgh et al. (2010) have evaluated long-term outcome of 124 dogs treated with either medical or surgical treatment. In this population, 110 dogs had an extrahepatic PSS and 14 an intrahepatic PSS. Ninety-seven dogs were treated surgically and 27 medically. The median follow-up time was 1936 days. The 1-, 2-, and 5-year survival rates were approximately 90%, 85%, and 75% for the surgically treated dogs and 80%, 60%, and 25% for the medically treated dogs. At 3000 days, approximately 70% of dogs with surgical treatment were still alive, while 15% of dogs with only medical treatment were still alive. The age and the shunt type did not have an effect on survival rate. The quality of life, as assessed by the frequency of clinical signs at home, for the surgically treated group was significantly better than the quality of life of the medically treated group at four and seven years after entering the study.

In a study on 25 dogs with an intrahepatic shunt, and 39 dogs with an extrahepatic shunt, Parker et al. (2008) reported a median survival time of 50.6 months for 64 dogs, with PSS treated surgically with a median follow-up time of 51.7 months. A 1-, 2-, and 5-year survival rate of 93%, 79%, and 29% were reported for the overall population. There was no significant difference in the median survival time between the dogs with extrahepatic PSS and intrahepatic PSS. No risk factors were identified in that study.

In a study on 32 dogs with intrahepatic shunt treated surgically, Papazoglou et al. (2002) reported a 61% survival rate at one year and a 55% survival rate at two years. All of the dogs were treated with partial suture ligation. Total protein (<4 g/dl) and PCV were two prognostic indicators for long-term survival.

In a study on 95 dogs with intrahepatic shunt treated with an endovascular approach and coils, Weisse et al. (2014) reported a median survival time of 6 years with a median follow-up time of 958 days. A partial attenuation was possible in 92 patients. Sixteen dogs had more than one intervention to further occlude the shunt. The outcome was considered excellent in 66% of cases.

In a multi-institutional study on 58 dogs with intrahepatic shunts (31 treated with cellophane banding and 27 treated with an endovascular approach), Case et al. (2018) reported 1- and 2-year survival rate of 89% for the dogs treated with cellophane banding and 87% and 80% for the dogs treated with endovascular approach. There was no significant difference between the two treatments. The 5-year survival rate was 75% for the dogs treated with cellophane banding and 80% for the dogs treated with endovascular approach.

In a study on 206 dogs with extrahepatic shunt treated with an ameroid ring, Falls et al. (2013) reported a 50% survival time of 12.6 years.

In a study on cats with extrahepatic PSS, Cabassu et al. (2011) reported a 66% survival rate, three years after surgery.

Havig and Tobias (2002), in a retrospective study on 12 cats, reported a 0% perioperative mortality rate, but 4 out of 9 cats with long-term follow-up were euthanized because of seizures. Kyles et al. (2002) in a retrospective study on 23 cats, reported a 4% preoperative mortality rate and a 77% complication rate (cortical blindness and seizures) after surgery. However, 75% of cats had an excellent long-term outcome with very limited clinical signs.

References

Adin, C.A. et al. (2006). Outcome associated with use of a percutaneously controlled hydraulic occluder for treatment of dogs with intrahepatic portosystemic shunts. *J. Am. Vet. Med. Assoc.* 229 (11): 1749–1755.

Besancon, M.F. et al. (2004). Evaluation of the characteristics of venous occlusion after placement of an ameroid constrictor in dogs. *Vet. Surg.* 33 (6): 597–605.

Breznock, E.M. and Whiting, P.G. (1985). Portacaval Shunts and Anomalies. WB Saunders.

Bright, S.R. et al. (2006). Outcomes of intrahepatic portosystemic shunts occluded with ameroid constrictors in nine dogs and one cat. *Vet. Surg.* 35 (3): 300–309.

Bristow, P. et al. (2017). Long-term serum bile acid concentrations in 51 dogs after complete extrahepatic congenital portosystemic shunt ligation. *J. Small Anim. Pract.* 58 (8): 454–460.

Bussadori, R. et al. (2008). Transvenous coil embolisation for the treatment of single congenital portosystemic shunts in six dogs. *Vet. J.* 176 (2): 221–226.

Butterworth, R.F. (2002). Pathophysiology of hepatic encephalopathy: a new look at ammonia. *Metab. Brain Dis.* 17 (4): 221–227.

Cabassu, J. et al. (2011). Outcomes of cats undergoing surgical attenuation of congenital extrahepatic portosystemic shunts through cellophane banding: 9 cases (2000–2007). *J. Am. Vet. Med. Assoc.* 238 (1): 89–93.

Case, J.B. et al. (2018). Outcomes of cellophane banding or percutaneous transvenous coil embolization of canine intrahepatic portosystemic shunts. *Vet. Surg.* 47 (S1): O59–O66.

Culp, W.T.N. et al. (2017). Prospective evaluation of outcome of dogs with intrahepatic portosystemic shunts treated via percutaneous transvenous coil embolization. *Vet. Surg.* 47 (1): 74–85.

Culp, W.T.N. et al. (2018). Prospective evaluation of outcome of dogs with intrahepatic portosystemic shunts treated via percutaneous transvenous coil embolization. *Vet. Surg.* 47 (1): 74–85.

d'Anjou, M.A. et al. (2004). Ultrasonographic diagnosis of portosystemic shunting in dogs and cats. *Vet. Radiol. Ultrasound* 45 (5): 424–437.

Falls, E.L. et al. (2013). Long-term outcome after surgical ameroid ring constrictor placement for treatment of single extrahepatic portosystemic shunts in dogs. *Vet. Surg.* 42 (8): 951–957.

Frank, P. et al. (2003). Helical computed tomographic portography in ten normal dogs and ten dogs with a portosystemic shunt. *Vet. Radiol. Ultrasound* 44 (4): 392–400.

Frankel, D. et al. (2006). Evaluation of cellophane banding with and without intraoperative attenuation for treatment of congenital extrahepatic portosystemic shunts in dogs. *J. Am. Vet. Med. Assoc.* 228 (9): 1355–1360.

Fryer, K.J. et al. (2011). Incidence of postoperative seizures with and without levetiracetam pretreatment in dogs undergoing portosystemic shunt attenuation. *J. Vet. Intern. Med.* 25 (6): 1379–1384.

Greenhalgh, S.N. et al. (2010). Comparison of survival after surgical or medical treatment in dogs with a congenital portosystemic shunt. *J. Am. Vet. Med. Assoc.* 236 (11): 1215–1220.

Greenhalgh, S.N. et al. (2014). Long-term survival and quality of life in dogs with clinical signs associated with a congenital portosystemic shunt after surgical or medical treatment. *J. Am. Vet. Med. Assoc.* 245 (5): 527–533.

Hardie, E.M. et al. (1990). Status epilepticus after ligation of portosystemic shunts. *Vet. Surg.* 19 (6): 412–417.

Havig, M. and Tobias, K.M. (2002). Outcome of ameroid constrictor occlusion of single congenital extrahepatic portosystemic shunts in cats: 12 cases (1993–2000). *J. Am. Vet. Med. Assoc.* 220 (3): 337–341.

Heldmann, E. et al. (1999). Use of propofol to manage seizure activity after surgical treatment of portosystemic shunts. *J. Small Anim. Pract.* 40 (12): 590–594.

Holford, A.L. et al. (2008). Adrenal response to adrenocorticotropic hormone in dogs before and after surgical attenuation of a single congenital portosystemic shunt. *J. Vet. Intern. Med.* 22 (4): 832–838.

Hottinger, H.A. et al. (1995). Long-term results of complete and partial ligation of congenital portosystemic shunts in dogs. *Vet. Surg.* 24 (4): 331–336.

Hunt, G.B. (2004). Effect of breed on anatomy of portosystemic shunts resulting from congenital diseases in dogs and cats: a review of 242 cases. *Aust. Vet. J.* 82 (12): 746–749.

Hunt, G.B. and Hughes, J. (1999). Outcomes after extrahepatic portosystemic shunt ligation in 49 dogs. *Aust. Vet. J.* 77 (5): 303–307.

Hunt, G.B. et al. (2004). Outcomes of cellophane banding for congenital portosystemic shunts in 106 dogs and 5 cats. *Vet. Surg.* 33 (1): 25–31.

Klopp, L. et al. (2013). Portosystemic shunts. In: Small Animal Soft Tissue Surgery (ed. E. Monnet), 409–440. Oxford: Wiley Blackwell.

Kummeling, A. et al. (2004). Prognostic implications of the degree of shunt narrowing and of the portal vein diameter in dogs with congenital portosystemic shunts. *Vet. Surg.* 33 (1): 17–24.

Kummeling, A. et al. (2006). Coagulation profiles in dogs with congenital portosystemic shunts before and after surgical attenuation. *J. Vet. Intern. Med.* 20 (6): 1319–1326.

Kummeling, A. et al. (2010). Hepatic volume measurements in dogs with extrahepatic congenital portosystemic shunts before and after surgical attenuation. *J. Vet. Intern. Med.* 24 (1): 114–119.

Kyles, A.E. et al. (2002). Evaluation of ameroid ring constrictors for the management of single extrahepatic portosystemic shunts in cats: 23 cases (1996–2001). *J. Am. Vet. Med. Assoc.* 220 (9): 1341–1347.

Landon, B.P. et al. (2008). Use of transcolonic portal scintigraphy to evaluate efficacy of cellophane banding of congenital extrahepatic portosystemic shunts in 16 dogs. *Aust. Vet. J.* 86 (5): 169–179; quiz CE161.

Lee, K.C. et al. (2006). Association of portovenographic findings with outcome in dogs receiving surgical treatment for single congenital portosystemic shunts: 45 cases (2000–2004). *J. Am. Vet. Med. Assoc.* 229 (7): 1122–1129.

Lipscomb, V.J. et al. (2007). Complications and long-term outcomes of the ligation of congenital portosystemic shunts in 49 cats. *Vet. Rec.* 160 (14): 465–470.

Maddison, J.E. (1992). Hepatic encephalopathy. Current concepts of the pathogenesis. *J. Vet. Intern. Med.* 6 (6): 341–353.

Mehl, M.L. et al. (2005). Evaluation of ameroid ring constrictors for treatment for single extrahepatic portosystemic shunts in dogs: 168 cases (1995–2001). *J. Am. Vet. Med. Assoc.* 226 (12): 2020–2030.

Mehl, M.L. et al. (2007). Surgical management of left-divisional intrahepatic portosystemic shunts: outcome after partial ligation of, or ameroid ring constrictor placement on, the left hepatic vein in twenty-eight dogs (1995–2005). *Vet. Surg.* 36 (1): 21–30.

Monnet, E. and Rosenberg, A. (2005). Effect of protein concentration on rate of closure of ameroid constrictors in vitro. *Am. J. Vet. Res.* 66 (8): 1337–1340.

Murphy, S.T. et al. (2001). A comparison of the ameroid constrictor versus ligation in the surgical management of single extrahepatic portosystemic shunts. *J. Am. Anim. Hosp. Assoc.* 37 (4): 390–396.

Papazoglou, L.G. et al. (2002). Survival and prognostic indicators for dogs with intrahepatic portosystemic shunts: 32 cases (1990–2000). *Vet. Surg.* 31 (6): 561–570.

Parker, J.S. et al. (2008). Histologic examination of hepatic biopsy samples as a prognostic indicator in dogs undergoing surgical correction of congenital portosystemic shunts: 64 cases (1997–2005). *J. Am. Vet. Med. Assoc.* 232 (10): 1511–1514.

Roy, R.G. et al. (1992). Portal-vein thrombosis as a complication of portosystemic shunt ligation in 2 dogs. *J. Am. Anim. Hosp. Assoc.* 28 (1): 53–58.

Swalec, K.M. and Smeak, D.D. (1990). Partial versus complete attenuation of single portosystemic shunts. *Vet. Surg.* 19 (6): 406–411.

Tisdall, P.L. et al. (2000). Neurological dysfunction in dogs following attenuation of congenital extrahepatic portosystemic shunts. *J. Small Anim. Pract.* 41 (12): 539–546.

Tobias, K. et al. (2004). A new dissection technique for approach to right-sided intrahepatic portosystemic shunts: anatomic study and use in three dogs. *Vet. Surg.* 33 (1): 32–39.

Traverson, M. et al. (2018). Comparative outcomes between ameroid ring constrictor and cellophane banding for treatment of single congenital extrahepatic portosystemic shunts in 49 dogs (1998–2012). *Vet. Surg.* 47 (2): 179–187.

Vogt, J.C. et al. (1996). Gradual occlusion of extrahepatic portosystemic shunts in dogs and cats using the ameroid constrictor. *Vet. Surg.* 25 (6): 495–502.

Wallace, M.L. et al. (2016). Assessment of the attenuation of an intra-abdominal vein by use of a silicone-polyacrylic acid gradual venous occlusion device in dogs and cats. *Am. J. Vet. Res.* 77 (6): 653–657.

Wallace, M.L. et al. (2018). Gradual attenuation of a congenital extrahepatic portosystemic shunt with a self-retaining polyacrylic acid-silicone device in 6 dogs. *Vet. Surg.* 47 (5): 722–728.

Weisse, C. et al. (2014). Endovascular evaluation and treatment of intrahepatic portosystemic shunts in dogs: 100 cases (2001–2011). *J. Am. Vet. Med. Assoc.* 244 (1): 78–94.

White, R.N. et al. (1998). Surgical treatment of intrahepatic portosystemic shunts in 45 dogs. *Vet. Rec.* 142 (14): 358–365.

Winkler, J.T. et al. (2003). Portosystemic shunts: diagnosis, prognosis, and treatment of 64 cases (1993–2001). *J. Am. Anim. Hosp. Assoc.* 39 (2): 169–185.

Wolschrijn, C.F. et al. (2000). Gauged attenuation of congenital portosystemic shunts: results in 160 dogs and 15 cats. *Vet. Q.* 22 (2): 94–98.

Worley, D.R. and Holt, D.E. (2008). Clinical outcome of congenital extrahepatic portosystemic shunt attenuation in dogs aged five years and older: 17 cases (1992–2005). *J. Am. Vet. Med. Assoc.* 232 (5): 722–727.

Yool, D.A. and Kirby, B.M. (2002). Neurological dysfunction in three dogs and one cat following attenuation of intrahepatic portosystemic shunts. *J. Small Anim. Pract.* 43 (4): 171–176.

Youmans, K.R. and Hunt, G.B. (1998). Cellophane banding for the gradual attenuation of single extrahepatic portosystemic shunts in eleven dogs. *Aust. Vet. J.* 76 (8): 531–537.

Zwingenberger, A. (2009). CT diagnosis of portosystemic shunts. *Vet. Clin. North Am. Small Anim. Pract.* 39 (4): 783–792.

Section IX

Pancreas

42

Surgery of the Pancreas

Daniel D. Smeak and Eric Monnet

Department of Clinical Sciences, College of Veterinary Medicine and Biomedical Sciences, Colorado State University, Fort Collins, CO, USA

42.1 Indications

Surgery for pancreatic disease in small animals is uncommon. Most procedures performed in small animal surgery are for biopsy purposes and partial pancreatectomy/nodulectomy for mass removal. More rarely, pancreatic drainage is performed for abscesses and cysts (Smith and Biller 1998; Allen et al. 1989; Coleman and Robson 2005). Surgery is generally contraindicated for treatment of acute pancreatitis except to provide temporary biliary diversion in patients with mounting biliary obstruction (covered in Chapter 37), or when a pancreatic abscess or persistent pseudocyst requires debridement and/or drainage.

Chronic low-grade pancreatic disease often must be differentiated from other causes of chronic gastrointestinal disorders. Biopsies are indicated to help determine the cause of diffuse pancreatic disease. Some pancreatic diseases are only apparent microscopically, for example in chronic pancreatitis in cats, while others may be grossly evident and multifocal in nature. Pancreatic biopsies with tissue culture are routinely obtained in cats suspected to have triaditis, cholangitis, pancreatitis, and/or inflammatory bowel disease, even if the pancreas appears overtly normal (Weiss et al. 1996; Bazelle and Watson 2014).

Partial pancreatectomy may be indicated for focal trauma, or the presence of an isolated neoplastic mass, pseudocyst, or abscess, provided these causes do not deeply involve the central body of the pancreas. When these conditions do affect the central body, other less aggressive procedures such as local nodulectomy, or focal debridement and drainage are generally recommended over aggressive resection to avoid significant clinical consequences resulting from permanent biliary diversion and exocrine pancreatic insufficiency (from pancreatic duct ligation).

Small accumulations of fluid pocketing within the pancreas (abscesses or cysts less than 4 cm) found during ultrasound in dogs and cats that have no associated clinical signs are not initially treated with surgery and are monitored by ultrasound. If the cyst increases in size or particularly if clinical signs occur and worsen, ultrasound-guided aspiration is considered first (Smith and Biller 1998). If clinical signs persist after aspiration, and the pseudocyst/abscess fails to resolve, open surgical intervention is considered.

For endocrine neoplasia (most commonly insulinoma), in all areas except the angle of the pancreas, partial pancreatectomy (removal of the distal portion of the pancreatic lobe containing the focal lesion) is recommended versus simple nodulectomy. In the rare instance when the surgeon cannot locate an insulinoma during exploration, a left pancreatic lobectomy has been recommended for biopsy purposes and to hopefully capture an undetected mass in the left lobe. This lobe was chosen because the left lobe is easier to remove without interfering with blood supply of surrounding viscera. Currently, the recommendation is to obtain multiple biopsies in several areas of the pancreas, and regional lymph node and liver sampling when no identifiable pancreatic nodule is found (Cornell and Tobias 2018). In any case with suspected pancreatic neoplasia, regional lymph nodes are examined and removed for biopsy.

Total pancreatectomy is rarely, if ever, indicated for diffuse pancreatic disease. It is generally not indicated to perform pancreaticoduodenectomy for aggressive pancreatic or duodenal conditions (such as diffuse necrotizing pancreatitis or neoplasia) because of the associated high rate of morbidity and mortality (Cornell and Tobias 2018).

Gastrointestinal Surgical Techniques in Small Animals, First Edition. Edited by Eric Monnet and Daniel D. Smeak.
© 2020 John Wiley & Sons, Inc. Published 2020 by John Wiley & Sons, Inc.
Companion website: www.wiley.com/go/monnet/gastrointestinal

Pancreatic carcinoma in cats and dogs is a highly invasive disease with early metastasis, so it does not make sense to recommend total pancreatectomy without expecting a significant improvement in survival.

42.2 Surgical Procedures

42.2.1 Pancreatic Biopsy

In dogs and cats with diffuse disease, the site for surgical biopsy is chosen at the distal aspect of the right or left lobe of the pancreas. These sites are preferred because they can be exposed adequately, and they are located well away from the pancreatic and biliary duct system and major blood supply.

42.2.1.1 Suture Fracture Technique

A "suture fracture" technique is the standard technique, particularly when a lobule of the gland extends out away from the pancreas. The mesoduodenum or omentum is incised on either side of the proposed biopsy site base. A 4-0 monofilament absorbable suture strand is passed through the incisions and around the isolated lobule (Figure 42.1). The suture is slowly tightened, crushing the pancreatic parenchyma and occluding peripheral ducts and vessels. Tissue distal to the ligature is incised, leaving a few millimeters of the pancreatic stump past the ligature. Larger defects in the omentum or mesoduodenum are closed with similar suture. Alternately, small samples of the pancreas can be obtained by simply "shaving off" a shallow piece of pancreas with a #15 BP blade.

When it is necessary to take biopsies in the body of the lobes, if possible, a free margin of tissue is chosen rather than the central portion to avoid vascular or ductal damage.

42.2.1.2 Laparoscopic Pancreatic Biopsy

Laparoscopic pancreatic biopsy can be accomplished with the patient in dorsal or left lateral recumbency using 2 or 3 ports depending on the location of the preferred biopsy site and the need for manipulation of adjacent organs for exposure (Monnet and Twedt 2003; Cosford et al. 2008; Webb and Trott 2008; Mayhew 2009). Laparoscopic pancreatic biopsies are taken at similar sites as open biopsies, and are obtained with a 5 mm punch biopsy instrument (Figure 42.2) (Harmoinen et al. 2002; Monnet and Twedt 2003; Freeman 2009).

42.2.2 Nodulectomy (Enucleation) Via Blunt Dissection

Nodulectomy may be elected for focal lesions anywhere in the pancreas, but it is chosen primarily for excision of small isolated lesions in the central or mid-body regions. For right mid-lobar lesions, the cranial pancreaticoduodenal artery branches are carefully identified and bluntly dissected from the pancreatic lesion to protect the shared blood supply with the duodenum. The lesion is isolated by incising overlying mesoduodenum and meticulous blunt separation between the lobules of pancreas adjacent to the nodule with fine mosquito hemostatic forceps or sterile cotton-tipped swabs. Main pancreatic ducts when identified are isolated and preserved and associated smaller duct branches and vessels are ligated with fine absorbable sutures. Ideally a margin of normal tissue should be removed with the nodule. The resulting mesoduodenal defect is closed with fine absorbable monofilament suture.

42.2.3 Partial Pancreatectomy

Partial pancreatectomy refers to removal of most of one lobe. Dissection of the distal portion of the lobe is begun by incising the mesoduodenum (right lobe) or the dorsal

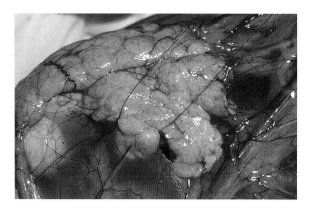

Figure 42.1

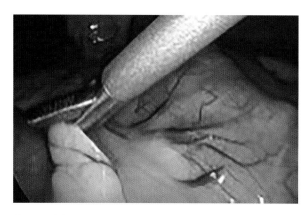

Figure 42.2

leaf of the greater omentum (left lobe). To ensure complete removal of endocrine tumors, a minimum of a 0.5–1 cm margin of normal-appearing pancreas should be included in the excised sample if possible. For pancreatic endocrine neoplasms, it is generally recommended that the nodule and the lobe distal to the nodule be removed *en bloc*. In Figure 42.3 an insulinoma is shown in the mid-distal portion of the right limb. In this case a partial pancreatectomy would be performed on the free portion of the distal right limb (see dotted line). In addition, regional lymph nodes and the liver are sampled to obtain prognostic information, and, when there are identifiable nodules, these are excised to help reduce functional tumor burden. Metastatic liver nodules typically appear as single or multiple well-circumscribed raised pale to tan nodules. For partial pancreatectomy on the left side, the omentum is dissected off from the portion of the pancreas to be excised. Any vasculature supplying the affected portion is ligated with fine absorbable suture. A major pancreatic vessel branch from the splenic artery provides blood supply to the

middle and distal third portion of the left lobe. This major branch is carefully dissected well away from the main splenic artery to help avoid damage to this important vessel. A splenectomy may be required if the splenic artery is damaged during the dissection. When the splenic branch is ligated, for example when a splenic torsion is removed, the more medial portion of the remaining left lobe will receive adequate blood supply from branches coming from the central body region (cranial pancreaticoduodenal and small common hepatic branches).

If the pancreatic lesion is strongly adhered to the wall of the stomach (white arrows) (Figure 42.4a), a partial gastrectomy is required with a TA stapler (black arrows) (Figure 42.4b) to able to complete the partial gastrectomy. A splenectomy is also performed because the splenic artery cannot be preserved.

For the right lobe, starting distally and moving cranially, the pancreas is carefully dissected from the duodenum and closely attached pancreaticoduodenal vessel with cotton-tipped swabs or fine hemostatic forceps. The caudal pancreaticoduodenal artery and branches to the descending duodenum are carefully preserved when dissecting between intestine and right pancreatic lobe (Eloy et al. 1980). After all attachments to the affected portion of the lobe have been removed, the pancreatic stump can be occluded by the same methods mentioned in the Section 42.2.1 (suture fracture, and blunt dissection and ligation). Alternately, some surgeons use a vessel sealant device to seal and incise along the base of the lobe (Hartwig et al. 2010; Wouters et al. 2011). If the area of pancreas resection is quite thick, the stump can be sealed with a 30 mm thoraco-abdominal stapler V-3 (Bellah 1994).

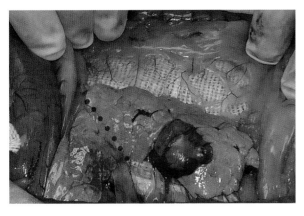

Figure 42.3

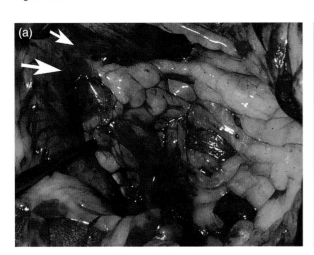

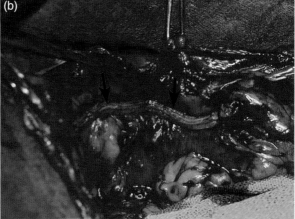

Figure 42.4

42.2.4 Total Pancreatectomy

The most challenging part of total pancreatectomy is preserving blood supply to the descending and proximal duodenum (Rosin et al. 1972). If the blood supply cannot be preserved, pancreaticoduodenectomy may be considered (Figure 42.5). This is rarely elected in small animals because of the associated high rate of morbidity and mortality (Cornell and Tobias 2018). If the distal aspect of the common bile duct is removed with the pancreas, some form of biliary diversion needs to be performed to allow free drainage of bile into the intestine (see Chapter 37 on biliary diversion techniques). As described for partial pancreatectomy, the dissection is started at the distal aspect of the left lobe. Omental attachments are removed, and the branch of the splenic artery entering in the body of the left lobe is ligated. The main splenic artery is preserved, otherwise, if this is not possible, a splenectomy is required. Dissection is continued to the angle of the pancreas, and branches of the gastroduodenal and common hepatic arteries are ligated and transected as they enter the parenchyma. If exposure is limited at that point, dissection of the right limb of the pancreas is performed next. The caudal pancreaticoduodenal artery and branches to the descending duodenum are carefully preserved when dissecting between intestine and right pancreatic lobe. This is best accomplished by recognizing an anatomic cutting line between the two peritoneal layers overlying the duodenum and pancreas as mentioned in Section 42.2.3. When only one peritoneal layer is carefully incised, this allows separation of the two organs and selective ligation of branches between the two structures (Eloy et al. 1980). When dissecting the pancreas from the proximal duodenum, the recurrent duodenal branch of the right gastroepiploic artery should be identified and preserved (Cobb and Merrell 1984). If it is not possible to

identify and preserve the recurrent duodenal branch of the right gastroepiploic artery during total pancreatectomy, the author bluntly dissects the pancreatic tissue from the pancreaticoduodenal vessels with cotton-tipped swabs, and focuses on preserving any observable blood supply to the duodenum in that area.

Finally, the pancreatic ducts are transected as they are identified close to the mesenteric border at the angle of the pancreas and proximal duodenum. If possible, the common bile duct is preserved during the dissection, or a biliary diversion is planned if the duct is damaged or needs to be removed with the pancreatic lesion. The mesoduodenal and omental defects are closed routinely.

42.2.5 Pancreatic Drainage

Open drainage of a cystic inflammatory pancreatic disease condition (abscess, pseudocyst) is indicated when the lesion cannot be safely resected *en bloc* via partial pancreatectomy, or by local resection with blunt dissection. The goals of most pancreatic drainage procedures are to resect as much of the free wall of the cavitary lesion as possible ("deroofing"), obtain tissue for histopathologic analysis and culture, and provide either local active suction drainage and/or "physiologic drainage" with omentalization (Jerram et al. 2004; Johnson and Mann 2006). After the free wall of the lesion is resected, several layers of healthy omentum are tacked to the interior of what is left of the cavitated lesion wall with fine absorbable monofilament sutures. Either open peritoneal drainage or active suction drainage may also be used for adjunctive abdominal drainage in some cases (Salisbury et al. 1988; Johnson and Mann 2006; Anderson et al. 2008). If enough viable omentum is not available for "physiological drainage," an internal means of drainage can be considered if the capsule of the cavitated lesion is thick and complete, and the lesion cannot be readily resected or drained to the outside. The affected pancreatic area is isolated with laparotomy pads, and a similar-sized incision in the cavitated lesion and adjacent stomach or duodenum is created. The two incisions are anastomosed with monofilament absorbable suture or with a gastrointestinal stapler connecting the lumen of the duodenum or stomach to the cyst or abscess lumen. This conduit allows continuous internal drainage of the cystic mass (Bellenger et al. 1989).

42.3 Tips

It is recommended to consider enteral feeding through a jejunal tube or J through G tube in unstable or malnourished patients that are not expected to eat for some time

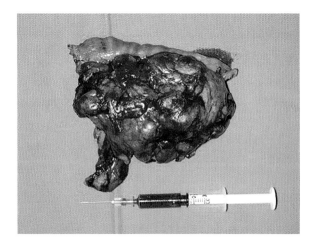

Figure 42.5

after surgery. If pancreatitis is present and if the patient is vomiting, use of a jejunostomy tube is paramount for nutritional support to the patient. If the patient is not expected to vomit, a simple gastrostomy tube may suffice.

During nodulectomy, the author prefers ligation or vascular clips versus electrosurgical means of occluding the fine ducts and vessels to help reduce collateral thermal damage.

To reduce manipulation of the pancreas and improve exposure, multiple stay sutures in the duodenum or stomach are very useful to maintain retraction during dissection. Broad malleable ribbon retractors are helpful to safely retract around the proposed excision site.

For partial pancreatectomy, it is helpful to first gently grasp the distal portion of the affected lobe with forceps or preplaced stay sutures to lift the isolated pancreas away from surrounding tissues to obtain better exposure of the blood supply entering the affected gland.

To preserve the pancreaticoduodenal vessels and vasculature to the descending duodenum, an "anatomic cutting line" can be found between the two peritoneal layers of the mesoduodenum overlying the mesenteric border of the duodenum and pancreas. When only one of the peritoneal layers is carefully incised, this allows separation of the two organs and facilitates selective ligation of branches between the two structures.

The "deroofing" and omentalization technique are the preferred method for most cavitated pancreatic lesions unless the cavitated lesion is at the terminal aspect of the pancreas. In that instance, the author prefers to remove the cavitated lesion via partial pancreatectomy. The omentum used for internal drainage should be healthy, and it should be gently folded into layers before being packed into the cavitated lesion. It is then carefully fastened to the inside of the lesion with sutures, avoiding damage to its blood supply.

42.4 Post-Operative Care and Complications

Complications from pancreatic surgery include pancreatitis, hemorrhage, ischemia of the duodenum, and peritonitis (Matthiesen and Mullen 1990; Cornell and Tobias 2018). Pancreatic biopsy should not be expected to cause significant clinical signs or biochemical abnormalities in dogs and cats (Allen et al. 1989; Lutz et al. 1994; Barnes et al. 2006). However, pancreatitis is not uncommon after nodulectomy, particularly around the angle of the pancreas and occasionally after partial pancreatectomy (Matthiesen and Mullen 1990; Yotsumoto et al. 1993). The animal is monitored closely for development of nausea, vomiting, cranial abdominal pain, and systemic inflammatory syndrome. Oral feeding is restricted in the immediate 24–36 hours after major pancreatic surgery until the patient is interested in food and has no signs of gastrointestinal reflux or vomiting. When feeding is tolerated, small volumes of bland, low-fat food are offered several times daily. Fluid, electrolyte balance, and vascular oncotic pressure are maintained after surgery to help support the patient and prevent post-operative pancreatitis. Necessary analgesic and antiemetic drugs are administered. Intravenous antacid therapy is administered to help reduce gastrointestinal ulceration and esophageal damage secondary to gastric acid reflux (Cornell and Tobias 2018).

References

Allen, S., Cornelius, L., and Mahaffey, E. (1989). A comparison of two methods of partial pancreatectomy in the dog. *Vet. Surg.* 18: 274–278.

Anderson, J.R., Cornell, K.K., Parnell, N.K. et al. (2008). Pancreatic abscess in 36 dogs: a retrospective analysis of prognostic indicators. *J. Am. Anim. Hosp. Assoc.* 44: 171–179.

Barnes, R.F., Greenfield, C.L., Schaeffer, D.J. et al. (2006). Comparison of biopsy samples obtained using standard endoscopic instruments and the harmonic scalpel during laparoscopic and laparoscopic-assisted surgery in normal dogs. *Vet. Surg.* 35: 243–251.

Bazelle, J. and Watson, P. (2014). Pancreatitis in cats. Is it acute, it is chronic, is it significant? *J. Feline Med. Surg.* 16: 395–406.

Bellah, J.R. (1994). Surgical stapling of the spleen, pancreas, liver, and urogenital tract. *Vet. Clin. North Am. Small Anim. Pract.* 24: 375–394.

Bellenger, C., Ilkiw, J., and Malik, R. (1989). Cystogastrostomy in the treatment of pancreatic pseudocyst/abscess in two dogs. *Vet. Rec.* 125: 181–184.

Cobb, L. and Merrell, R. (1984). Total pancreatectomy in dogs. *J. Surg. Res.* 37: 235–240.

Coleman, M. and Robson, M. (2005). Pancreatic masses following pancreatitis: pancreatic pseudocysts, necrosis, and abscesses. *Compend. Contin. Educ. Pract. Vet.* 27: 147–154.

Cornell, K. and Tobias, K.M. (2018). Pancreas. In: *Veterinary Surgery Small Animal*, 2e (eds. S.A. Johnston and K.M. Tobias), 1886–1901. St Louis: Elsevier.

Cosford, K., Carr, A., Schmon, C. et al. (2008). Evaluation of laparoscopic assisted pancreatic biopsies in 11 healthy cats. *J. Vet. Intern. Med.* 22: 813.

Eloy, R., Bouchet, P., Clendinnen, G. et al. (1980). New technique of total pancreatectomy without duodenectomy in the dog. *Am. J. Surg.* 140: 409–412.

Freeman, L.J. (2009). Gastrointestinal laparoscopy in small animals. *Vet. Clin. North Am.* 39: 903–924.

Harmoinen, J., Saari, S., Rinkinen, M. et al. (2002). Evaluation of pancreatic forceps biopsy by laparoscopy in healthy beagles. *Vet. Ther.* 3: 31–36.

Hartwig, W., Duckheim, M. et al. (2010). LigaSure for pancreatic sealing during distal pancreatectomy. *World J. Surg.* 34: 1066–1070.

Jerram, R.M., Warman, C.G., Davies, E.S.S. et al. (2004). Successful treatment of a pancreatic pseudocyst by omentalisation in a dog. *N. Z. Vet. J.* 52: 197–201.

Johnson, M.D. and Mann, F.A. (2006). Treatment for pancreatic abscesses via omentalization with abdominal closure versus open peritoneal drainage in dogs: 15 cases (1994–2004). *J. Am. Vet. Med. Assoc.* 228: 397–402.

Lutz, T., Rand, J., Watt, P. et al. (1994). Pancreatic biopsy in normal cats. *Aust. Vet. J.* 71: 223–225.

Matthiesen, D. and Mullen, H. (1990). Problems and complications associated with endocrine surgery in the dog and cat. *Probl. Vet. Med.* 2: 627–667.

Mayhew, P. (2009). Techniques for laparoscopic and laparoscopic-assisted biopsy of abdominal organs. *Compend. Contin. Educ. Pract. Vet.* 31: 170–176.

Monnet, E. and Twedt, D.C. (2003). Laparoscopy. *Vet. Clin. North Am. Small Anim. Pract.* 33: 1147–1163.

Rosin, E., Campos, R., Moberg, A.W. et al. (1972). Technique for total pancreatectomy of dog. *Am. J. Vet. Res.* 33: 1299–1302.

Salisbury, S., Lantz, G., and Nelson, R. (1988). Pancreatic abscess in dogs: six cases (1978–1986). *J. Am. Vet. Med. Assoc.* 193: 1104–1108.

Smith, S. and Biller, D. (1998). Resolution of a pancreatic pseudocyst in a dog following percutaneous ultrasonographic-guided drainage. *J. Am. Anim. Hosp. Assoc.* 34: 515.

Webb, C.B. and Trott, C. (2008). Laparoscopic diagnosis of pancreatic disease in dogs and cats. *J. Vet. Intern. Med.* 22 (6): 1263–1266.

Weiss, D., Gagne, J., and Armstrong, P. (1996). Relationship between inflammatory hepatic disease and inflammatory bowel disease, pancreatitis, and nephritis in cats. *J. Am. Vet. Med. Assoc.* 209: 1114–1116.

Wouters, E.G., Buishand, F.O., Kirk, M. et al. (2011). Use of a bipolar vessel sealing device in resection of canine insulinoma. *J. Small Anim. Pract.* 52: 139–145.

Yotsumoto, F., Manabe, T., Ohshio, G. et al. (1993). Role of pancreatic blood flow and vasoactive substances in the development of pancreatitis. *J. Surg. Res.* 55: 531.

Index

Page numbers in *italic* refer to figures.
Page numbers in **bold** refer to tables.

Gastrointestinal Surgical Techniques in Small Animals, First Edition. Edited by Eric Monnet and Daniel D. Smeak.
© 2020 John Wiley & Sons, Inc. Published 2020 by John Wiley & Sons, Inc.
Companion website: www.wiley.com/go/monnet/gastrointestinal